More Praise for
Ashtanga Yoga — The Intermediate Series

"I was pleased to find that once again Gregor Maehle has done an excellent job of presenting the traditional method of Ashtanga Yoga. This book provides a wealth of background information essential for building the context needed to fully benefit from this profound method of yoga — to prepare the soil so the practice bears the intended fruit. Students need to do the work of reading and studying the ancient texts in order to fully appreciate the practice, to have a context in which it can fit. This book helps to fill in many of those blanks. I salute Gregor for his hard work and his studiousness and thank him for helping to maintain the authentic, traditional practice, thus enabling students to have the intended experience of this great form of yoga."

— Chuck Miller, Ashtanga Yoga teacher,
senior student of Shri K. Pattabhi Jois since 1980

"Gregor Maehle presents a carefully crafted and thoroughly researched view of the Ashtanga Yoga Intermediate Series. The first available book on the topic, this is a great guide for students of Ashtanga Yoga and a valuable resource for all yoga practitioners wishing to study the Intermediate Series in more detail. The anatomical explanations, illustrations, and technical assistance will be very beneficial for many students and teachers alike."

— Kino MacGregor, founder of Miami Life Center and creator of
instructional Ashtanga Yoga DVDs

"I wish this book had been around when I was introduced to the Intermediate Series. It is immensely informative — a must-read for every practitioner who would like to look beyond the form. When embarking on the journey of the Intermediate Series, one intuitively understands that there is a depth to this practice that is beyond words. This book has given me great insight into the richness and interconnectedness of our practice and helped me understand why I have always felt this way."

— Angelika Knoerzer, director of North Sydney Yoga

ASHTANGA YOGA

The Intermediate Series

ASHTANGA YOGA
The Intermediate Series

Mythology, Anatomy, and Practice

Gregor Maehle

with Dr. Monica Gauci, chiropractor

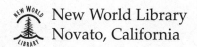
New World Library
Novato, California

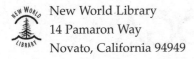 New World Library
14 Pamaron Way
Novato, California 94949

Photographs by Adrian Kat
Illustrations by Toby Gibson
Composition by Tona Pearce Myers

Library of Congress Cataloging-in-Publication Data
Maehle, Gregor.
 Ashtanga yoga—the intermediate series : mythology, anatomy, and practice / Gregor Maehle with Dr. Monica Gauci, chiropractor.
    p.   cm.
Includes bibliographical references and index.
ISBN 978-1-57731-669-5 (pbk. : alk. paper)
1. Astanga yoga. I. Gauci, Monica. II. Title.
RA781.68.M343 2009
613.7'046--dc22   2009038441

First printing, November 2009
ISBN 978-1-57731-669-5
Printed in Canada on 100% postconsumer-waste recycled paper

New World Library is a proud member of the Green Press Initiative.

10   9   8   7   6   5   4   3

To our ancient mother, India — origin of civilization
long before our written history dawned,
abode of the noble ones (*aryas*),
land who brought forth an endless stream of sages
and liberated ones (*rishis*), who produced the manifold sciences (*vidyas*)
and the language of wisdom (*sanskrita*), and who does not cease
to provide paths for those who dare.
May there dawn a new age that reveals again your original splendor.

CONTENTS

ACKNOWLEDGMENTS

Many thanks to the modern master of Ashtanga Vinyasa Yoga, Shri T. Krishnamacharya, and those who studied under him and continue his work. Without their contributions, this beacon of light would have been extinguished.

Thanks also to my wife, Monica, for contributing valuable information in the fields of anatomy and *asana* and for her relentless pursuit of knowledge.

PREFACE

After my first book, *Ashtanga Yoga: Practice and Philosophy*, was published, many readers approached me requesting that I write a book on the intricacies of the Intermediate Series of Ashtanga Yoga.

During the writing of this new book, which took more than two years, it became apparent to me that so much that we know today about yoga goes back to the late Shri T. Krishnamacharya. Although I never studied with the great master, I had the great fortune of working with four of his students, B. N. S. Iyengar, K. Pattabhi Jois, B. K. S. Iyengar, and A. G. Mohan.

In this book I am attempting to present the original, integrative yoga that became fractured following Krishnamacharya's demise in 1989. You will find ever present in this book T. Krishnamacharya's emphasis on learning scripture, devotion, understanding Sanskrit, adapting the practice to the individual, and doing whatever is reasonable and beneficial to the student.

Although I made every effort to present this yoga in its original true form, I am aware that my representation does not even come close to the master's learning and understanding.

INTRODUCTION

My aim in writing this book is to supply Ashtanga Yoga practitioners and teachers with the information they need to practice the Intermediate Series of this yoga safely and effectively. To this end, I have included extensive descriptions of all the postures that make up this series and in-depth discussions, in Western anatomical terms, of the main themes.

This book also informs the reader of the larger context in which the Intermediate Series and Ashtanga Yoga in general exist, which consists not only of the mythological basis of the Intermediate Series but also the relationship of Ashtanga Yoga to other forms of yoga. It explains the role of *asana* practice — specifically that of the Intermediate Series — in relation to the spiritual path of the practitioner.

The book is divided into three parts. Part 1 covers the spiritual and mythological foundations of this yoga; part 2 discusses the anatomical and other practical issues of the practice; and part 3 provides a detailed description of the postures of the Intermediate Series. With its varied content, this book will interest not only intermediate practitioners but also those who would like to learn more about Ashtanga Yoga in general and Ashtanga Vinyasa Yoga specifically.

Regardless of the use to which you put this book, I encourage you to consult my first book, *Ashtanga Yoga: Practice and Philosophy*. It describes the Primary Series of Ashtanga Yoga, which needs to be mastered before undertaking the Intermediate Series. It also contains a commentary on Patanjali's *Yoga Sutra*, the defining text of yoga philosophy, as well as an essay on yoga history.

Origins of Ashtanga Yoga

Most Indians identify the ancient seer Patanjali as the father of all yogas. Traditionally, they have viewed Patanjali as a semi-divine being, a manifestation of Ananta, the serpent of infinity.

Patanjali displayed an incredible level of mastery in compiling the *Yoga Sutra*; he also published texts on Sanskrit grammar and Ayurvedic medicine. Thus you can think of Patanjali as a master of advanced yoga techniques, a professor of various branches of classical knowledge, and a mythological, semi-divine being all wrapped in one. The Indian masters I have studied with report that Patanjali lived six thousand years ago, though some Western scholars claim that he lived more recently.

Ashtanga Yoga can be traced all the way back to Patanjali. Ashtanga Yoga is mentioned in many ancient texts, such as the *Mahabharata*, the longest Indian epic. These references make it clear that the term *Ashtanga* was always used to refer to Patanjali's yoga. *Ashtanga* is derived from the Sanskrit words *ashtau*, meaning "eight," and *anga*, meaning "limb." These words describe the essence of Ashtanga Yoga — a discipline built of eight distinct practices, or limbs. The postures, or *asanas*, that most Westerners associate with the term *yoga* make up only one of these eight limbs.

The following are the eight limbs as described by Patanjali:[1]

1. Restraints (*Yamas*)
2. Observances (*Niyamas*)
3. Postures (*Asanas*)
4. Breath extension (*Pranayama*)
5. Internal focus (*Pratyahara*)
6. Concentration (*Dharana*)
7. Meditation (*Dhyana*)
8. Ecstasy (*Samadhi*)

I say more about these limbs in short order.

One of the outstanding features of Indian spiritual traditions such as yoga is that through the ages their practices have adapted to meet the changing requirements of an evolving society.

1   *Yoga Sutra* II.29.

Ashtanga Yoga is no different, and in the past few millennia it has taken many forms. For example, a fairly recent form, only about one thousand years old, is Hatha Yoga, a Tantric yoga that focuses on the body and proper execution of elaborate techniques. One of Hatha Yoga's defining texts, the *Hatha Yoga Pradipika*, calls the practice a "ladder" for those who want to reclaim the heights of Ashtanga Yoga.[2]

Another school or mode of Ashtanga Yoga is Ashtanga Vinyasa Yoga — the practice that is the subject of this book. Today this school is often called simply Ashtanga Yoga. This abbreviated form of the name is a bit confusing because it could refer to either Ashtanga Yoga as a whole or the subdivision that is Ashtanga Vinyasa Yoga. The term *Ashtanga Yoga* is now universally accepted, and that's the one I use in this book. The reader will have to judge from context whether *Ashtanga* refers to the general mantle of Patanjali's yoga or the specific discipline of Ashtanga Vinyasa Yoga.

Ashtanga Vinyasa Yoga was founded by the seer Vamana, who according to my Indian preceptors lived four thousand years ago. During that period, cities in India were growing rapidly, and as a result the people felt increasing demands on their time.[3] The society needed a practice that encompassed all the elements of Patanjali's original yoga but took up less time. Rishi Vamana fulfilled this need by introducing the concept of *vinyasa* in his text *Yoga Korunta*.

In *vinyasa*, postures (*asanas*, the third limb) are combined with internal muscular contractions (*bandhas*) and breath control or extension (*pranayama*, the fourth limb) to form what are called "seals" (*mudras*). The postures are performed in particular sequences and further combined with focal points (*drishtis*) for the eyes. These modifications "turbo-charge" the postures. When practiced correctly with the fifth and sixth limbs (*pratyahara*, the sense withdrawal technique, and *dharana*, the concentration technique that involves listening to the breath), the postures lead to a meditative state (*dhyana*, the seventh limb). Over time the regular

practice of these integrated limbs purifies the mind and body and eventually leads to ecstasy (*samadhi*, the eighth limb).

The following section presents an overview of the eight limbs of Ashtanga Yoga; a more detailed exploration appears in chapter 1.

The Eight Limbs

Patanjali had achieved the state of *samadhi*, which refers to an experience of oceanic or divine ecstasy. Today the term *ecstasy* often connotes a drug-induced state of euphoria or the peak of sexual pleasure, but there is a passage in the scriptures wherein *samadhi* is said to have about a trillion times the intensity of sexual pleasure.[4] In other words, it is far beyond anything you can imagine in normal experience. Because he existed continually in this state of absolute freedom, Patanjali described a path that could lead all of us to it. He asked himself, Which state immediately precedes divine ecstasy? The answer was meditation (*dhyana*). *Samadhi* is our true nature, but we cannot receive it if our minds are too busy to listen, he reasoned; therefore, the path to *samadhi* lies in quieting the mind, which is accomplished when one achieves the state of relaxed openness that occurs in meditation.

Patanjali then asked himself, Which state immediately precedes *dhyana*? The answer was concentration (*dharana*). Concentration is the state that enables one to stay in meditation (or in any other state, for that matter). Many people achieve a spontaneous meditative state for split seconds only. The goal is to perpetuate that state, and that is made possible by *dharana*.

What does one need for concentration to arise? One needs inward focus (*pratyahara*), answered Patanjali; concentration is destroyed by outward distractions.

Patanjali then inquired, What state is the prerequisite for inward focus? The answer was easy. Since the mind goes wherever the breath or its subtle equivalent, *prana*, goes, one needs breath regulation (*pranayama*) to achieve inward focus.

Which state is necessary for one to practice breath regulation? asked Patanjali finally. Since

---

2 *Hatha Yoga Pradipika* I.1.
3 The oldest excavated Indian city, Mergarh, is now confirmed as being eight thousand years old. It had 25,000 inhabitants.

4 *Brhad Aranyaka Upanishad* 4.3.33.

breath and *prana* are dispersed in an unhealthy body, and health is produced by the practice of postures, the answer was *asana*.

Patanjali saw that these six steps had to be placed on a foundation of ethical guidelines governing one's inner and outer life. On this basis he stipulated the first two limbs, the restraints (*yamas*) and observances (*niyamas*). Without these limbs as the foundation for the others, all the benefit accrued by practicing the other six limbs would likely be lost.

Although Patanjali conceived of the eight limbs from the top down, we must practice them from the bottom up, starting with the ethical precepts of *yama* and *niyama*.

The Russian-Doll Model of the Eight Limbs

Patanjali portrayed the eight limbs of yoga as sequential in nature, which can be understood through the following metaphor: Conditioned existence was likened to confinement in a prison tower, with yoga as the means of escape; practicing the first limb was like dangling a silken thread from the tower, practicing the second like tying a thicker cotton thread to the silken one, practicing the third like following the cotton thread with a cord, and so on until the strong rope of the seventh limb allowed you to descend. In this metaphor, which I introduced in *Ashtanga Yoga: Practice and Philosophy*, the limbs of yoga are introduced sequentially and shown to work one after the other. This is a workable model, but it has its limitations; in particular, it insinuates that each limb of yoga is abandoned once the next one is achieved. But one cannot abandon any of the limbs until one has achieved all of them and is about to enter objectless *samadhi*, the highest form of *samadhi*. Those of us who haven't yet achieved objectless *samadhi* need to practice the lower limbs as we progress through the higher ones.

A useful way to understand this aspect of the limbs is to think of the limbs as a set of Matryoshka dolls. These Russian nesting dolls are usually painted wooden figures, each of which can be pulled apart to reveal another, smaller figure of the same sort inside. When the outermost doll is opened, we find another doll in it; that second doll opens to reveal another inside it; and so on. If we think of yoga's eight limbs as similar to these Russian dolls, the outermost doll would be the first limb, *yama*, and the last, innermost one would be the concluding limb, *samadhi*. Each successive doll is contained within the dolls outside it, just as each successive limb is supported by the already perfected limbs that lead to it. As you progress in your practice, each new limb brings you further along your path only if you adhere to it within the context of the earlier limbs or stages.

The Importance of *Asana*

Modern (and particularly modern Western) practitioners of yoga can easily jump to the conclusion that yoga postures are mere gymnastic exercises, without spiritual or philosophical significance. One purpose of this book is to correct this misconception, to make it very clear that the *asanas* are part of a spiritual culture that aims at nothing short of bringing practitioners to a state of complete and absolute freedom in which they realize their innermost divine potential.

For the majority of modern people, mere sitting in meditation is not sufficient to achieve any lasting spiritual progress or transformation. If you practice only sitting meditation or self-inquiry or the study of scripture, you can easily fool yourself about your state of attainment. True knowledge is not something that occurs in one's mind alone; it has a physical dimension as well. The Armenian mystic George I. Gurdjieff expressed this in the words, "True knowledge is of a chemical nature."[5] What he meant is that authentic knowledge has a biochemical and bioelectrical component; it has substance. This component is what traditional yogis called *siddhi*, which is sometimes translated as "supernatural power" or "proof." *Asana* lays the groundwork for achieving the biochemical and bioelectrical changes in our bodies that are necessary for gaining true knowledge.

Sitting in meditation is sufficient only for those fit to practice Jnana Yoga. The term *Jnana Yoga* is

5 My translation, from P. D. Ouspensky, *Auf der Suche nach dem Wunderbaren* [In Search of the Miraculous] (Munich: Otto Wilhelm Barth Verlag, 1982), p. 52.

more closely investigated in chapter 1, but in a nutshell it refers to gaining freedom by the mere contemplation of the fact that one's true self is identical with the infinite, pure consciousness, without resorting to any other techniques. Jnana Yoga and the associated seated meditation (that is, sitting upright with the head, neck, and spine in one line) can be practiced only if one's intelligence is completely freed from the stains of *rajas* (frenzies) and *tamas* (dullness).[6] If you are not tainted by these states, go right ahead and try to achieve *samadhi* through sitting. If, however, your intellect oscillates, as mine does, between frenzy and dullness (with some bright moments in between), then the practice of *asana* will be useful for you.[7]

Richard Freeman, in his collection of discourses called *Yoga Matrix*, likened the practice of postures to going through your body with a fine-tooth comb. Thoughts and emotions that are powered by *rajas* or *tamas* leave imprints in your bodily tissue that make it more likely that *rajasic* or *tamasic* states will be repeated. These imprints are released through posture practice, thus forming the bedrock for higher yogic technique.

Putting Technique in the Proper Context

Those who practice Ashtanga Vinyasa Yoga (or any of the many other forms of Karma Yoga, a term that is explained in chapter 1) face a certain danger: becoming attached to technique. They can get comfortable with repeating techniques that they have already mastered without ever relating them to the ultimate purpose of the techniques, which is to allow the practitioner to abide in infinite

consciousness. The yogic techniques become empty of meaning and an end in themselves. In modern Ashtanga Vinyasa practitioners, this may surface as a one-sided emphasis on *asana* practice and a refusal to invest any time or energy in the higher limbs. It is unlikely that this is what Patanjali wanted to see in students when he compiled the *Yoga Sutra*.

Ironically, it is often those yogis who have become very proficient at what they do who are most strongly attached to their techniques. Their breathtakingly athletic skill in practicing postures has become the basis of their self-image, and they are reluctant to progress to stages in which proficiency in *asana* is no longer the point. Understandably, they don't want to surrender their abilities and knowledge. But this surrender is necessary if one wishes to progress along the spiritual path. According to Patanjali, one must undergo *paravairagya* (a complete letting go) to achieve super-cognitive (objectless) *samadhi* and through it liberation.

In this book I try to counteract the tendency to get caught up in technique, by reminding you that the purpose of *asana* is to recognize yourself as infinite consciousness (*jnana*) and as a child of God (*bhakti*). The purpose of chapter 1 is to convince you that the essence of all modes of Karma Yoga — everything you do to become free and yourself, including *asana* — is still just *jnana* and *bhakti*, which are one. In chapter 4, you will learn that the essence of each posture is its underlying divine form.

An effective way to avoid an attachment to technique is to place yourself right from the beginning in the service of one of the aspects of the Supreme Being. You need to continually remind yourself that the ultimate purpose of the eight limbs is not to become good at their execution. Their purpose is to realize the *Brahman*. As Shri T. Krishnamacharya expressed it, "The eight limbs are the eight limbs of Bhakti."

The Intermediate Series of Postures

The Intermediate Series in Ashtanga Vinyasa Yoga serves as an important part of the discipline that

---

6　According to yoga, the intellect is made up of three *gunas* (qualities), which are *tamas* (dullness), *rajas* (frenzy), and *sattva* (wisdom). The first two qualities need to be reduced through practice, study, and devotion.

7　Some modern teachers claim that when Patanjali wrote about *asana*, he was referring only to the sitting posture of meditation. But the Rishi Vyasa has spelled out in his commentary on the *Yoga Sutra* that posture in yoga is not just sitting with one's head, neck, and back in a straight line but is the practice of a complete course of yogic *asanas* (Swami Hariharananda Aranya, *Yoga Philosophy of Patanjali*, Albany: State University of New York Press, 1983, p. 228).

may lead to mastery of the eight limbs and, ultimately, to liberation. Let's now look briefly at the structure of the Intermediate Series, which I cover in detail in chapter 6 and, of course, in part 3.

The Intermediate Series is constructed of the following elements:

1. An opening consisting of some twisting (*Pashasana*) and forward bending (*Krounchasana*)
2. An extensive backbending sequence consisting of eight postures (*Shalabhasana, Bhekasana, Dhanurasana, Parshva Dhanurasana, Ushtrasana, Laghu Vajrasana, Kapotasana,* and *Supta Vajrasana*)
3. A forward-curling arm balance (*Bakasana*) to counteract the backbends, combined with some more twisting (*Bharadvajasana* and *Ardha Matsyendrasana*)
4. A leg-behind-head sequence consisting of three postures (*Ekapada Shirshasana, Dvipada Shirshasana,* and *Yoganidrasana*)
5. A dynamic forward bend (*Tittibhasana*) to link the preceding and subsequent postures
6. An arm-balance section consisting of four postures (*Pincha Mayurasana, Karandavasana, Mayurasana,* and *Nakrasana*)
7. A wind-down consisting of a hip opener (*Vatayanasana*), another forward bend (*Parighasana*), a hip and shoulder opener (*Gaumukhasana*), another twist (*Supta Urdhva Pada Vajrasana*), and a sequence of headstands (*Mukta Hasta Shirshasana* and *Baddha Hasta Shirshasana*)

The three essential parts of the series are the backbends, leg-behind-head postures, and arm balances (items 2, 4, and 6 above); the other four sections function mainly to connect and prepare. The Intermediate Series strongly differs from the Primary Series, which is made up of forward-bending postures and hip rotations.

The Benefits of Practicing the Intermediate Series

Practicing the Intermediate Series yields many benefits to the gross body — that is, the body that is perceptible to the senses. Your body will become healthier, stronger, leaner, and athletic, much like that of a racehorse. And yes, of course, the shape of your derriere will also improve. (You see, I know what motivates many modern yogis.) But let's leave jokes aside and focus on what's really important: the effect of the Intermediate Series on the subtle body.

The subtle body is chiefly made up of chakras (energy centers), pranic currents called *vayus* (vital airs), and the receptacles of the *vayus*, the *nadis*. *Nadis* are the conduits, or energy channels, of the subtle body, along which the various forms of life force (*prana*) move. The *nadis* are clogged in most people and must be purified if one is to progress to the higher limbs. The Intermediate Series serves this function of purification; in Sanskrit it is called *Nadi Shodhana*, which means "purification of the *nadis*."

Some have translated the term *Nadi Shodhana* as "purification of the nervous system," but this translation is problematic. The *nadi* system is much subtler than Western anatomy's nervous system. The nervous system refers to part of the gross body, which is obviously very different from the subtle *nadi* system. Many nerve ganglions of the gross body are several millimeters in diameter and can easily be seen by the naked eye. *Nadis*, on the other hand, are considered to be one one-thousandth the diameter of a hair. As part of the subtle body, they cannot be perceived by the senses.

As one practices the Intermediate Series, and later the Advanced Series and meditation exercises, the *nadis* are gradually purified. Since *prana* ascends through the body via the *nadis*, this purification clears the way for *prana* to ascend all the way to the crown chakra, a culmination that marks the physical dimension of divine revelation or, in other words, of the state of liberation.

The *nadis* also require balancing, so that *prana* can flow through them evenly. The three primary *nadis* are the *pingala* (the right, or solar, nostril), the *ida* (the left, lunar nostril), and the *sushumna* (the central energy channel). When the breath flows predominantly through the *pingala*, the mind tends to adopt a solar or fundamentalist attitude, which means adhering to one truth while overlooking the many other truths.[8] When the breath flows predominantly through the *ida*, the mind tends to adopt a lunar or relativist attitude, which means that one is attracted by many truths but unable to pick the one that is most appropriate in a given circumstance. During a *samadhic* state, there is no such imbalance, because either the *prana* flows in the *sushumna* or, as some authorities maintain, there is no *pranic* movement at all.

When a race car driver prepares for a championship race, he or she makes sure that the car is in perfect condition, ready for peak performance. The car is taken apart to make sure that all its parts are clean and in working order. If there are any blockages in the fuel ducts, air intakes, hoses, combustion chambers, exhaust pipes, or manifolds, the parts are cleaned to unclog them; otherwise they will impinge on the optimal flow of energy. In a similar way, if you see *samadhi* as the peak human experience and want to achieve it as much as the race car driver wants to win the race, you must make sure your *nadi* system is in top condition. If it isn't, you either won't have the mystical experience or won't be able to put it into context and integrate it into your life. This necessary cleansing and fine-tuning of the *nadi* system is achieved by becoming proficient in the practice of the Intermediate Series of postures. Thus the practice of this series helps lay the foundations for higher yoga.

Prerequisites for Practicing the Intermediate Series

Practicing the Intermediate Series is incredibly beneficial. However, just as a farmer must till and fertilize the soil before yielding the harvest, you can reap the many benefits of the practice only if your ground — your mind and body — is properly prepared. Before starting the Intermediate Series, you need to fulfill the following three conditions:

- Be able to correctly practice all the postures of the Primary Series (as explained in *Ashtanga Yoga: Practice and Philosophy*).
- Attain *Yoga Chikitsa* (yoga therapy), the goal of the Primary Series, by practicing the Primary Series for a sufficient length of time.
- Have built a sufficient amount of strength and endurance.

Let's look at each of these conditions separately.

PROFICIENT PERFORMANCE OF POSTURES

Attempting the Intermediate Series too soon is like building a second story on a house before the concrete in the supporting pillars of the first story has cured. Inevitably, your building will soon show cracks. The cardinal postures of the Primary Series are *Pashimottanasana* and *Baddhakonasana*, and you should display sufficient proficiency in these two postures. It is difficult, however, to define the required level of proficiency. You need to be flexible enough in both forward bending and hip rotation so that you can satisfactorily perform the three energetically most effective and important postures of the Primary Series, namely *Marichyasana D*, *Supta Kurmasana* (which includes *Kurmasana*, a vinyasa of *Supta Kurmasana*), and *Garbhapindasana*. You can read about the importance of these three postures in *Ashtanga Yoga: Practice and Philosophy*.

ATTAINMENT OF YOGA CHIKITSA

Yoga Chikitsa means "yoga therapy" and refers to the process of eliminating the basic causes of diseases and balancing the *doshas* in the body (*vata*, *pitta*, and *kapha*) and *gunas* in the mind (*tamas*, *rajas*, and *sattva*) through regular practice of postures. Some dancers, gymnasts, and very flexible people can do the postures of the Primary Series right at the beginning. But this is not enough. They need to practice the Primary Series until the health and balance of *Yoga Chikitsa* is achieved.

Patanjali lists the obstacles to yoga.[9] The first,

8 Terminology courtesy of Richard Freeman.

9 *Yoga Sutra* I.30.

sickness, results primarily from an imbalance of the *doshas*; *Yoga Chikitsa* improves this balance. Attaining *Yoga Chikitsa* does not mean that you will never become sick again, since disease stems primarily from its root cause, the mind, and also from the environment and from karmic influences. *Yoga Chikitsa* will, however, improve your health and increase your resistance to disease and your capacity to recover quickly.

Yoga Chikitsa can be obtained by practicing the complete Primary Series every day for approximately one year. Please note that this is only a rough guideline, and the time required varies from person to person. Only a qualified teacher can determine if you have achieved *Yoga Chikitsa*.

Patanjali states that practice can succeed only when it is sustained uninterruptedly, for a long time and with a devotional attitude.[10] So, as indicated previously, the Primary Series needs to be performed daily and in an uninterrupted fashion for an entire year. If the student is not able to practice daily in a devoted fashion, then she or he is not ready to commence the Intermediate Series.

ATTAINMENT OF STRENGTH AND ENDURANCE

The final condition that one must fulfill before starting the Intermediate Series is to possess a sufficient amount of strength and endurance. The Intermediate Series is much more demanding than the Primary and requires more lengthy practice. You will need to have ample reserves built up before embarking on the long trek through the Intermediate Series.

You probably have adequate strength if you can cleanly jump from *Dandasana* to *Chaturanga Dandasana* and move from Downward Dog to *Dandasana* in a controlled fashion. Sufficient endurance is indicated by the ability to sustain indefinitely a six-day-per-week practice of the full Primary Series. In addition, you should be able to perform the Primary Series with ease on your worst days, energetically speaking.

Before you commence the Intermediate Series, ask yourself whether you have the extra time and

10 *Yoga Sutra* I.14.

energy to invest in your practice. If you are not confident that the answer is yes, staying with the Primary Series for another year until you have made the space in your life is a safer bet.

A Final Word on Readiness

Each person begins his or her practice at a different level of readiness and progresses at a unique pace. This concept is central to Vedic teaching. One needs to practice that stage (*bhumika*) of practice that one is fit or ready for (*adhikara*). The term *adhikara* is formed from the verb root *kri*, "to do," and the prefix *adhi-*, meaning "on either side" (as opposed to above or below). *Adhikara*, therefore, means to do that which is at your level and not something that is beyond your understanding or capability (or not challenging enough).

Indian scriptures generally state who is qualified to perform the actions described therein. Such an injunction may consist of only one stanza or even only one word. For example, the *Yoga Sutra* starts with the statement "*atha yoga anushasanam*," which can be translated as "Here starts the discourse of yoga for the benefit of those who have realized that the objects of this world cannot quench their thirst." Much of this message is encrypted in the important word *atha*. The author, Patanjali, wishes to express that those who still believe that they can achieve freedom merely by becoming smart, sexy, powerful, and wealthy are not qualified (*adhikarin*) to receive this instruction. Other texts devote several lengthy stanzas — usually titled *adhikarin* or *adhikara* — to the recitation of an entire catalog of conditions that the yogi needs to meet before embarking on his or her practices.

In days past, many yogic disciplines severely limited their audiences by imposing hard-to-meet conditions. The schools were concerned with not the quantity but rather the quality of the students. Many yogic schools targeted a very particular bandwidth of students, and all applicants above or below that bandwidth were sent off to look somewhere else. In the ancient days, teachers did their best to drive students away rather than collect them. It is a modern phenomenon for teachers to project the idea that their teaching suits everybody's needs.

Traditionally, it was the teacher who chose what type of practice the student was ready for.

In days of yore, teachings were categorized according to *bhumika*. *Bhumika* means step, degree, or stage. As there were people of many different stages of evolution, there were many different teachings to suit the various stages. The right teaching for a particular person was considered the teaching that accommodated the person's present stage and was capable of lifting him or her to the next higher stage. Nowadays, influenced by the democratization of society, everybody wants to have the highest teaching, whether it is suitable or not. The highest teaching is generally accepted to be Jnana Yoga (also called the *Brahma Vidya*), the discipline in which only pure knowledge and no form of practice is used (see the more detailed discussion in chapter 1). For this reason Jnana Yoga has gained many fans in Western society. However, according to the traditional view only a few are qualified (*adhikara*) for this highest path. Further, if you do not practice the path you are fit for, not only will you achieve no results; you will also waste your time and that of your teacher. To prevent this, you need to judge objectively which practice you are fit for (*adhikara*). Once you have reached a certain stage, you then progress to the next higher stage (*bhumika*) without attempting to skip ahead.

Patanjali provided an easy way of navigating this problem when he created the eight limbs, which are neatly organized according to stage. That he adhered to the *bhumika* doctrine becomes clear when we read "*tasya saptada pranta bhumih prajna.*"[11] This *sutra* says that complete and authentic knowledge of objects (*prajna*) is arrived at in seven stages.

If you have the time and energy to continue your journey through Ashtanga Vinyasa Yoga by embarking on the Intermediate Series, you will find that you have an incredible tool at your disposal. Although the Intermediate Series initially requires a great deal of energy, time, and determination, the outcome is worth the effort. The daily practice of the full Intermediate Series deepens your quality of life so much that once you are established in this regimen, you simply will not want to live in a body that does not undergo this type of yogic training.

11 *Yoga Sutra* II.27.

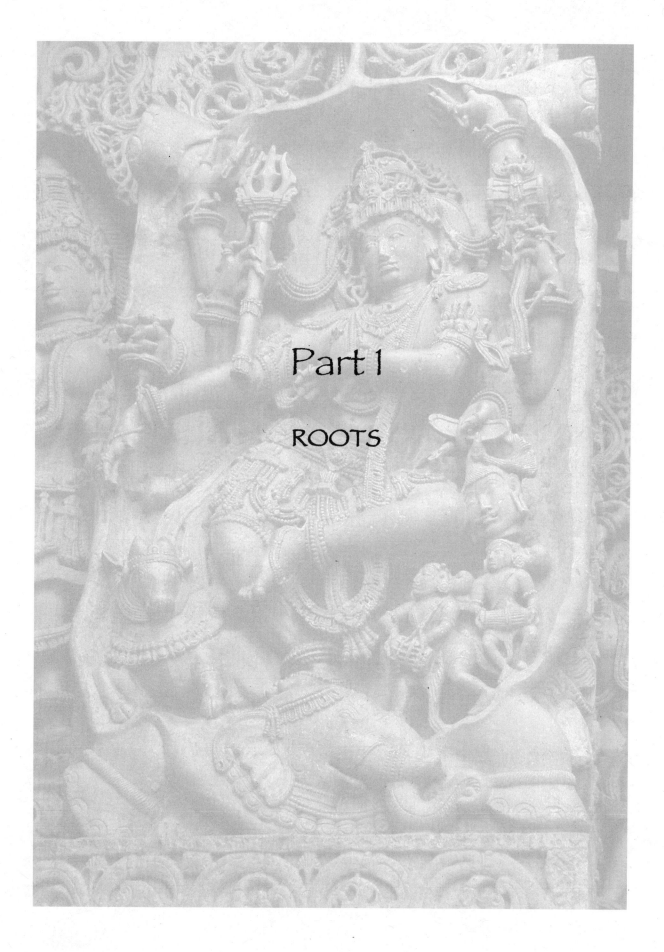

Part 1

ROOTS

Chapter 1
Jnana, Bhakti, and *Karma:* The Three Forms of Yoga

In this chapter we look at the three basic forms of yoga — Jnana, Bhakti, and Karma — exploring how they differ and what they share in common. Essentially, Jnana Yoga is the yoga of knowledge; Bhakti Yoga is the yoga of devotion; and Karma Yoga is the yoga of action. All modes or expressions of yoga can be classified under these three disciplines. The yogi needs to understand that they are complementary. They suit different temperaments; some people may practice one form for a period of their lives and then switch to another. The subject of this book, Ashtanga Yoga, falls under the umbrella of Karma Yoga, but it incorporates certain aspects of the other two forms.

We also look at the different modes of Karma Yoga, the form of yoga most widely known and practiced in the West. This includes a more detailed look at the eight limbs of Ashtanga Yoga. This knowledge will enable you to sift through all the diverse information you hear about yoga and put it into the context of your own practice.

Yoga in its various forms crystallized out of the *Vedas*, the oldest scriptures known to humankind. The *Vedas* are considered to be of divine origin. They contain eternal knowledge (the term *Veda* comes from the root *vid*, "to know"), which is revealed anew during each world age to those who are open to hearing it. Those who receive this knowledge and record it are called Vedic seers, or *rishis.*[1]

Because the *Vedas* are voluminous, they are divided into categories to make them more accessible. Well known are the four main Vedic texts, the *Rigveda, Samaveda, Yajurveda,* and *Atharvaveda;* each of these categories represents a set of family lines (*gotra*) that was entrusted to preserve that particular set of scriptures. The *Vedas* are also commonly divided according to the subjects the passages deal with. These divisions are called *kandas* (portions). The three *kandas* are the *Karma kanda,* which pertains to performing actions; the *Upasana kanda,* which concerns itself with worship of the divine; and the *Jnana kanda,* the portion pertaining to self-knowledge. As you may have guessed, the *Karma kanda* became the basis for Karma Yoga, the *Upasana kanda* led to Bhakti Yoga, and the *Jnana kanda* laid the foundation for Jnana Yoga.

Jnana Yoga

The term *Jnana* comes from the verb root *jna,* to know. In fact, both the Greek word *gnosis* and the English word *know* have their origin in the Sanskrit *jna.* Jnana Yoga is the most direct path to recognizing yourself as a manifestation of divine consciousness, but it is considered to be the most difficult. In the days of the *Bhagavad Gita,* Jnana Yoga was called *Buddhi Yoga* (the yoga of intellect) or the yoga of inaction, because one practices it through contemplation alone. This form of yoga is the one predominantly taught in the ancient *Upanishads,* the mystical and philosophical section of the *Vedas.* In the *Brhad Aranyaka Upanishad* this yoga is described as consisting of three steps: *shravana* (listening), *manana* (contemplating), and

---

1 The term *rishi* is inextricably linked to Veda. You won't find a Buddhist *rishi* or a Tantric *rishi.*

nidhidhyasana (being established).[2] The practitioner first listened to a teacher who had attained the illustrious self-knowledge that all is in fact nothing but *Brahman* (consciousness). He then let go of all his desires, such as wealth, success, pleasure, fame, and family; retired to a quiet place; and contemplated the words of the teacher. After due consideration, he recognized the eternal truth of the teaching and was then permanently established in that truth.

From this short description, you may understand why this path is considered short and direct but also very difficult. It is short because there are very few steps involved. After finding a teacher, there is really only one step: the contemplation, in a solitary place, of your unity with the Supreme Self. It is a difficult path for many reasons. It requires that a self-realized teacher accept you as a student. Such teachers were considered hard to find even in the ancient days, and they are much rarer today. It then requires that you *completely* let go of all attachments to wealth, success, pleasure, fame, family, and so on. Modern Western teachers who prefer to communicate to their students that they can "have it all" do not drive this point home enough. Traditionally this highest path was taught only to renunciates and ascetics, those who had taken a vow to forsake all the worldly attachments mentioned. The reasoning was that one had to let go of all external attachments if one was to surrender all one's inner attachments in the process of merging with the Supreme Self.

Also, the path of Jnana Yoga requires an intellect so pure, powerful, and intense that from the mere instruction of a self-realized teacher it can understand and accept the truth and become permanently established in it, free of duality. Such intellects are exceedingly rare. Understanding is easy, but what about remaining grounded in the truth even in moments of doubt, when one faces one's inner demons?

For this reason the path of Jnana Yoga is considered fit for only a select few. As the ancient Vedic text the *Samkhya Karika* puts it, only those whose intellects are entirely free of erroneous cognition can attempt it.[3] There are only a few Indians today who consider themselves fit for Jnana Yoga, and we may take this as a sign of the great humility and maturity of the Indian culture. On the other hand, many modern Western practitioners believe they deserve everything, including spiritual liberation, immediately and without having to give up anything. Thus they tend to view as a nuisance the preparations and qualifications that are asked of traditional Indian students.

Jnana Yoga was popularized mainly by the great Shankara, who lived some two thousand years ago.[4] Shankara is considered a *jagat guru* (world teacher), a name given to rare teachers of high stature who appear every few centuries or once in a millennium to reinterpret the scriptures and restore their original meaning. This had become necessary in Shankara's time; even though Jnana Yoga had been taught long before Shankara by *rishis* (seers) such as Vasishta, Yajnavalkya, and Vyasa, it was no longer understood properly because of changes in society and conventional language. Shankara wrote many great treatises and commentaries to present the ancient teachings again in their proper form. From today's perspective, Shankara's achievements look so gargantuan that many view him as a semi-divine or divine manifestation; in fact, he is often seen as a manifestation of the Lord Shiva himself.

In the twentieth century, Jnana Yoga was again popularized through the great example of Ramana Maharshi. Because Ramana was such an exceptional individual, he, too, was seen by many Indians as a divine manifestation — this time of Lord Skanda, the second son of Lord Shiva.

---

2 The *Brhad Aranyaka Upanishad* is the oldest, largest, and most important of the *Upanishads*. The genealogy of teachers listed in this *Upanishad* spans approximately 2,500 years.

3 *Samkhya Karika* of Ishvarakrishna, stanza 64. The *Karika* is today considered the most important text of *Samkhya*, as all of the older texts are lost. *Samkhya* is the most ancient Indian philosophy, one of the six orthodox systems of Vedic thought (*darshanas*).

4 Western scholars date him from 788 to 820, but this view is increasingly criticized. Indian tradition holds that he lived well before that date. His birth name was Adi Shankara. In India he is known as Shankaracharya (the teacher Shankara). In the colophon of his texts he often called himself Shankara Bhagavatpada, after his teacher Govinda Bhagavatpada.

The ancient teacher Shankara and the modern teacher Ramana had many things in common. Both held that true knowledge (*Jnana*) can be attained only through Jnana Yoga. However, both taught that those who cannot attain Jnana directly — which includes all but a few individuals — can go through a possibly lengthy preparation period and emerge ready to undertake Jnana Yoga. This preparation could consist of either of the other two paths of yoga, Bhakti Yoga or Karma Yoga.

Bhakti Yoga

Bhakti Yoga is the path of devotion that grew out of that portion of the *Veda* that deals with worship (*Upasana kanda*). It is based on the realization that most people have an emotional constitution rather than the cool, abstract, intellectual one that lends itself to Jnana Yoga. Also, it accepts the fact that it is much more difficult to realize consciousness as the impersonal absolute (called *nirguna Brahman*, the formless *Brahman*) than to surrender to a divine form (called *saguna Brahman*, *Brahman* with form).

Bhakti Yoga's path to freedom is reasonably direct but somewhat lengthier than that of Jnana Yoga. The term *bhakti* is created from the Sanskrit root *bhaj*, to divide. Unlike Jnana Yoga, which views the self of the individual and that of the Supreme Being as one and the same, Bhakti Yoga accepts the eternal division between the self of the devotee and the omnipotent self of the Supreme Being.

Our modern understanding of this difference in thought between these two branches of yoga originated from a teacher named Ramanuja. Many centuries after Shankara had brought about a renaissance of the ancient Vedic teaching, the essence of his teaching was again lost. Shankara had emphasized the complete identification of the individual self (*atman*) with the infinite consciousness (*Brahman*). Although this teaching is enshrined in the *Upanishads*, its opposite — the essential separation between *atman* and *Brahman* — is also enshrined. Some of Shankara's followers, taking his teachings to the extreme, had started to portray them as merely an analytical, philosophical, and scholastic path that was bereft of devotion and of compassion for the toiling masses of the population. Ramanuja arose as a great new teacher who could correct this misconception and reconcile the two views. Ramanuja taught the *beda-abeda* doctrine, which means "identity in difference." He agreed with Shankara that the individual self was consciousness and thus was identical with the Supreme Being. However, he added that the *atman* (individual self) was always limited in its power, knowledge, and capacity, whereas the Supreme Being (*Brahman*) was not, and in that regard *atman* and *Brahman* were different, hence the name "identity in difference."

Since according to this view there is an eternal division between the individual self and the Supreme Being, Ramanuja held that the right way to approach the Infinite One was not through knowing but through the path of devotion called Bhakti Yoga. Taking this path, the followers of Ramanuja developed an intense love for and devotion toward the Supreme Being and its many divine manifestations.

Today, the Hare Krishna movement, as an example, claims that Bhakti Yoga is the fastest, safest, and most direct way to freedom. However, this path is not as simple as it appears at first sight. Bhakti Yoga will not lead you to freedom unless you practice it with utmost and total surrender, as teachers like Ramanuja have done. It is also not without danger. The danger consists of the fact that devotees may attach egoic notions to the form of the Supreme Being that they worship. They start to believe that their God is better or more divine, and that their devotion to this one true God makes them superior to others. They may even despise followers of other religions and view them as inferior. Sadly, this is far from what Bhakti Yoga at its outset desired to achieve.

Bhakti can work only if you can see the Lord, the Goddess, the infinite formless consciousness (*Brahman*) — whichever form of the Divine you worship — in every being you encounter as well as in your own heart. The Supreme Being is infinite consciousness, love, and intelligence; it is your divine core. Around this core, which is your true self, various layers such as ego, mind, and body crystallize and form the human being. Since the

Supreme Being is undividable, we carry the wholeness of God in our hearts, and all of us are children of God. True Bhakti Yogis see all beings as their Lord and themselves as the servants of all beings. God is not in stone houses with stone images inside. Those houses and images may be helpful for the purpose of meditation, but true religion, true Bhakti, consists in worshiping the Divine in the hearts of all those we meet.

If you misunderstand Bhakti Yoga, you can believe that the Krishna you read about is more sacred and true than the Krishna in the heart of the being across from you. You may then conclude that this being is inferior because he or she worships the Supreme Being not in the form of Krishna but rather as Shiva, Allah, Jehovah, Yahweh, or some other deity. Certain devotees of the Lord Vishnu in India, for example, profess widespread contempt for the Lord Shiva, although the scriptures teach that Vishnu and Shiva are one and the same. A truly strange world this is. In cases such as this, the interest has shifted from recognizing the Supreme Being behind its manifold forms to taking pride in oneself based on the particular form that one's own devotion takes.

Bhakti Yoga requires not only fervor but also the self-reflectiveness of a clear intellect. Otherwise the intensity of one's experience of the Divine can easily lead one to be less compassionate toward others. Indian folklore is full of warnings of such erroneous views. For example, the learned Narada, a full-time attendant of the Supreme Being in the form of the Lord Vishnu, was once jealous of the Lord's love of a particular peasant. Narada asked the Lord what was so special about this peasant who was pronouncing the Lord's name only once per day, just before he fell asleep. The Lord asked Narada to fill a cup to the brim with oil and then carry it around his throne without spilling a drop. As Narada did so, he focused completely on the task. When he had completed it, he called out proudly, "Done! And no drop wasted!" The Lord then asked him, "And how often did you think about me? That peasant has to toil all day to extract from the soil a meager life for his family. But however hard his day is, he never

fails to remember me just before he falls asleep in exhaustion." Narada realized that his devotion had caused him to be prideful, a potent danger on the Bhakti path.

One of the great advantages of Bhakti Yoga is that it generally enables one to continue with most of everyday life; it changes only one's focus. After choosing the Bhakti path you no longer perform your daily duties striving for gain or advantage; instead, you surrender or offer all your actions, including their results, to your chosen image of the Divine.

Generally all forms of yoga contain a Bhakti component, emphasizing service to the Supreme Being. Patanjali states, "*samadhi siddhi ishvara pranidhanat*," or, "The power of *samadhi* can be obtained by surrendering to the Supreme Being."[5]

Karma Yoga

The term *karma* comes from the verb root *kru*, "to do," and *Karma Yoga* in the original Vedic sense means simply "path of action." The *Karma Kanda* of the *Veda*, which probably goes back more than ten thousand years, contains instructions for actions and rituals that one can perform with a particular goal in mind, such as obtaining wealth or the object of one's passion, becoming a good person, or achieving spiritual goals.

Approximately five thousand years ago, the Lord Krishna introduced a new form of Karma Yoga to Arjuna on the battlefield of Kurukshetra.[6] He described it as surrendering the fruit of one's actions to the Supreme Being. Note the difference between this definition of Karma Yoga and the idea of *karma* presented in the *Karma Kanda*. Krishna tells us not to be interested in the result of our actions but instead to "surrender the fruit of your action to me." In the *Vedas*, on the other hand, action (*karma*) is always used to achieve a particular effect. Lord Krishna actually criticizes the stance of the *Vedas* when he says, "*traigunya vishaya veda nistraygunyo bhavarjuna*," which loosely translates as "The *Vedas*

5 *Yoga Sutra* I.23.
6 *Bhagavad Gita* III.3 ff.

deal with accumulation only; be you without desire for gain."[7] Today, following on this idea, the term *Karma Yoga* is commonly used to refer to selfless service to others, such as going to an *ashrama* and chopping the veggies without pay.[8] In this book I will use the term *Karma Yoga* only in its original Vedic sense and not in its more recent meaning as taught by the Lord Krishna.

An important difference between Karma Yoga and the other two forms of yoga revolves around this issue of renouncing gain. The path of Jnana Yoga is traditionally taught only to those who have renounced the desire for any form of gain or success. Similarly, Bhakti Yoga requires one to internally renounce any gain that may accidentally come one's way and surrender it to one's chosen divine form. Karma Yoga, in contrast, requires its followers to give up the idea of gain and success only once the state of "discriminative knowledge" or "knowledge of the difference between self and nonself" is attained. This state is reached only after approximately 95 percent of the journey has been completed.[9] Although many of its higher techniques are difficult and demanding, in this regard Karma Yoga is a more "novice" type of yoga; it has lower entry requirements than Jnana and Bhakti Yoga and addresses those who are not yet ready to give up the pursuit of gain for themselves. (It is important here to remember that spiritual gain stands in the traditional Indian view on the same level as material gain; it is still just an attempt to get ahead.)

Seen from the lofty heights of Jnana or Bhakti Yoga, which aim at recognizing the infinite *Brahman* either with or without form, Karma Yoga is a modest path dealing with modest achievements in the relative world, such as acquiring a healthy body,

a steady mind, and a luminous intellect — all with the goal of gradually removing the barriers to spiritual liberation. Practitioners achieve these aims by performing the eight limbs of Patanjali's Ashtanga Yoga. Ashtanga Yoga, then, is the underlying structure or architecture of Karma Yoga.

Although Karma Yoga is a practical, mundane approach to realizing liberation, the concepts essential to Jnana and Bhakti Yoga lie at its core. When practicing the many elaborate techniques of Karma or Ashtanga Yoga, we need to remember that we do this only because we are in essence both infinite consciousness (the heart of Jnana Yoga) and children of God (the essence of Bhakti Yoga). These three paths are, after all, different routes to the same destination.

The Many Modes of Karma Yoga

Whereas there is only one type of Jnana Yoga and one type of Bhakti Yoga, Karma Yoga has differentiated into many different modes with different names, according to precisely what actions and techniques are suggested. Kriya Yoga, Kundalini Yoga, Hatha Yoga, Mantra Yoga, Tantra Yoga, Laya Yoga, Dhyana Yoga, Samadhi Yoga, and Raja Yoga are all different modes of Karma Yoga. In all these modes of yoga, the practitioner performs certain yogic actions intending to derive a direct benefit, such as a stronger, healthier body, a longer life, a smooth flow of *prana* (and eventually its arrest in the central energy channel), a powerful intellect that can concentrate at will, a penetrating insight that can be directed at objects normally hidden, the ability to know whatever one wishes — and the list goes on.

Western students are often confused by this apparent multiplicity of yogic teachings, which is replicated in the multiplicity of India's many divine forms and images. We may understand this fact by likening yoga to medicine — as, for example, the Rishi Vyasa did in his commentary on the *Yoga Sutra*. In medicine we have many different remedies addressing the various ailments that patients can develop. In a similar way, the many different forms of Karma Yoga have developed to address different problems.

---

7 *Bhagavad Gita* II.45. The *Vedas'* chief concern is here said to be the accumulation of material or spiritual merit. The Lord, however, wants Arjuna to abide in *Brahman*, beyond loss or gain.

8 The Cambridge scholar Elizabeth De Michelis's excellent study *The History of Modern Yoga* reveals how and through whom many of our modern ideas of yoga were introduced from Western and Christian sources.

9 Discriminative knowledge (*viveka khyateh*) is the result of the last and highest cognitive (objective) *samadhi*. Cognitive *samadhi* is, however, superseded by the still higher super-cognitive (objectless) *samadhi*.

Although all people are essentially the same at their divine cores, they vary greatly in their outer layers: the body, mind, ego, and intellect. Because people have very different bodies and minds, different approaches have been developed to remove the different obstacles located therein. Karma Yoga has developed its many modes because it targets these variable aspects of human individuals. Jnana and Bhakti Yoga, in contrast, have not had to differentiate because they address the divine consciousness or true self, which does not vary among individuals.

Ashtanga Yoga: The Architecture of Karma Yoga

The universally accepted form and structure that Karma Yoga takes is the eight-limbed yoga of Patanjali called Ashtanga Yoga. All of the eight limbs are in one form or another represented in all modes of Karma Yoga. The reason for using eight sequential steps may be understood through the following metaphor: Let's assume for a moment that the goal of yoga, called liberation, is located on the moon and its opposite, the state called *bhoga* (bondage) is here on Earth. Jnana and Bhakti Yoga hold out the possibility — not a realistic one for most people — of reaching your goal with one giant step. Eight-limbed Karma Yoga, on the other hand, provides you with a spacecraft that you can use to reach your destination, a spacecraft similar to the *Saturn V* rocket that powered the *Apollo 11* mission to the moon. The *Saturn V* had several stages. The first stage lifted the spacecraft to a certain height, and once its fuel had been exhausted the next stage was fired up. With the final stage the spacecraft had reached a distance far enough from the Earth that it could now "fall" toward the moon, attracted by the moon's gravitational field. In a similar way, Karma Yoga offers eight successive stages, each one carrying you successively higher toward the natural state of *yoga* (freedom) and away from the gravitation of *bhoga* (bondage).

Karma/Ashtanga Yoga gives you the opportunity to take small steps first. When you have done those steps successfully, you feel ready to take the slightly bigger steps that come next. Each step slightly modifies your body, mind, ego, and intellect, preparing them for the next, bigger step. Once you have taken the prescribed eight steps, you are then ready to take the plunge. That plunge is the same one the Bhaktas and Jnanis take, but the Ashtanga approach helps you prepare, organically and holistically, for it.

Let's take a closer look at the various steps or limbs of Karma/Ashtanga Yoga, focusing mainly on the higher limbs, as they are usually neglected in descriptions. For this purpose we return to the Russian-doll metaphor introduced in the Introduction.

YAMA — *RESTRAINT*

Yama comprises five restraints. Along with the second limb, *niyama* (observance), those restraints form the base of Karma Yoga. The five restraints are as follows:

1. Do not harm.
2. Be truthful.
3. Do not steal.
4. Have intercourse only with your lawful partner.
5. Do not give in to greed.

If your resolve to stick to these restraints is not firm, you may abuse the very great powers you gain through yoga. These are not just empty words. A significant number of practitioners in the long history of yoga have gone down that path.

NIYAMA — *OBSERVANCE*

Once you have made the transforming commitment to adhere to the *yama*, you adopt the following five *niyamas* (observances):

1. Inner and outer cleanliness
2. Contentment
3. Simplicity
4. Study of sacred texts
5. Surrender to the Supreme Being[10]

Of course, *niyama* will bring you progress only if it is adhered to within the context of the first limb, *yama*.

10 For a detailed description of each of these observances, please see *Ashtanga Yoga: Practice and Philosophy*, pp. 216–17.

ASANA — *POSTURE*

Once the practitioner has integrated *yama* and *niyama* into her life, she can begin the practice of *asana* (posture). There are hundreds of yoga postures; practicing them makes the body strong and supple, prepares it for the ascent of *prana*, and restores the natural balance of the body's three constitution types, or *doshas*: *vata*, *pitta*, and *kapha*.[11] It thereby removes the various obstacles listed by Patanjali, such as sickness and rigidity.[12] *Asana* coupled with *pranayama* removes even more obstacles, such as doubt, negligence, laziness, and sense indulgence. Most important, though, *asana* serves as the bedrock of meditation proper: performing the postures prepares the body for extensive sitting in the main yogic meditation postures, which are *Padmasana* (lotus posture), *Siddhasana*, *Swastikasana*, and *Virasana* (note that the names of these postures differ slightly among the different schools of *asana*). *Padmasana* is by far the most important of these postures — see the sidebar above titled "*Padmasana*: Seat of Power."

PRANAYAMA — *BREATH CONTROL AND EXTENSION*

Once the yogi is proficient in *asana*, breath extension can occur within the context of posture. In other words, the two are not separate practices; we assume *asana* to practice *pranayama*. The very significant effects of *pranayama* can be classed into three main groups:

1. *Prana*, which previously was scattered, is concentrated.
2. Pranic flow between the lunar and solar parts of the *nadi* system is harmonized.
3. *Prana* is arrested in the central channel of the *nadi* system, which leads to reabsorption of the mind into the heart.

PRATYAHARA — *INTERNAL FOCUS*

Pratyahara consists of a catalog of techniques used to focus the mind inward, thus forming the essential prerequisite for the arising of the higher limbs. It is ideally practiced in *Padmasana* or a similar potent *asana* and within the state of *kumbhaka* (breath retention). During *kumbhaka* we focus initially on locations within the gross body, which constitutes stage 1. Stage 2 is reached when we visualize the chakras of the subtle body and the mind is made to rest on them. This process is strongly intensified if it occurs within the framework of *asana* and *pranayama*. During this time of practice, the senses are prevented from "logging on" to their usual objects of desire, thus establishing inward focus.

The practice of *pratyahara* is based on the following concept: When the senses come into

11 For a description of the *doshas*, see David Frawley's *Ayurvedic Healing: A Comprehensive Guide* (Delhi: Motilal Banarsidass, 1992), p. 3.
12 *Yoga Sutra* I.30.

contact with objects in the external world (*object* being defined as anything that can be experienced by means of the senses), the objects arouse in the beholder reactions such as desire or repulsion, which all tend to ripple the surface of the lake of the mind. Some objects when presented to the mind will even bring about a downright storm. Once this has happened, it is difficult or impossible to use the mind as a tool for meditation. In *pratyahara*, you avoid the disturbances of the external world by settling the mind on something that is not in the outer world; you withdraw your senses into yourself "like a turtle withdraws its limbs."[13]

There are several categories of suitable *pratyahara* objects, which are principally categorized according to subtlety. The practitioner starts with gross objects, those that are perceptible to the senses. Typically these are the so-called *drishtis* (focal points), such as the tip of the nose, the eyebrow center, the big toes, the tip of the tongue, the nostrils, the highest point of the palate, the navel, the ankle, or other body parts; and of course the *bandhas*, principally the *Mula Bandha* (pelvic lock).

Once the yogi's focus is established on the gross level, subtle objects are chosen. The typical subtle objects used for *pratyahara* are the chakras. One starts by clearly visualizing the *muladhara* chakra; once attention is established there, one goes on to *svadhishthana* chakra, and so on. At this early point, you visualize only the following dimensions of the chakra: number of petals, color, and position (in case of the *Muladhara*, that would be four petals, dark red color, and a location near the tailbone). You have established proficiency in *pratyahara* when your focus during *kumbhaka* can be kept on the chakras, one after the other, without the senses grasping external objects.

DHARANA — CONCENTRATION

The ancient texts describe more than one hundred forms or techniques of *dharana*. They generally agree on the following point, however: *dharana* is practiced once proficiency in *asana*, *pranayama*, and *pratyahara* is gained and not before. Yogis achieve

13 *Bhagavad Gita* II.58.

dharana once they can use willpower to focus on the chosen object. But because this concentration is powered by a willful effort, it may be frequently interrupted, much as an Internet connection is sometimes interrupted when you are using an old-fashioned dial-up connection.

Practically, *dharana* is done in the following way: You assume *Padmasana*, *Siddhasana*, *Swastikasana*, or *Virasana* and commence *pranayama* until breath retention (*kumbhaka*) is reached. Once in *kumbhaka*, you rest the mind on your chosen location, beginning with the base chakra (*muladhara*). Rather than just visualizing the chakra in its location close to the coccyx (tailbone) and stopping there, you concentrate now on a particular aspect of that chakra. The first aspect would be the solidity of the earth element (*prithvi*). You then go on to the Sanskrit letters that are associated with the four petals of this chakra — that is, *va, sa, sha* (retroflex), and *sha* (palatal). The next aspect may be the root syllable (*bija akshara*) of the base chakra, *lang*. After that you may concentrate on the subtle essence or quantum (*tanmatra*) of the chakra, which in the case of the base chakra is smell (*gandha*). At this point you may conclude concentration on the base chakra and go on to the water chakra (*svadhishthana*). It is not specified how many breath retentions one has to spend on each aspect of the chakra.

DHYANA — MEDITATION

Dhyana, or meditation, can flourish only once concentration is mastered. Whereas concentration relies on willpower, meditation occurs effortlessly. The difference between the two is like the difference between a dial-up Internet connection and a high-speed broadband connection. In meditation, there is a continuous flow of awareness from the meditator toward the chosen meditation object and a constant stream of information or data from the object to the meditator — very much like what occurs on an Internet connection with fast upload and download speeds.

Let's assume that you have sufficiently practiced concentration and are therefore ready to embark on the exciting practice of meditation proper. I use the word *exciting* because once you have properly concentrated and thus "seen" the underlying truth of the various aspects of the chakra (that is, form, location, Sanskrit letters, root syllables, color, gross element, mandala, subtle essence), you can put them all together. At this depth of concentration, effort suddenly falls away and you get a direct line to the underlying reality of the chakra.

The fascinating opening that happens when you get to this stage is that you can "download" or "log on" to the *deva*, or divine form, that resides in or presides over each respective chakra (Lord Brahma for the *muladhara* chakra, for example).[14] The view of the divine form instills you with confidence in your progress and devotion. The *deva* is a manifestation of its mantra, the root syllable. In fact, the chakra, the associated element, and the presiding divine form are all manifested by the mantra, which in itself was a part of the creation of the universe by means of sound or vibration.

In *dhyana*, due to the permanent "logging on" to the object of contemplation, you no longer switch your attention from one aspect of the chakra to another (location to color to number of petals to root syllable to gross element, and so on); instead, you become able to see them all together as an interconnected, reciprocal whole. For the base chakra, for example, the divine form (Lord Brahma) is understood as a psychological representation of the root mantra, and the root mantra as an acoustic representation of the Lord Brahma; at the same time, the Earth element is seen as a material representation of the Lord Brahma and the Lord Brahma as a divine or celestial representation of the Earth element; in addition, the sense of smell appears as a subtle representation of the Earth element, and the Earth element as the subtle

equivalent of the sense of smell. The Earth element is also represented in the *yantra* (geometrical representation of the sacred) of the *Muladhara*, which is a square, and in the number of petals, which is four. All of these represent themselves in the microcosm of the human being on a subtle level as the *muladhara* chakra. This underlying reality at the foundation of *dhyana* needs to be deeply contemplated or spontaneously understood, whichever suits your temperament.

Unlike with *asana* and *pranayama*, it is difficult for an outside observer (that is, a teacher) to ascertain whether *pratyahara*, *dharana*, or *dhyana* have been attained. It is possible to quantify *asana* and *pranayama* — you can say that you practiced for two and a half hours and during that time you held eighty postures and forty breath retentions — but the practice of the inner limbs is not so easily measured.

SAMADHI — *ECSTASY*

Placing the innermost nesting doll of *samadhi* within the context and framework of the previous seven limbs is important; in Patanjali's view it is with *samadhi* that yoga becomes really interesting. Patanjali devoted the overwhelming majority of his *sutras* to this final limb. *Samadhi* denotes a deep state of meditation or the culmination thereof. Its pronounced fruit is the revelation of deep reality as such. For this reason a good translation for *samadhi* is "ecstasy" rather than the more puritan "bliss" or the bland "absorption." But the term *ecstasy* has its limitations also. It is derived from the Greek word *ekstasis*, meaning to stand beside oneself or be beside oneself (with joy). In *samadhi*, however, one does not stand beside oneself but rather deeply *within* oneself.[15]

The ecstasy of *samadhi* does not happen all at once. In *samadhi* we work through many substages, first using easy gross objects in meditation and later complex subtle objects. And once *samadhi* is mastered, we are met with a paradox. The final fruit of *samadhi*, liberation, is bestowed through complete

---

14 The term *deva* (divine form) unfortunately has been translated as "god." The *devas* are not gods, and India is not polytheistic. The superficial so-called polytheism of Hinduism is only a veiling of the deeper monotheism to which all the authoritative texts subscribe. The divine forms or celestials, which we see when success in meditation arises, are nothing but manifestations of aspects of the one Supreme Being. There may be a multiplicity of divine forms for the purpose of meditation, but there is only one *Brahman*, as the *Upanishads*, the *Bhagavad Gita*, and the *Brahma Sutra* teach in manifold passages.

15 To correct this problem, Mircea Eliade has suggested using the term *enstasy*, meaning "standing within," but this term still has not been widely accepted. See Mircea Eliade, *Yoga: Immortality and Freedom* (Princeton, NJ: Princeton University Press, 1969), p. 77.

surrender and divine grace and cannot be acquired by means of effort and willpower.

HOW INTENSE IS THE ECSTASY OF *SAMADHI*?

The great Rishi Yajnavalkya, the most prominent of the *rishis* (seers) of the *Upanishads*, explained the intensity of the ecstasy of *samadhi* thus:

Imagine the highest joy a human being is capable of experiencing through the combined attainment of wealth, power, and sexual pleasure. Multiplying this ecstasy by the factor of one hundred, we arrive at the ecstasy that can be experienced by those of our ancestors who have attained a heavenly existence. Multiplying their ecstasy by one hundred, we arrive at the level of ecstasy of the divine nature spirits known as *gandharvas*. Multiplying their ecstatic state again by one hundred, we arrive, according to Yajnavalkya, at the maximum ecstasy experienced by one who has attained a state of divinity by virtuous action (*karmadevah*). One hundred times greater than this state of ecstasy is that of one who has attained divinity by birth or knowledge. Again one hundred times greater than that ecstasy is the state of one who has studied the scriptures and is free from desires. One hundred times greater than that, however, is the ecstasy of one who has realized the state of consciousness identified by Patanjali as "seedless *samadhi*."

This highest level of ecstasy is the result of multiplying by one hundred six times, which means that — according to Yajnavalkya, who, historically speaking, was one of the greatest authorities on the matter — *samadhi* confers one trillion times the ecstasy that an ideal human life could possibly provide. Indian texts sometimes exaggerate the states that they describe, a tendency called *stuti* (praise, advertising, glorification). However, Yajnavalkya doesn't appear to share this tendency, and judging from the recorded dialogues and texts he left behind, there is no doubt that he knew and researched each of the ecstatic states mentioned.

Samadhi is the limb through which the mind and subconscious are deconditioned — and this is a

process that takes time. The conditioning (*vasana*) that we undergo during our lives creates fears, desires, expectations, prejudices, and so on, and these prevent us from seeing reality as such because they are superimposed on what we see. Once all this dross of the ages is removed, for the first time one can see the world and the self as they really are.

If we call meditation (*dhyana*) a broadband connection to our meditation object, we need to call *samadhi* the ability to download a holographic image of our meditation object in real time.[16] In other words, the moment the *samadhic* mind (that is, the mind in *samadhi*) fixes itself to an object, the mind is capable of reproducing an identical representation of the object. Being able to exactly duplicate objects in the mind means for the first time ever it is possible to see the world as it really is and not just some pale, dusty, warped, and twisted replica of what one believes or estimates it could be. This is effectively the most complete revolution that can possibly happen to a human mind. It means that the content of the mind has become identical with reality. In other words, what is in the mind is now as real as reality outside, effectively eliminating the distinction between inside and outside.

Once the mind has achieved this quality of stainlessness it becomes capable of creating reality. This is due to the fact that at this level of concentration what is in the mind becomes so real that it will manifest as reality. This explains the various powers of the yogis, *siddhas*, and *rishis* that Patanjali describes in the third chapter of the *Yoga Sutra*.

The yogi, however, applies this newfound power not to hocus-pocus but to the raising of *kundalini*, which produces divine revelation. It is here that ethics become fundamental. If you are not firmly grounded in the first and second limbs, you

16 *Object* here does not mean "thing." A meditation object is any object suitable for meditation. *Suitable* here means an object that neither excites nor dulls the mind but rather stimulates its wisdom and intelligence; such an object is *sattvic* (sacred). The scriptures list many *sattvic* objects; they include the *Om* symbol or sound, a lotus, the moon, a star, a chakra, the sound or light in the heart, a *tanmatra* (subtle essence), the instruments of cognition such as mind, ego, intellect, and the various manifestations of the Supreme Being. Excluded, by definition, is the consciousness itself, which is the subject and therefore can never be an object.

may at this point fall for the dark side. It is for this reason that yoga insists on *Ishvara pranidhana*, a personal devoted relationship to one of the aspects or manifestations of the Supreme Being, whichever one it may be. This close intimate devotion is what will save you when the dark night of your soul arises or when the Prince of Darkness appears on your doorstep to tempt you. Devotion to the Supreme Being will keep you firmly focused on developing the highest within yourself.

When the day arrives and you may look directly into the blinding light of infinite consciousness, you need to be prepared. It is not easy to get a direct view of the supreme self. When Arjuna received the celestial eye that allowed him to behold the Supreme Being in the form of the Lord Krishna, his hair stood on end, his breath became rapid, his heart almost burst — and he could not hold the gaze.[17] If you have duly practiced the eight limbs of yoga and the various types of *samadhi*, the final *samadhi* will show you what Arjuna saw on that fateful day five thousand years ago on the eve of the battle of Kurukshetra. But here comes the problem: like Arjuna on that day, you will be mightily challenged not to close your eyes before that divine glory and look in the opposite direction. This, in fact, is what we are doing every moment of our lives to sustain our own individual, insignificant, and isolated existences. We are expelling the Supreme Being from our hearts in order to stay in control because to keep looking could mean the end of our personalities as we know them. Yogic training, however, will enable you to keep your inner eyes wide open when the day arrives for you to be shown the intense light of infinite consciousness.

It is possible to have a glimpse of this light in the form of a spontaneous temporary mystical experience and come out the other end unchanged. If you have not read the ancient texts or prepared yourself in ways that allow you to put the experience in context, you can come out of such a mystical experience even more confused than before, wanting to repeat the experience by pursuing sex, power, wealth, and so on. This is one of the dangers of pursuing the "instant

enlightenment" path. As long as the mind is not purified of its innate tendency to jump from thought to thought like a monkey from branch to branch, you likely will leave the mystical experience, dropping out of it to follow the next whim of the mind.

Because the mind tends to attach itself to the next object that arises, it cannot without training stay focused on the subject, consciousness. The mind will go after tangible or experiential objects (wealth, power, sex, fame, and so forth), because the subject, although the giver of infinite ecstasy, is intangible. This means that the untrained mind will abandon the mystical experience, even though this is the opposite of what must happen. You need to stay in this state with your eyes wide open, your hair standing on end, and your brain on fire for at least several hours. Some texts hint at a minimum of three hours. Buddha sustained his mystical experience for a whole night; it was more than a decade before Ramana Maharshi could speak and act conventionally after his experience.

Understanding *Samadhi* through Indian Spirituality

The eternal state of infinite consciousness and deepest level of reality is called *Brahman*. The *Brahman* has two poles, Shiva and Shakti. Shiva, which we may call the male pole, is pure consciousness. Shiva stays forever uninvolved, witnessing the world from Mount Meru (Kailasha), not unlike a distant father who watches with bewilderment his wife running a household consisting of six kids, two cats, and a dog. Mount Meru is represented in the microcosm of the individual as the crown chakra. On an individual level, Shiva represents consciousness, which looks down from the crown chakra (the Mount Meru of the individual), witnessing and being aware of thought and action. We cannot reduce Lord Shiva to this metaphorical meaning, however. He is all that we can imagine him to be, all that we cannot imagine, and both together; he is also none of these and all of what is beyond.

Lord Shiva's consort, the goddess Shakti, has a different temperament. She creates, sustains, and reabsorbs the entire creation through her various movements. The movement of creation is her descent from consciousness into matter, a movement that is called *evolution*. She descends from consciousness (her union with Shiva) into intelligence (*buddhi*), which is represented in the body as the *ajna* chakra (third eye). From there she descends into the space/ether element, which is located in the throat chakra (*vishuddha*). From here she crystallizes through air, fire, water, and earth, which manifest in the microcosm of the individual as the heart (*anahata*), navel (*manipuraka*), lower abdomen (*svadhishthana*), and base (*muladhara*) chakras, respectively.

When she dissolves and reabsorbs creation, Shakti is called *Kundalini*, and her ascent is called *involution*. The yogi lets *Kundalini* rise to the crown chakra, where the original unity of Shiva and Shakti is experienced, yielding the ecstatic state of *samadhi*.

When the goddess descends she leaves a particular trail, along which we can follow her back home. She does this by using the essence (*tanmatra*) of the previous chakra to create the next lower one. By taking this essence and reabsorbing it into the higher one, we lift Shakti up from chakra to chakra. This process is referred to in the scriptures as *bhuta shuddhi* (elemental purification). It can be performed in two ways, either in meditation or in *samadhi*. The meditative *bhuta shuddhi* is a typical daily ritual performed even nowadays by many devotional Indians. If it is performed in *samadhi* by a mind that has become able to create reality, the purification of the elements results in an involution back up

through the chakras that leads to divine revelation in the *sahasrara* (crown chakra) — the realization of pure consciousness. When this state is finally made firm through repeated application, it is then called *kaivalya*, or liberation. It is so called because it frees us from the bondage of conditioned existence, allowing us to abide in the limitless ecstasy of infinite consciousness.

Only then, when all eight limbs are mastered in simultaneous application, are they finally discarded, and all exertion abandoned. As mentioned earlier, Patanjali calls this process *paravairagya* — complete letting go. We also find this process enshrined in the *Bhagavad Gita*, where Lord Krishna states that by knowing the Supreme *Brahman* all one's duties are discharged.[18] Once the divine view is had, there is no more plan or structure. From here, life is infinite freedom and unlimited spontaneity.

Until that point, however, effort and willpower are the means by which you progress. This means keeping one's ethical precepts (*yama* and *niyama*) in place, assuming *Padmasana* or similar suitable postures (*asanas*) in the technically correct fashion, entering *kumbhaka* (*pranayama*), drawing one's senses inward (*pratyahara*), concentrating on one's meditation object (*dharana*), receiving a permanent stream of information from it (*dhyana*), and finally establishing an authentic duplication of that object in one's mind (called objective or cognitive *samadhi*). In this traditional way yogis have practiced for thousands of years. Only today do people believe that one can discard or shortcut any lengthy preparation.

18 *Bhagavad Gita* XV.19–20.

Chapter 2
Using Indian Myth and Cosmology to Deepen Your Practice

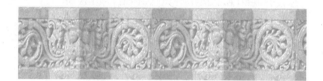

In this chapter I explain the importance of studying the mythological tradition that underlies all yogic practice.[1] In the course of this discussion, I show how the study of myth can change the way you practice yoga and live your life. I also explain how, through myth and divine forms, you can create your own private hotline to and from the Supreme Being.

In chapter 1, I explained that for the majority of modern people, Karma/Ashtanga Yoga — the yoga of techniques and actions — is the most promising method to pursue. I also showed that those who practice this yoga face the danger of getting completely absorbed in techniques such as practicing *asana*, forgetting that the underlying purpose of all yoga is either to obtain self-knowledge (*Jnana*) or to realize yourself as a child of God (*Bhakti*) — which ultimately become the same thing once the mind is transcended in the state of infinite consciousness.

The best way to keep one's practice whole, to avoid the pitfalls of obsession with technique and

neglect of the ultimate purpose of yoga, is to connect deeply with the spiritual roots of yoga. The modern Ashtanga Yogi has two pathways available by which he or she may integrate the ancient spiritual roots of yoga into his or her practice. Path 1 — studying Indian philosophy — will connect you with your Jnanic roots. Path 2 — studying Indian myth — will connect you with your Bhaktic roots. Although these are different paths, they share the same origin and destination. For this reason, it is also possible for the Karma yogi to follow both paths simultaneously, creating an approach with three prongs — Karma, Bhakti, and Jnana Yoga — like the trident of the Lord Shiva.

What is the right path for you? That depends on your pranic constitution. The study of philosophy is the tool of choice if you have an academic and intellectual inclination, which is usually the case if your subtle body has a preponderance of *prana* flowing in the solar *nadi*. Philosophy often consists of causal chains in which arguments and positions are strung on a logical thread, as flowers are strung together to form *malas* in India. Practitioners grasp it slowly by means of rational understanding. Mythology, in contrast, is for those more intuitively endowed, those who have a preponderance of *prana* flowing in the lunar *nadi*. Myth expresses complex, multilateral connections. Often multiple paradoxes are encrypted in myth; the listener or reader grasps them spontaneously by means of intuition.

My first book, *Ashtanga Yoga: Practice and Philosophy*, discusses in detail the subject of Indian philosophy as well as the ancient branch of Indian psychology. Readers who have a solar, or rational, constitution may refer to that work. The present chapter, which focuses on Indian myth, is for those readers who have a lunar, intuitive constitution, those who want at least an introduction to the fascinating world of Indian mythology, and those who want to benefit from the fact that reading myth

---

1 Some traditional authorities consider the Western term *myth* derogatory when used to describe ancient Indian tales. This is because in modern usage, *myth* is also used to refer to an untrue but commonly believed notion. But this is not the primary definition of *myth*, which is instead a traditional story about the early history of a people or civilization, often including deities or other supernatural beings. The terms *myth* and *mythology* are used here strictly in the primary sense of the term.

helps develop the intuitive, right side of the brain, which allows you to spontaneously understand connections.

As philosophy was compiled in terse texts called *sutras*, mythology was collected in extensive tales called *Puranas*. *Purana* means "ancient." Today, eighteen main *Puranas*, called *Maha Puranas*, and eighteen ancillary *Puranas*, called *Upa Puranas*, exist. Since there was no tradition established to preserve their accuracy, as was the case with the *Vedas*, the *Upanishads*, and many of the *sutras*, much material was added to the *Puranas* over time. Although their cores are ancient, the *Puranas* are interspersed with modern, occasionally dubious material. For this reason, they need to be taken with a grain of salt. Nevertheless, they constitute a rich encyclopedia of the myths of India.

Myth and the Development of the Higher Self

The ancient spiritual practice of retelling, listening to, reading, and reliving myths is integral to Indian culture, and it continues today. Myths were and are still considered important because reading sacred texts stimulates the *sattvic*, or spiritual and noble, aspects of the psyche. This is why Patanjali identified the reading of sacred texts as *svadhyaya* (self-study) and made it a part of both *niyama* and Kriya Yoga (yoga of action, preliminary yoga). Even in Patanjali's time, people engaged their minds for much of the time in activities that stimulated the *tamasic* and *rajasic* forces of their personalities, and Patanjali recognized that reading sacred texts was an effective way of engaging and developing the higher aspects of the psyche instead. Reading the myths in the sacred texts was the pursuit of an *arya*, somebody who strives to develop qualities of his noble, higher, and sacred self.[2]

Today, we are tempted even more to indulge the lower urges of our psyches, surrounded as we are by mass media, digital entertainment, advertising,

2 The Sanskrit term *arya* means "noble." It does not refer to ethnicity but denotes people who have a spiritual outlook on life and who accept that in the heart of every person, however foolish he or she may appear, is an eternal, divine self.

and the like. If Patanjali were alive today, he would want us to read holy books instead of watching reality shows or soap operas. How much time do you spend watching television, listening to radio and music, and reading newspapers and trash novels? If you keep feeding yourself with this material, you may invest a lot of effort into your daily *asana* practice and be surprised by how little you actually change.

If you are currently a media consumer, try an experiment: for a predetermined time frame such as one complete moon cycle (twenty-eight days) or one year, instead of consuming various forms of entertainment promulgated through the mass media, read passages from the sacred texts, even if just for thirty minutes every day. If you reclaim some or ideally all time and energy you spend on mindless entertainment and invest it into reading holy books, you will be surprised by how much your life will change in a short time.

Myth and Your Meditation Deity

Aside from imparting a generally beneficial influence, reading sacred texts carries with it a specific and crucially important effect: it is fundamental for realizing one's *ishtadevata*, or meditation deity. This is because the sacred texts, in relating the many myths, describe in detail the many divine forms from which your *ishtadevata* may be drawn. The concept of *ishtadevata* is for those who want to understand the Indian mind, are interested in Indian spirituality, and want to integrate Indian spirituality into their lives.

The ancient Indian sages recognized that people are very different and that what works for one person does not necessarily work for another. People may have intellectual, devotional, emotional, or physical constitutions. And within these categories we find still many more subdivisions and combinations. Due to this fact, many different meditation images were developed so that there was one to suit each of the many different constitutions. These meditation images have human aspects that we can recognize in ourselves, but they also have divine aspects, which are usually worshiped outside of ourselves.

Meditation deities are derived from the many divine forms called *devas*. The term *deva* is often translated as "god," and as such it has acquired much unfortunate baggage.[3] It is best to use the original Sanskrit word, with its far more complex meaning, which has the great advantage of continually reminding us that we may not understand the term completely. The terms *divine form* and *divine image* are also acceptable because they are somewhat less loaded than *god*, although they do not have the richness of *deva*, with its many nuances.

To understand the significance of the concept of *deva*, we need to look at the relationship of the many *devas* (which is a lunar concept born of *prana* going through the left nostril) to the one *Brahman* (which is a solar concept born of *prana* going through the right nostril). The many Indian deities are only aspects of the one *Brahman*, and thus one is not different from another. The sacred texts that are considered the highest authority (the *Upanishads*, the *Bhagavad Gita*, and the *Brahma Sutra*; collectively referred to as *prashthana trayi* or the triple canon) all agree that there is only one Supreme Being but that this Supreme Being can be seen or understood in many different ways. For example, in the *Bhagavad Gita*, Lord Krishna says, "Whichever *deva* you worship you will always come to me." The *Skanda Purana* states, "Vishnu is nobody but Shiva, and he who is called Shiva is but identical with Vishnu."[4] The *Varaha Purana* says that Devi (the Great Goddess), Vishnu, and Shiva are one and the same and warns that those "idiots" who don't understand this fact will end up in hell.[5] These are very strong words, but it is obvious for all those who have truly breathed the spiritual air of India that all divine images are nothing but representations and manifestation of the one *Brahman*, the infinite consciousness and deep reality.

The *Brahman*, however, is for most people an abstract and intangible concept that is difficult to grasp. It is much easier to understand deities with forms and particular qualities. Another advantage of representing the *Brahman* with diverse deities is that it helps counteract dogma. Rather than specifying one correct path for approaching the realization of the *Brahman*, India accepted all paths as long as they led to divine revelation. How's that for practicality?

The *Brahman*

Let's take a closer look now at the term *Brahman*, which is never to be confused with Lord Brahma, who is only one of many divine images. *Brahman* is called truth or reality (*sat*) because it cannot be broken down into smaller constituents. Therefore we can also call it deep reality. Indian thought considers things that can be reduced to smaller parts as mere appearance (which does not necessarily mean they are unreal). Underneath mere appearance is that which is not further reducible to anything — and this is what Indian texts call the *Brahman*. It is also described as *chit*, infinite consciousness — infinite both in temporal and spatial senses. Our modern scientific knowledge of physical matter — that atoms are reducible to electrons, neutrons, and protons and that those are reducible to subatomic particles, which are in turn further reducible — makes this principle even more profound.

Brahman has limitless potential. It is considered to be the state before and after the Big Bang that produced the universe. It continues to exist during the unfolding of the universe because it is touched neither by space nor by time and it gives rise to an infinite number of universes. The realization of *Brahman* is thought to bestow limitless ecstasy (*ananda*).

The *Upanishads* talk about the *Brahman* either as *nirguna* (without quality) or *saguna* (with quality). This does not mean that there are two different *Brahmans* but rather that individual human beings will be better able to relate to one view or the other. Neither of the views is right; the only question is, By which view can you realize the *Brahman*?

According to the *nirguna* view, the *Brahman* is the formless, infinite absolute. Any quality that is

3 When Westerners first came to India they applied their knowledge of European culture to India. Since ancient European religions were polytheistic, Western observers projected this knowledge onto the Indian culture and called the Indians' *devas* "gods." This led to the belief that Indians worship many different gods.
4 *Skanda Purana*, I, 8, 20.
5 Arthur Avalon, *Shakti and Shakta* (Madras: Ganesh & Co., 1994), p. 288.

projected onto this formless consciousness is already part of the relative world of manifestation. No quality can be eternal, and therefore none can really describe the *Brahman*. This view is held by most schools of Buddhism (although they don't call it *Brahman*) and by Shankara's school of Advaita Vedanta. Islam can also be said to share this view; it forbids any depicting of the Supreme — or in fact any qualifying of the Supreme whatsoever — because it considers any human representation as a sullying of the infinite.

Strict adherents of *nirguna Brahman* reject beingness as a quality of *Brahman*. They consider the *Brahman* to be beyond being, beyond nonbeing, both being and nonbeing simultaneously, and none of the above. They wish to express that the *Brahman* is beyond any categories of the mind while also encompassing all categories the mind can think of and even those that the mind cannot think of. In other words, the followers of the Nirguna School, such as Shankara, consider being-ness as a "relative" category, while the *Brahman* is absolute.

For all those who ascribe to the *nirguna* view, the formless absolute is their *ishtadevata*, their meditation deity. There can be no other, because they reject the notion that the *Brahman* has form. This is the path of Jnana Yoga (the yoga of knowledge), which was discussed in chapter 1.

For all those who cannot or do not want to worship the formless absolute — which probably is the majority of modern people — there is the *Brahman* with form (*saguna*). If we add form to *Brahman* we arrive at the Supreme Being, often called Ishvara.[6] The name *Ishvara* usually does not imply a particular deity; it is also the name that Patanjali uses for the Supreme Being. He qualifies it as little as possible.[7] Nevertheless we do learn from Patanjali that the Supreme Being utters the sacred syllable *Om*, is a form of consciousness different from humans, is all knowing and unlimited by time, and is the author of yoga. This list gives us only a very vague idea of what the Supreme Being is and

leaves open the form one should use when meditating on the Supreme.

Let's now go deeper into the qualities in which Indian thought generally clothes the Supreme Being. In historical times Ishvara was often depicted as Trimurti, the three-faced one. A Trimurti statue will have one head with three faces looking into different directions, the three faces representing Lord Brahma, the creator; Lord Vishnu, the maintainer; and Lord Shiva, the cosmic destroyer.[8] The idea of the Trimurti is to show that all three are only various faces of the one Supreme Being. Interestingly, however, Lord Brahma is not worshiped at all in India; there is only one temple related to Brahma, and even that temple is devoted to Brahma's wife and not directly to him.

The more commonly worshiped three deities, or forms of the Supreme, are Lord Shiva, who stands for the pure consciousness within us; Lord Vishnu, representing the true self; and Devi Shakti, the Mother Goddess, who represents the entire world of creation (*prakrti*), our breath and life force (*prana*), and the ascending energy current in the central channel of the *nadi* system (*kundalini*).

These three forms of the Supreme Being are the three main meditation images. They have been broken down into many sub-images, which are so manifold that they may seem as numerous as the people on the planet. Since one's *ishtadevata* (meditation deity) needs exactly to meet one's emotional needs, there could theoretically be as many *ishtadevatas* as there are people.

An Intimate Relationship with the Divine

Your relationship to your *ishtadevata* needs to become as intimate as possible. A well-known passage of the *Upanishads* states, "In the core of your body is a lotus flower in which is situated a triangular shrine. In this shrine resides the true self, in which miraculously is assembled this entire vast universe with all its mountains, rivers, trees, oceans, stars and suns."[9] Since the entire universe is thought

---

6 *Ishvara* is also listed as one of the 1,000 names of Lord Shiva, but the term is not used here with that meaning.
7 Grammatically the *Brahman* is masculine, feminine, and neuter simultaneously.

8 Not to be mistaken with the *Brahman*, the formless absolute.
9 *Chandogya Upanishad* 8.1.

to be located inside the Supreme Being, this passage states that the Supreme Being resides in our hearts. From this point of view, the many different so-called gods are only devices that enable our individual psyches, which differ so much from one individual to another, to meditate on and identify with the one Supreme Being in our hearts. This brings us back to the purpose of mythology: when we listen to the myths and tales of ancient India and start to read the texts that describe them, we become more and more familiar and intimate with the various divine images. In due time our *ishtadevata* will be revealed.

Once you know your *ishtadevata*, you have your own private frequency through which you connect with the Supreme Being. There is no point in squabbling over which frequency — that is, which God — is better or more correct. The important point is that you find your frequency and enter into a relationship with the Supreme Being in which you find guidance and offer your service.[10]

There is great beauty and humility in the *ishtadevata* concept. Your *ishtadevata* is your way to access the Supreme Being, and its particularity reminds you that it is only your own limited view of the One. You cannot criticize or belittle somebody else just because you do not understand that person's view of the Supreme Being. Again, there are as many *ishtadevatas* and routes to infinite consciousness as there are people on Earth.

True Religion

In a larger context, this is the basis for the practice of what I call true religion. To practice true religion means to recognize all religions, and particularly those that appear alien to us, as an emanation of and true path to the Supreme Being. A person who claims that truth is to be found only in the religion of his or her tribe is not religious but merely sectarian. A sectarian has an agenda, which is mainly to prove that a particular approach or religion is right or wrong. The emphasis of a sectarian is on controlling the behavior of other people. A truly religious person, in contrast, is not interested in the path through which you reach the Supreme Being but rather in whether you get there and how fast. The emphasis is on the Supreme Being itself and its ecstatic revelation to the individual.

10 From time to time Indian authorities such as Shankara had to come forward and outlaw some of these meditation images because they had led to some bizarre forms of worship (such as the *thuggees*). Shankara, his advice obviously not followed by everyone, limited "correct" worship to six divine forms: the Lord Shiva; his two sons Ganesha and Kartikeya (often called Murugan, Ayeppa, Subramaniam, Kumara, or Skanda); the Lord Vishnu (represented by his many *avataras* such as Lord Rama and Lord Krishna); the Goddess (known by many names, including Uma, Parvati, Durga, and Devi); and finally Surya, the sun.

Chapter 3
Sanskrit: The Sacred Language of Yoga

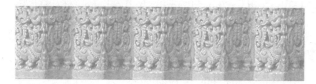

In this chapter I invite you to take a closer look at the Sanskrit language. Sanskrit is both the carrier of the most extensive spiritual tradition of humankind and the language that the Supreme Being created to teach yoga and to guide human beings in their return to infinite consciousness. Learning at least the basics of Sanskrit is a fundamental part of one's yoga practice and spiritual development; in this chapter I explain why this is so.

You may have heard of the great teacher Jiddu Krishnamurti, one of the few outstanding intellectual giants of the twentieth century. Krishnamurti spent most of his life circling the globe to lecture, never finding the peace and quiet he needed to realize a lifelong goal: to learn Sanskrit. Finally, at age ninety-five, knowing he had little time to live, he sat down to learn the language. Krishnamurti lived his life to the fullest, and while he proposed many provocative concepts, I'm sure that he died with a sense of satisfaction that he had given his all. The fascinating fact remains, however, that he did not just spend his final days gazing into the sunset but instead studied Sanskrit. It speaks volumes to us about the importance of this language.

Unfortunately, some modern Western yoga teachers have publicly stated that Sanskrit is of no relevance for modern yogis. This can be seen as another sad case of Westerners looting foreign cultures for anything that can be exploited for short-term gain — in this case, the practice of postures — and discarding in ignorance everything that seems too deep and difficult to understand. But the truth is that an ability to pronounce Sanskrit mantras properly is absolutely necessary for advanced yoga practice. Correct pronunciation requires at least some knowledge of the Sanskrit language, particularly of the fundamental relationship between sound and spirituality that is at its core.

Sanskrit is a mantric language, and it is nothing but the science of sound itself. *Mantras* are sound forms that contain encoded reality and have the power to alter and produce reality. Sound, according to the *Vedas*, is not just an audible sensation; it goes much, much deeper. Sound includes all forms of vibratory patterns, such as brain waves, the orbits of electrons around atomic nuclei, the movements of celestial bodies, and the reverberations caused by the Big Bang. It is therefore the essence of reality.

The Four Phases of Sound

According to Vedic science, there are four phases or states of sound: *para, pashyanti, madhyama,* and *vaikhari.* I know that's a lot of strange words in one sentence, but if you can wrap your mind around these four terms you will have understood the basis of much of advanced yoga. Only the last of the four, the *vaikhari* phase, is audible to the ear, because only *vaikhari* is a gross, physically manifested sound (included in this category are sounds that can be perceived only by an ear more sensitive than the human ear, such as that of a cat, dog, or bat). In other words, everything that Western science classifies as sound falls into this lowest category.

The unfolding of the four phases of sound is parallel to the unfoldment of the *gunas,* or qualities of nature, and is most easily understood in that context. So let's look at the *gunas* first. To get a quick handle on the *gunas,* liken them to the three elementary atomic particles of physics. Just as the electron, neutron, and proton form in varying combinations all atoms, elements, and compounds, the three *gunas* — *sattva, rajas,* and *tamas* — make up, in ever-varying combinations, all objects. With this analogy in mind, the late Sanskrit scholar Surendranath Dasgupta (1887–1952) labeled *tamas* as the mass particle, *rajas* as the energy particle, and *sattva* as the intelligence particle. Just as in Western elementary physics, these particles appear sometimes as particles and at other times as waves of energy.

The three *gunas* have four phases, called unmanifest, manifest, subtle, and gross. You might have guessed already that these phases are related to the four states of sound. These states and their results have been seen by the ancient *rishis*, and even yogis today can still see and verify them in *samadhi*.

THE UNMANIFEST STATE AND PARA

The first state is called the unmanifest state; in it *rajas, tamas,* and *sattva* are in equilibrium. There is no manifestation — no objects or phenomena — because the *gunas* cancel each other out. In Western science we call that the state before the Big Bang. Indic thought calls this state *prakrti*. This beautiful Sanskrit term, which gave rise to such important English words as *procreation* and *practical*, can be translated as "procreativity" or simply "nature."

Yoga sees *prakrti* as an unconscious (*acetanam*) matrix.[1] The Supreme Being in the form of the Lord Krishna describes the very same *prakrti* as a machine operated upon by Him,[2] and the Agama Shastra describes it as the Great Goddess Uma Parvati herself.[3] We need not be disturbed by these differences, as all three views are correct and describe aspects of *prakrti*. What is important is that during the *prakrti* state all phenomena are unmanifest. There is no universe, only the infinite eternal consciousness called *Brahman*.

In the unmanifest state, in the *Brahman*, there

exists already a potential, a divine intention to bring forth the entire creation. This divine intention is called *shabda Brahman,* or the vibration aspect of infinite consciousness. Thus the unmanifest state has a sound, called *para* (beyond). *Para* is a divine sound that has no physical manifestation; only in the most advanced states of *samadhi* can it be heard. Sound at the *para* stage can be perceived only from the *sahasrara* chakra — the crown energy center, which lies not within the body but above the crown of the head — where consciousness is realized. The *para* sound can be "heard" in the highest state of *samadhi*, when *shakti* (life force) ascends all the way to the *sahasrara* chakra. Through the "hearing" of the *para* sound, the yogi travels "beyond" relative existence and enters the state of *Brahman*.

THE MANIFEST STATE AND PASHYANTI

From the unmanifest state, the *gunas* are stirred into action through the mere presence of consciousness, which functions as a catalyst. Like a chemical catalyst, consciousness is present and necessary for the "reaction" of manifestation to take place, but it is not changed or altered in the process at all. This second *gunic* state is called the manifest state, and during it the only category of manifestation that the *gunas* bring forth is cosmic intelligence (called *mahat* in its universal form and *buddhi* in its individual form). The sound during this state is called *pashyanti* and it consists of only one syllable, the sacred syllable *Om*.

The importance of *Om*, the primordial sound and mightiest of all mantras, cannot be overestimated. Says the *Mandukya Upanishad*: "*Om* is all there is, all that has been, and all that will be. And all that is beyond these three is also *Om*."[4] This sacred and foremost sound can be heard during *samadhi*, and focusing on its perception is the principal meditation technique advocated in the *Upanishads*.

Also coming into existence during the manifest state of the *gunas* is the *karana sharira* of the various beings. The *karana sharira*, which exists within cosmic intelligence, is called the "causal body";

1 *Samkhya Karika* of Ishvarakrishna XI.
2 *Bhagavad Gita* IV.6.
3 Arthur Avalon, *Introduction to Tantra Shastra* (Madras: Ganesh, 2004), pp. 4ff.

4 *Mandukya Upanishad* I.1.

however, it is very different from what we generally understand the term *body* to mean. The *karana sharira* consists of eternal or extremely long-lived conditioned patterns (*vasanas*) and subconscious imprints (*samskaras*).

During the manifest state of the *gunas* and the *pashyantic* state of sound, ego does not yet exist, and as such we cannot really say, "It is I who is reborn" — an expression that the Buddha rightly criticized. Nevertheless, some form of subconsciousness, which at this point is not attached to any egoic notions, does exist. Therefore, as something disappears, something else must reappear. The force and information behind this "something" is the *karana sharira*, the causal body.

When through yogic effort *shakti* is made to rise to the *ajna* chakra (third eye center), the sacred *Om* is heard, cosmic intelligence is realized, and the causal body is cleansed, which enables the yogi to let go of or disassociate from karma. The *shakti* can be made to ascend by means of chanting, meditating on, and finally "hearing" the sound *Om*. Paradoxically, although *shakti* needs to have reached the *ajna* chakra for *Om* to be heard, *Om* really is heard — or, more accurately, manifests — in the *anahata* chakra (heart center).

THE SUBTLE STATE AND MADHYAMA

As the process of creation continues, the *gunas* now swing from the manifest into the subtle state. During the subtle state of the *gunas*, the sound state of *madhyama* is produced. The *madhyamic* state brings forth the fifty letters of the Sanskrit language, which are composed of sixteen vowels and thirty-four consonants. This is significant for the following reason: During the subtle state the *gunas* bring forth egoity (*ahamkara*), and only from this moment on can we strictly speak from I-thought, I-awareness, or I-consciousness. Then the *gunas* produce the subtle elements/essences (*tanmatras*). Finally, both together — egoity and subtle elements — produce the subtle or energy body (*sukshma sharira*), which is sometimes also called the yogic body or energy body. The subtle body consists of *pranas* (vital currents), *nadis* (energy channels), *bindus* (energy points), personal *vasana*

(conditioning) and *samskaras* (subconscious imprints), and, importantly, chakras. As a result, the subtle body understands and reacts to Sanskrit. You can chant your mantras in English or any other language as long as you wish; they will not transform the subtle body. To use an information-technology analogy, Sanskrit is the programming language that has been used to write the operating system of the subtle body. If you want to reprogram your operating system, you have to enter your new instructions in Sanskrit. Otherwise you will talk only to your conscious mind, which can be useful but is not nearly as effective.

Let's have a look now at how information is encrypted into the subtle body. Each chakra is related to certain Sanskrit letters and certain root syllables, or *bija aksharas*. The *bija aksharas* are mantras that are used to activate, open, and energize their respective chakras. They are also used in an important technique called *bhuta shuddhi*, the purification of the elements, which was described in chapter 1. During *bhuta shuddhi*, each element represented in and manifested through its respective chakra is dissolved into the next higher chakra. This process is called *involution*. It reverses the descent of *shakti*, which during the process of evolution crystallized down through all the elements until she came to rest in the *muladhara* chakra — at which point we lost awareness of the Divine within us. *Bhuta shuddhi* is not possible without using the root mantras of each chakra and element. This is because the Great Goddess/*prakrti*/*shakti* manifested and programmed the chakras and elements by emitting the root mantras during the *madhyama* state of sound. In this process lies the secret of many yogic techniques.

All phenomena are made up of vibrational patterns called *shabda*. Divine intention uses *shabda* in the form of mantra to shape reality. The ancient seers heard these mantras in deep *samadhi* and related them down to us. We now can use these precious mantras to shape our reality. The *rishis* have taught us mantras so that we could ultimately realize the divine intention that stood behind their initial use. Through the correct application of mantras we can raise *shakti* up through the six lower chakras to *Sahasrara*, where *shabda Brahman* is realized.

THE GROSS STATE AND VAIKHARI

During the final state of the *gunas*, called the gross state, the fourth state of sound, called *vaikhari*, emerges. The term *vaikhari* comes from the root *vac*, or "speech," which also gave rise to the English terms *word* and *verb*. *Vaikhari* is audible sound, and during the *vaikhari* state all nonmantric languages emerge, as do all other audible sounds. Sounds that happen to be outside the range of human hearing, such as those with an extremely high or low frequency, are also called *vaikhari*.

The languages that developed during the *vaikhari* state are nonmantric; these include all the Indo-European languages (such as English, Spanish, French, German, Italian, Russian, Iranian, Greek, Hindi, and Marathi). Although these nonmantric languages have Sanskrit roots, they are fundamentally different from Sanskrit, in that all nonmantric languages change over time. Words lose their original meanings and take on new ones. In Sanskrit, however, words have a fixed meaning because they are constructed from fixed elements. If a word is lost, it can be reconstructed from precise grammatical and phonetic rules, which are the same today as they were thousands of years ago. Also, whereas modern languages have a limited number of expressions, a nearly endless number of Sanskrit words can be created or reconstructed by following these exact, fixed rules and laws. These rules were defined by the ancient Sanskrit grammarian Panini, whose grammar is known as *Ashtadhyayi*.

Sanskrit as a Spiritual Discipline

Learning and using Sanskrit is a spiritual practice in itself. The Sanskrit language is designed in such a way that you must use your entire brain capacity if you want to understand and speak it reasonably well. Further, the way in which Sanskrit is pronounced can spawn important changes in the brain itself. Westerners often smile at the "strange" way Indians pronounce words. Indians seem to speak more from the back of the head, which reflects the fact that they tend to contemplate for a long time before they take action. Westerners, on the other hand, speak mainly through their incisors, which may correlate with a tendency to act quickly and without deep thought.

The way Indians think and their outstanding contributions in the areas of religion, philosophy, and art are deeply related to how Sanskrit is pronounced. Indians articulate sounds using five locations in the mouth: lips, teeth, hard palate, soft palate, and throat. This way of producing sounds involves the entire skull and encourages the

ENGLISH VERSUS SANSKRIT

English, like most other modern, nonmantric languages, has a strongly simplified grammar compared to that of Sanskrit. There are fewer grammatical cases, often no case endings, and fewer tenses (time modes). This has made it easier for English to jump boundaries and establish itself as an international trade language.

Another apparent virtue of the English language is its function as a vehicle of the idea of democracy. A complicated and sophisticated language such as Sanskrit, which requires a decade or more of intense study to master, will generally be spoken only by a small group whose members have the means to invest this time. (The ancient Indian sages solved this problem by reducing their needs and thereby precluding the need to work.) A democratic society is more likely to develop in a population that cannot so easily use language to differentiate between the privileged and the unprivileged.

While English has outdone all other languages in these fields, it falls significantly short in accurately portraying metaphysical and mystical concepts with a minimum of ambiguity. English simply does not have enough grammatical cases, tenses, or words for this task. Sanskrit is the language of choice when philosophy and mysticism are the subjects. It is no wonder that more than 150,000 treatises still exist in Sanskrit, and many times that number have been lost.

activation of the half-dozen energy centers in the head; these include the *lalana* or *talu* chakra, the *manas* chakra, the *indu* or *soma* chakra, the *brahmarandhra* or *nirvana* chakra, and the *guru* chakra. All these chakras are located in the area of the soft palate, especially at the rear and higher end, or in the direct vicinity of the palatal region and the cerebrum.

The presence of so many energy centers near the soft palate makes this part of the body the most vital and powerful for the purpose of yoga. It also explains the significance of three *mudras* (energetic seals): the *Nabho Mudra*, the *Manduka Mudra*, and the *Kechari Mudra*. In *Nabho Mudra,* the tongue is inverted and placed as far up as possible against the soft palate. It is used for the purpose of "milking" the *amrita* (nectar) oozing from the *soma* chakra. *Manduka Mudra* is similar to *Nabho Mudra* except that the tongue is actively moved left and right to make the nectar flow. In *Kechari Mudra*, the tongue is first massaged and lengthened, a process that can be drawn out and uncomfortable. Finally it is pressed up against the entire length of the soft palate and used to close the throat, thus achieving breath retention, while the gaze is fixed to the third eye. The *prana* is thus forced to enter *sushumna* (the central energy channel), and the *brahmarandhra* chakra (one of the palatal chakras) is opened.

The proper pronunciation of Sanskrit requires similar though less extreme movements of the tongue. The effects on the energy centers of the head are also similar but more subtle and spread over a longer time period. Sanskrit pronunciation of the simple word *Ashtanga*, for example, is completely different from how Westerners pronounce it. To make the *sh* and *t* sounds, Indians place the tongue in retroflex / cerebral position, and to make the various *n* sounds they place it in palatal position, which means that both the hard and the soft palates are receiving vibrational or mantric input when the word is pronounced. The same is true for many other Sanskrit words. Because of this, speaking Sanskrit permanently stimulates the cerebral chakras. Sanskrit is therefore the most cerebral of all languages in terms of not only structure and content but also pronunciation.

This is one of the reasons why most of the

spiritually liberated people have emerged in India. If there were a map that showed the origins of the spiritually completed people of the past five thousand years, it would display only a few dots in Europe; a few more in the Middle East; a formidable concentration in Tibet, China, and Japan; and a vast sea of dots in India.

The Sanskrit Tradition

The oldest piece of literature available in any language is the *Rigveda*, which was composed and recorded in Sanskrit. The *Rigveda* contains stanzas describing astronomical events that occurred more than eleven thousand years ago. The entire text is not necessarily that old, but certainly its oldest layers are.

But let's go back to the very beginning. In the traditional view, all knowledge existed in an eternal and uncreated state in the intellect of the Supreme Being before the advent of time. According to the Rishi Yajnavalkya (as recorded in the oldest and most important *Upanishad*, the *Brhad Aranyaka Upanishad*), the Infinite Being breathed forth, like the smoke from a fire that penetrates everywhere, the *Rigveda, Samaveda, Yajurveda,* and *Atharvaveda*; the *Itihasas* (*Ramayana* and *Mahabharata*); the *Puranas*; the sciences (*Vidyas*); the *Upanishads*; the Sanskrit grammar (*shloka*); and the *sutras* and commentaries.[5] At the same time, in order to give this knowledge form, the Supreme Being (in the form of Lord Shiva) produced the fifty letters of the Sanskrit language from the primordial sound *Om*. Then from these fifty letters, the Lord Shiva created the first Sanskrit grammar as a manifestation of that which was already eternal and perfect.

The Sanskrit language came forth in two different forms, now called Vedic and Classic Sanskrit. Western scholars claim that Classic Sanskrit evolved from Vedic,[6] but according to tradition the Supreme Being authored both forms at the same time, each for a different purpose.[7] Vedic Sanskrit was to be used for recording mantras,

5   *Brhad Aranyaka Upanishad* II.4.10.
6   William Dwight Whitney, *Sanskrit Grammar* (Delhi: Motilal Banarsidass, 1962), p. xii.
7   Swami Prakashanand Saraswati, *The True History and Religion of India* (Delhi: Motilal Banarsidass, 2001), p. 236.

chanting, and mystical communion. Classical Sanskrit was to be used to record philosophical teachings and to stimulate intellectual discussion.

Because all the knowledge contained within the various scriptures (*shastras*) was not created by a single human mind but seen only by those who were open to perceiving it in each historical phase, it is called the eternal teaching, *Sanatana Dharma*. Even at the end of this world cycle, this teaching will not be destroyed but will be breathed forth again in the next world cycle and again be seen by liberated ones.

Despite the eternal perfection of Sanskrit, we are losing more and more ancient treatises as time progresses. We have lost most Ayurvedic texts, more than twenty ancient grammar treatises, and even the founding text on philosophy, Kapila's *Shashti Tantra*. This loss of knowledge is due to the fact that entropy (disorder) increases as the universe gets older (we look at this phenomenon in detail in the next section of the chapter).

Sanskrit is not only the language in which the entire body of Vedic science, the eternal teaching, was composed; it is also a defining adjunct of the *Veda* itself. There are six so-called *Vedangas* (limbs or adjuncts) of the *Veda*. They are *Vyakarana* (grammar), *Jyotisha* (astrology), *Nirukta* (etymology), *Shiksha* (phonetics), *Chandas* (meter), and *Kalpa* (ritual). Of these a staggering four relate directly to the Sanskrit language.

Vyakarana is Sanskrit grammar. Since the first twenty treatises have been lost, we use now the grammar of sage Panini, called *Ashtadhyayi*. Panini lived prior to Patanjali, and Patanjali wrote his great commentary (*Mahabhashya*) on the *sutras* of Panini's grammar.

Nirukta is etymology. With its help, the exact meaning of each Sanskrit term can be arrived at. *Nirukta* is used to deconstruct words and trace them back to their original roots. From the verb root, which was used by the ancients to construct the word in the first place, the word's original meaning can still be derived. *Vyakarana* and *Nirukta* together facilitate *Jnana* (divine knowledge).

Shiksha, the next limb of the *Veda*, constitutes phonetics. It is the science of proper pronunciation of the Sanskrit words. Vedic teaching considers the whole world to be made up of sound (*shabda*). All knowledge is also expressed through sound. When mantras and stanzas are pronounced properly, the knowledge encrypted in them is transmitted. Again, many treatises of *Shiksha* have been lost and with them a great deal of precious knowledge.

Chandas is the section of the *Vedangas* that explains meter. The *Chandas Sutra* was authored by the Rishi Pingala. Meters are divided into either three or four lines called *pada*. Each pada is divided into eight to twelve syllables (*aksharas*). The well-known *gayatri* meter has three *padas* of eight *aksharas* each. The most common meter is the *trishtubh* meter, which has four *padas* of eleven *aksharas* each. *Chandas* and *Shiksha* are the *Vedangas* that facilitate *bhakti* (divine devotion).

The remaining two *Vedangas*, *Jyotisha* (astrology) and *Kalpa* (ritual), are related to karma yoga (divine action). See Table 1 for a summary of the relationships between limbs of the *Vedanga* and the forms of yoga.

TABLE 1. RELATIONSHIPS BETWEEN THE LIMBS OF THE *VEDA* (*VEDANGA*) AND THE BASIC FORMS OF YOGA	
Vedanga	**Form of Yoga**
*Vyakarana** (Grammar)	Jnana Yoga
*Nirukta** (Etymology)	(Divine knowledge)
*Shiksha** (Phonetics)	Bhakti Yoga
*Chandas** (Meter)	(Divine devotion)
Jyotisha (Astrology)	Karma Yoga
Kalpa (Ritual)	(Divine action)

* Directly related to Sanskrit

Reading *Shastra*

Recall Rishi Yajnavalkya's description of the *Brahman* breathing forth the *Vedas*, the *Upanishads*, the epics, the *Puranas*, all *sutras*, commentaries, and sciences and with them the Sanskrit language. This statement implies a unity of the many classes of *shastras* (scriptures) and their vehicle or carrier, the Sanskrit language. In other words, Sanskrit is inseparable from true knowledge (*vidya*) of yoga and the scriptures. It follows, then, that an understanding of Sanskrit will give you the ability not only to practice mantra correctly but also to interpret *shastra*. With some knowledge of Sanskrit, you will be able to determine when English translations of Sanskrit texts are erroneous, which is very often the case because the translators are not mystics and yogis but scholars. You will also be able to determine when "twilight language" is used in scriptures — when a superficial meaning is used to hide a deeper meaning from non-yogis. In this way your understanding of yogic technique will be vastly improved.

Shastra is important because it preserves much more accurately than modern texts and teachers the original knowledge of Vedic teaching. The original teaching of yoga was and is contained as divine intention in the state of *shabda Brahman*. From there it was brought forth as the mantra *Om*, which can be heard in meditation. The sacred syllable then broke up into the fifty Sanskrit letters, which you can still experience when meditating on the chakras. The fifty letters were also used to compose the many *shastras*. After that many more languages arose, and with them greater confusion about the true meaning of the original knowledge.

The history of the universe and the history of human civilizations can easily be understood when we apply to them the second law of thermodynamics. This law states that with the passage of time, the amount of entropy (disorder) in the universe increases. With the amount of disorder increasing, available energy slowly decreases until the system becomes defunct and breaks down. This tendency can be observed in all entities, including the universe as a whole, galaxies, stars and planets, civilizations, empires, religions, companies, plants, animals, and the human body. Over thousands of years, Indian thought and spiritual culture have evolved according to this law.

In line with this principle, Indians believe that Vedic civilization (and human society in general) started from an ideal, noble, and spiritual ideal and

from there it slowly descended into disorder. (Certainly in spiritual matters humankind has gone downhill since the time of the *Vedas*. We may have invented science and technology, but with accelerating environmental destruction it is yet to be seen whether coming generations will view our presumed progress as a blessing or as a scourge.) Accordingly, we are now in the grip of the dark age called *Kali Yuga*. *Kali Yuga* can be recognized by three facts: there is constant warfare in one place or another, people are identified with their bodies and wallets rather than with their divine selves, and, finally, corrupt teachers and teachings abound. You can make up your own mind whether this sounds like an accurate description of the world we live in.

I find myself reading fewer books on yoga written by modern authors and listening less often to modern and contemporary teachers. Instead I rely more and more on the original teachings encrypted in *shastra*. In this day and age it is necessary for all of us to take personal responsibility for our spirituality and obtain the advice and teaching of the ancient sages who lived during the Golden Age (*Satya Yuga*). This advice is readily available in the *shastras*.

The more *shastras* you have read and internalized, the less likely you are to become lost in the jungle of different opinions that exist in the world today. Despite our great progress, this jungle appears to have become denser as our history has progressed. I recommend that you find your way back to the original roots and sources of yoga. Try not to read modern interpretations of the *shastras*, which are creations of the *Kali Yuga*; instead read the *shastras* in the original, direct translations. Make sure that the direct translations include the original Sanskrit script type (called *devanagari*). While reading, keep an open mind, and when you come to passages that do not seem to make much sense, scan over the Sanskrit. Usually the obscurity or ambiguity arises through the translator's choice of English terms. Start to develop your own alternative choices of English terms. More often than not, there are no direct translations of Sanskrit terms, as there are so many more words in Sanskrit than in English. You need to understand that each choice of an English term constitutes an interpretation. Once you get used to this method of trying to understand the Sanskrit rather than accepting an ambiguous interpretation, you will quickly find that the voices of the ancient teachers find a direct road to your heart.

Two major pitfalls await you when you read the scriptures directly. The first pitfall may occur when you try to get an overview of the many types of *shastra*. Because each scripture says something different, you may get confused and not see the forest for all the trees. Remember that there is one common truth underlying all the scriptures, but it is clothed in many different ways. The second pitfall may occur if you read only one *shastra* or one class of *shastra*. Because you have no other points of reference, you can quickly come to the conclusion that what you are reading contains the whole of the truth, when in fact there are many *shastras* and all of them contain a wealth of wisdom.

These pitfalls exist primarily because of the way the *shastras* were written. They use exaggerated language called *stuti* to glorify the methods they present, while at the same time they critique the opposing school of thought with equally exaggerated language. This style of writing was employed mainly to attract followers, not to denigrate other teachings. *Stuti* often takes the form of stating that success can be had only by following the set of practices outlined in the present *shastra*. The *Hatha Yoga Pradipika*, for example, states that as long as the life force is not moved into the central channel (*sushumna*), all rambling about liberation is only the useless jabber of idiots.[8] This does not necessarily mean that the Jnana Yoga (which does not explicitly deal with moving *prana* into the *sushumna*) is idiocy. The stanza also advises those who practice Hatha Yoga to diligently proceed with their techniques and to not be concerned that the Jnanis (practitioners of Jnana Yoga) meditating next door are saying that they will soon leave the Hatha practitioners behind spiritually. Boasting about the prowess of one's school was as popular among ancient yogis as it is among supporters of modern football teams.

Similarly, some Vedanta texts advise against practicing yoga techniques. For example, Shankara, in his *Aparokshanubhuti*, says those who still practice *pranayama* are ignorant and should know better.[9] To interpret this statement accurately, you need to know that it is addressed not to just anyone, but to those who have already reached the stage of merely meditating on *Brahman*. Once this stage is reached, the *shastras* strongly advise against reverting to the practices that led to this stage. They do this for obvious reasons. Before you wear a particular garment, you will wash it if it has become dirty. Once it is clean, however, there is no point in continuing the washing process, as every time you will want to wear it, you will find it wet on the clothesline. One of my Indian teachers repeatedly used this analogy when referring to Westerners who limited their yoga practice to *asana*. The washing here is the preparatory practice such as *asana* or *pranayama*, while the wearing of the garment represents the realizing of consciousness (*Brahman*).

Luckily enough, Shankara sets the record straight in a treatise called *Yoga Taravali*, which was written for the benefit of the "dim-witted" yogis who were incapable of following him to the lofty heights of instant enlightenment.[10] In *Yoga Taravali* he advocates *pranayama*, the very practice he criticizes in *Aparokshanubhuti*. This tendency to have it both ways is typical of many great Indian teachers and may be seen as the wisdom to point different students in different directions.

Glorification (*stuti*) of the approach taught in a particular *shastra* often takes the form of grossly overstating the effects of practice. Patanjali, for example, states that merely abstaining from greed will lead to a shower from the diamond-spewing celestial mongoose. The wise will take such exaggerations with a grain of salt. When reading *shastra*, it is a good idea to visualize the author as a wise Indian sage dispensing advice with a twinkle in his eye.

---

8 *Hatha Yoga Pradipika*, IV.113.

9 Swami Vimuktananda, *Aparokshanubhuti of Sri Sankaracharya* (Kolkata: Advaita Ashrama, 1938), p. 65.
10 He uses the Sanskrit term *mudha*, which can also be translated as "idiot."

Chapter 4
The Mythology of the Intermediate Postures

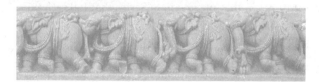

The postures of the Intermediate Series have been given names with spiritual or mythological significance to stir devotion in the heart of the yogi. When you study the myths related to each posture, you deepen your practice of yoga and thereby develop a personal relationship to the divine powers and ancient sages of yoga.

In this chapter I first explain the various categories of posture names and provide a table (see p. 31) that shows which category each Intermediate Series posture falls into. (You may notice that a few postures fall into more than one category, which reflects the richness of Indian mythology, wherein many terms have more than one meaning or connotation.) Then I provide some mythological context for each of the postures of the Intermediate Series.

The Categories of Postures

There are four categories of posture names: postures dedicated to lifeless forms, postures representing animals, postures representing human forms, and postures representing divine forms. Each category has its own unique *gunic* makeup, as explained below. Postures of the Primary Series tend to represent *tamas guna* (mass particle), those of the Intermediate Series are generally an expression of *rajas guna* (energy particle), and Advanced Series postures appear to be permeated by *sattva guna* (intelligence particle).

POSTURES DEDICATED TO LIFELESS FORMS

Lifeless forms are primarily made up of *tamas guna*. Most of the postures of the Primary Series are dedicated to lifeless forms, while the Intermediate Series (consisting of twenty-seven postures) includes eight *asanas* that fall into this category. Seven of these represent ancient forms of weaponry: the noose (*Pashasana*), the weapon of Yama (the Lord of Death) and Varuna (the Lord of the Ocean); the thunderbolt (three variations of *Vajrasana*), the weapon of Indra; the iron beam (*Parighasana*), a weapon used by Lord Hanuman; and the bow (*Dhanurasana* and *Parshva Dhanurasana*). Only *Vatayanasana* (window posture) represents a lifeless form that is not a weapon.

POSTURES REPRESENTING ANIMALS

This category is the dominant one in the Intermediate Series, with twelve postures. Animals tend to be *rajasic*.[1] Many of the animals from which postures take their names are related to *asuras* (demons) of the same name. For example, *Krounchasana* takes its name from *krouncha*, the Sanskrit word for heron, but *Krouncha* is also the name of an *asura*. Both animals and demons are thought to identify primarily with the body (whereas humans have the capacity to access and identify with their divine selves). Like animals, *asuras* are primarily of *rajasic* nature. In animals the *rajas* tend to manifest as fear, whereas the *asuras* tend to make anger their downfall.

POSTURES REPRESENTING HUMAN FORMS

A third category of yoga postures includes those dedicated to human forms. We find in this category postures named after parts of the human anatomy

---

1   There are exceptions. The cow, for example, as a manifestation of the cosmic feminine giving principle, is considered *sattvic*.

LIGHT ON *ASURAS*

Although the Sanskrit word *asura* is generally translated as "demon," this is, of course, problematic. Alternative translations are *demigod*, *titan*, and *devil*. Like the so-called gods (*devas*) and humans, the *asuras*, or anti-gods, are subject to the law of karma. Not all *asuras* cast negative figures; some of them have been outstanding spiritual beings. The *asura* king Prahlada, for example, was a great devotee of the Supreme Being in the form of Lord Vishnu, and the *asura* Vibhishana was a devotee of Lord Rama. The *asura* Baka was a devotee of the Supreme Being in the form of the Lord Krishna. The *asura* Ghattotkatcha, son of Bhima, was one of the greatest fighters on the side of the Pandavas during the Mahabharata war, and consequently shed his life for them.[2]

The *Ramayana*'s description of the *asura* fortress Lanka reads like that of a modern, sophisticated metropolis: Lanka is described as incredibly wealthy, beautiful, clean, and orderly, and its citizens learned, intelligent, and brave. The demons of Lanka, however, tend to make the wrong choices and follow a corrupt leader.

We need to understand *asura* metaphorically as having the potential for negative traits; for us humans it is important to recognize *asura* as our own dark side, our shadow that is always there. Conversely, *deva* is the light within us. We should not smirk at the naïveté of ancient societies and their talk about demons; instead we should consider that our own demonic potential can surface in many ways in the course of one day. There is no point in seeing the dark side only in others, either. Each human being has in each moment the choice to follow his or her demonic or divine potential. Only if we can acknowledge our own *asuric* potential can we overcome it. If we deny our dark side, it will only get stronger and stronger and surface in the most unlikely and most unwanted situations.

and after ancient human masters. Human beings are at various times under the sway of *tamas*, *rajas*, or *sattva*. For this reason, *asanas* are named only after those humans who have gone beyond their animalistic and demonic natures and have awakened to their inherent divinity. These are typically Vedic *rishis* or in some cases illustrious Tantric yoga masters. The purpose of this category of postures is to remind us of the sacred exploits of these masters and also to remind us of the divine potential inherent in every human. There are six postures in the Intermediate Series that fall into this category, with two of them named for sages (*Bharadvajasana* and *Ardha Matsyendrasana*), but we will find many more in later sequences.

POSTURES REPRESENTING DIVINE FORMS

The final category of postures is those named after divine forms. No postures in the Intermediate Series are named directly for a divine form, but several postures are related to celestial beings. These include *Pashasana* (the noose being the weapon of Varuna and Yama), *Kapotasana* (Kapota being one of the hundred names of Lord Shiva), the three *Vajrasanas* (the thunderbolt or *vajra* being the weapon of Lord Indra), and *Yoganidrasana* (which refers to the child form of the Lord Vishnu during the great deluge, Mahapralaya). There are many postures named after divine forms in the later, more advanced sequences.

Table 2 summarizes the categories and locates each Intermediate Series posture within its category.

Next we will take a closer look at the mythology behind the name of each posture.

Mythology of Posture Names

PASHASANA (NOOSE POSTURE)

The Sanskrit term *pasha* means "noose." *Noose* refers here to the position of the arms, which are thrown like a noose around the legs. Pasha is also one of the thousand names of the Lord Shiva, who is also called Pashaye, Lord with the noose.[3] The *Hatha*

---

2 The Pandavas were the five sons of King Pandu: Yudhishthira, Bhima, Arjuna, Sahadeva, and Nakula.

3 S. Sorensen, *An Index to the Names in the Mahabharata* (Delhi: Motilal Banarsidass, 1904), p. 522.

TABLE 2. THE INTERMEDIATE SERIES *ASANAS* CATEGORIZED

Category of Posture	Dominant *Guna*	Representative *Asanas* in the Intermediate Series
Lifeless Forms	*tamas*	*Pashasana* (noose posture) *Dhanurasana* (bow-shaped posture) *Parshva Dhanurasana* (side bow posture) *Laghu Vajrasana* (little thunderbolt posture) *Supta Vajrasana* (reclining thunderbolt posture) *Vatayanasana* (window posture) *Parighasana* (iron cage posture) *Supta Urdhva Pada Vajrasana* (reclining thunderbolt posture with one foot upward)
Animals/*Asuras*	*rajas*	*Krounchasana* (heron posture) *Shalabhasana* (locust posture) *Bhekasana* (frog posture) *Ushtrasana* (camel posture) *Kapotasana* (pigeon posture) *Bakasana* (crane posture) *Tittibhasana* (insect posture) *Pincha Mayurasana* (feathers of the peacock posture) *Karandavasana* (waterfowl posture) *Mayurasana* (peacock posture) *Nakrasana* (crocodile posture) *Gaumukhasana* (cow face posture)
Human Forms	*tamas, rajas,* and *sattva*	*Bharadvajasana* (posture dedicated to Rishi Bharadvaja) *Ardha Matsyendrasana* (posture dedicated to Matsyendranath, half-version) *Ekapada Shirshasana* (one-leg-behind-head posture) *Dvipada Shirshasana* (two-legs-behind-head posture) *Mukta Hasta Shirshasana* (free hands headstand) and *Baddha Hasta Shirshasana* (bound hands headstand)
Divine Forms	*sattva*	*Pashasana* (noose posture) *Kapotasana* (pigeon posture) *Laghu Vajrasana* (little thunderbolt posture) *Supta Vajrasana* (reclining thunderbolt posture) *Yoganidrasana* (yogic sleep posture) *Supta Urdhva Pada Vajrasana* (reclining thunderbolt posture with one foot upward)

THE UNFATHOMABLE DIVINE

Divine forms, also known as *devas* or celestials, are sometimes called gods, but as mentioned in chapter 2, this term is slippery and simplistic. As the *Upanishads* and *Brahma Sutra* convincingly state, there is only one *Brahman*. However, this abstract, formless *Brahman* is difficult to understand. For this reason, the pragmatic approach of the Vedic teaching is to form a close, intimate, personal relationship with one of the aspects or manifestations of the Divine.

Divine forms are meditation images of the Supreme, but their function and importance do not end there. They are also aspects of our higher nature. Here deities are not so much independent beings but rather forces within ourselves that determine our actions as aspects of ourselves. By meditating on a divine image we invoke its qualities. This process of bringing forth the divine qualities within us is very different from what is depicted in today's mass media, which continually portray the more demonic aspects of human nature and thereby provoke the audience to enact further demonic behavior.

Divine forms, of course, are ruled by *sattva*. However, as our demonic side is not always evil, our divine side is not necessarily always noble. The downfall of divine forms or celestials can be their attachment to pride and pleasure, as has been the downfall of many a noble human being.

Deities also represent forces of nature. Indra, for example, represents thunder and rain; Varuna represents the ocean; and Agni represents fire. Last but not least, they also often represent celestial bodies, such as Brihaspati representing Jupiter, or Varuna representing Uranus. Divine forms can also be much more than just deities; they can be *Brahman* with form. This is particularly true of Lord Shiva in his many manifestations, Lord Vishnu and his *avataras* (incarnations), and Devi, the Goddess.

Vedic divine images are so complex that we need to admit that we don't know exactly what they are, and we can only learn more about them as we go along. The list of characteristics given of the phenomenon *deva* is by no means complete. Everything that I have said so far about the Divine says more about my ignorance than about the Divine.

Yoga Pradipika starts with the assertion that it was the Lord Shiva (known in this case as Adinatha, or "primeval master") who first taught yoga.[4] What could be more befitting than to start the Intermediate Series with an homage to the moon-crested Lord who is held to be the author of yoga?

The term *pasha* is derived from the Sanskrit verb root *pash*, meaning "to bind." According to the nineteenth-century American linguist William Dwight Whitney, *pash* is inferable from the noun *pashu*, which is again listed as one of the thousand names of the Lord Shiva.[5] Monier Monier-Williams, a nineteenth-century linguist noted for compiling one of the most widely used Sanskrit-English dictionaries, translated *pashu* as "animal," but he pointed out that the term can also be applied derogatively to humans who are unevolved in sacred matters. He explained that the *Pashupatas* (an ancient school of Shiva worshipers) used the term *pashu* to refer to the individual consciousness or self, distinct from the consciousness of the Supreme Being. Human beings were labeled beasts (*pashus*) because they were commonly enmeshed in conditioned existence and unaware of their higher divine nature. The *Pashupatas* professed that those who do not evolve from this conditioned state are still "animals in sacred matters."[6]

The *Pashupatas* called the Supreme Being *Pashupati*, which is commonly translated as "Lord of the Beasts." The so-called *Pashupati* seal, a terracotta seal that was excavated on a site related to the Indus-Sarasvati culture, supplies us with the oldest known archaeological evidence of yoga. The seal depicts an ithyphallic figure with a bovine head, sitting in *Siddhasana*, surrounded by animals. The

---

4 Pancham Sinh, trans., *The Hatha Yoga Pradipika* (Delhi: Sri Satguru, 1991), p. 1.

5 William Dwight Whitney, *The Roots, Verb-Forms and Primary Derivatives of the Sanskrit Language* (Delhi: Motilal Banarsidass, 1963), p. 95.

6 Monier Monier-Williams, *A Sanskrit-English Dictionary* (Delhi: Motilal Banarsidass, 2002), p. 611.

figure is thought to represent the Lord Shiva, the bovine head representing his *vahana* (vehicle), the bull Nandi.

In Kathmandu, Nepal, an ancient Shiva temple called Pashupati Nath still exists today. Pashupatism is thought by some to be the oldest religion on Earth. Although this religion is generally thought to be extinct, there are still *sadhus* in India who regard themselves as *Pashupatas*.

In the *Mahabharata* we find numerous references to the term *pashupata*. *Pashupata* is an adjective meaning "belonging to Pashupati" (Shiva). It is also the name of the most terrible weapon of the Lord, called the *Pashupata* missile, the arrow that he unleashed from his bow to destroy the three aerial demon cities, called Tripura.

The *Puranas* describe this most destructive of all missiles as having Vishnu (the Supreme in its function as sustainer) as its shaft, Agni (the Supreme in its function as fire) as its tip, and Vayu (the Supreme in its function as wind) as its feathers. The *Skanda Purana* states that the *Pashupata* missile was created from the backbone of the Rishi Dadhicha, who also gave his skull for the manufacturing of the *vajra*, the weapon of the Lord Indra.

In the *Mahabharata*, Arjuna realizes that he needs this missile to win his brother's empire back. He performs austerities in the forest and finally receives the *Pashupata* missile as a boon from Lord Shiva.

Similarly, the performance of this first posture in the Intermediate Series must be seen (if the practitioner is of devotional character) as asking a boon of the trident-bearing Lord (Shiva). The boon being requested is, as usual, immortality — not the immortality of the body, however, but that of recognizing oneself as consciousness, which is eternal and uncreated and therefore immortal. The Lord Shiva is a personification of infinite consciousness.

Pashasana also symbolizes the noose that the Lord throws around the yogi to save him from the fangs of Yama, the Lord of Death. Apart from Lord Varuna, Lord Yama is the other famous carrier of the noose. He is thought to cast the noose at the moment of death to usher the spirit of the departing away.

KROUNCHASANA (HERON POSTURE)

Krouncha means "heron." A pair of herons figure prominently in the incident that not only gave rise to Indian poetry but also triggered the composition of the oldest epic, the *Ramayana*.

At the outset of the *Ramayana* we find sage Valmiki accompanied by his disciple Bharadvaja in the forest.[7] When Valmiki wants to take a bath, he suddenly becomes aware of two *krounchas* engaged in love play. Just then a hunter appears and strikes down the male *krouncha* with an arrow. As the male bird lies on the ground in his blood, the female cries out in agony at the loss of her mate. Valmiki is intensely touched by this tragedy and in the midst of his passion curses the hunter for killing the bird. He then realizes that his outcry was spontaneously forged into metrical quarters, each containing the same number of syllables. Because it was produced by the sentiment grief (*shoka*), he calls his creation *shloka*. Later on, Valmiki is visited by Lord Brahma, who explains that what the seer discovered was in fact poetry, and he assigns him to cast into verse the entire tragedy of the life of Rama (the king of Ayodhya and sixth *avatara* of Lord Vishnu), which today we know as the *Ramayana*, the first and foremost of all poems.

Krouncha also refers to a famed *asura* who is the antagonist in a tale about the Rishi Agastya, who brought the eternal teaching (*sanatana dharma*) to South India and Indonesia. The story commences with Agastya visiting Mount Kailasha in order to obtain a boon from Lord Shiva. Agastya asks for the boon to install a *tirtha* (sacred bathing site) in South India. For this purpose, the Lord turns the goddess Kaveri, who is attending him at the time, into a river and places her in Agastya's water pot (*kumbha*) for easy transport.

On his way to South India, Agastya finds a huge mountain obstructing his way. After several attempts to walk around the mountain, which are thwarted by the mountain repositioning itself, Agastya eventually realizes that the mountain is the *asura* Krouncha. Krouncha wants to prevent

7   Robert P. Goldman, trans., *The Ramayana of Valmiki*, vol. I (Delhi: Motilal Banarsidass, 2007), pp. 127ff.

Agastya from installing the sacred site, because it would block Krouncha from further defiling the country.

Agastya curses the *asura* to forever remain a mountain, called Krouncha Mountain, until a divine force frees him. This divine force would eventually arise in the form of Lord Shiva's second son, Skanda, the Lord of War, who splits open Mount Krouncha with an arrow.

Agastya, upon finding the correct location for his sacred site, releases the waters of his vessel, and the River Kaveri is born. This river is still well known today, as it flows through the entire Indian state of Karnataka. The *ashrama* of the *rishi* is said to have been located at the source of the Kaveri, in the Western Ghats. The Kaveri is considered so sacred that even the goddess Ganga, whose material manifestation is the River Ganges, bathes there once a year to cleanse herself from the degradation she has to absorb as a bathing site.

SHALABHASANA (LOCUST POSTURE)

Shalabha means "locust" or "grasshopper." The term is derived from the root *shal*, which is an exclamation denoting suddenness, the kind of movement typical of a locust.

In the *Adi Parva* of the *Mahabharata*, the *asura* Shalabha is listed as the previous embodiment of the demon emperor Prahlada.[8] After Shalabha breathed his last breath, he was reborn with the name Prahlada, son to the mighty demon king Hiranyakashipu.

Hiranyakashipu is a very prominent figure in the *Puranas*. He was a son of the Rishi Kashyappa, of Kashyappasana fame. Kashyappa himself was a son of the Rishi Marichi, to whom as many as eight *Marichyasanas* are dedicated. We met the Rishi Kashyappa already in *Ashtanga Yoga: Practice and Philosophy*, as the father of Garuda, the king of the eagles.

Hiranyakashipu had a brother named Hiranyaksha, and as the sons of Kashyappa and his

8 The *Mahabharata* has eighteen chapters. Since many of these chapters are hundreds of pages long, they are called *parvas* (books). The first chapter is the *Adi Parva*, Book of the Beginning.

wife, Diti, they were born with an extraordinary destiny. To understand the significance of the two brothers we have to go back many, many millennia to a fateful day, the events of which not only triggered the two greatest wars of India's ancient history but also caused a conflict that spanned three world ages.

Jaya and Vijaya were both gatekeepers at Vaikuntha, the celestial abode of Lord Vishnu. Both were absorbed in Bhakti Yoga, the yoga of devotion to their master. One day the rishis Sanaka and Sanatkumara, along with other *rishis*, approached the gate wishing to address the Lord. Jaya and Vijaya were in an arrogant mood that day and, wishing to keep the Lord's glory to themselves, refused entry to the *rishis*.

The group of *rishis* pronounced a terrible curse on Jaya and Vijaya, condemning them to spend their lives roaming the Earth as *asuras* (demons) engaged in acts of hatred against their master, the Lord Vishnu.

In despair, Jaya and Vijaya turned to Lord Vishnu and asked him to modify the curse of the *rishis*. Lord Vishnu pointed out that he could not do so and didn't want to as they had acted wrongly, but he told them that since all their thoughts had always been bent only on him, from now on they would practice Krodha Yoga. Krodha Yoga is the practice of reaching an intense state of concentration on a chosen object, not through love but through hatred. (Krodha Yogis, like Bhakti Yogis, eventually become what they focus on, with the important difference that during the process Krodha Yoga bestows incredible pain, whereas Bhakti Yoga bestows bliss.) Lord Vishnu then promised his two devotees that they would hate him with such fervor that inevitably they would be drawn toward him like moths into the flame of a candle, only to be killed by his hand and thus again become one with him.

The curse ran its course, and the words of the *rishis* came true as Jaya and Vijaya were born as fierce demons in three consecutive ages. The wars and conflicts that arose through their insatiable hatred of the Lord stimulated the latter to manifest ever-greater *avataras* to quell the activities of his former devotees. They also gave rise to the greatest

Indian tales and epics, the *Bhagavata Purana*, the *Ramayana*, and the *Mahabharata*.

The point of this story about Jaya and Vijaya is that the brothers Hiranyaksha and Hiranyakashipu were Jaya and Vijaya reborn. Both grew up into very powerful warriors and lived for the sole desire of destroying the Lord. Hiranyaksha eventually challenged the Lord when the latter lifted the Earth from the bottom of the primordial ocean, assuming his mighty Varaha (celestial boar) *avatara*.[9] After an arduous fight, Hiranyaksha met his end at the tusks of the Varaha.

Hiranyakashipu did not take very well to the news of his brother being killed by his archenemy. His hatred grew even stronger. He performed intense austerities to such an extent that eventually Lord Brahma had to descend from heaven and ask him which boon he wanted to obtain.[10] Like every true demon before him, Hiranyakashipu asked for his present body to be immortal, since identification with the body is known as the demonic teaching.[11] Significantly, Lord Brahma answered that he could not bestow this boon since even he himself was not immortal.

Hiranyakashipu then asked for the second best boon he could think of: to be killable neither by man nor by beast, neither during day nor at night, neither in a house nor outside a dwelling, neither on the ground nor up in the air, and by no weapon of any kind. Brahma happily granted this boon, since although quite comprehensive it was still finite.

With renewed vigor, Hiranyakashipu then tackled the pursuit of the Lord's peril. Since he was

invincible, he easily became the king of the *asuras* and amassed a mighty army. He soon embarked on his various campaigns of looting and ransacking the three worlds (earth, heavens, and netherworld) with the aim of finally meeting and challenging his chosen enemy, Lord Vishnu.

One day when Hiranyakashipu was away, his own city was attacked and looted by Lord Indra and his army of *devas* (the Indian *devas* are not averse to the pastime of ransacking and pillaging). Hiranyakashipu's wife, Kayadhu, was dragged away as booty but subsequently rescued from Indra's humiliation by the celestial Rishi Narada. Narada is described as having the gifts of eternal youth and flattering speech and being most handsome and a great musician and singer. It is said that by the time Kayadhu left Narada's *ashrama* and returned to Hiranyakashipu, the love-smitten demon queen was pregnant.

Hiranyakashipu was too engaged in wreaking destruction to notice that his first son, Prahlada, who was none other than a reincarnation of the *asura* Shalabha, nevertheless had many traits unworthy of a demon and was rather like a celestial. While Hiranyakashipu was abroad to practice pillaging and ransacking, Prahlada was trained in the demonic arts to be a worthy successor to the demon king. On returning, Hiranyakashipu inquired about Prahlada's progress, only to find his son spontaneously bursting into praises of the much-despised Lord Vishnu. Hiranyakashipu at this point developed serious stomach ulcers. After several attempts to retrain Prahlada in the demonic arts failed — he tried to get him to devour pious devotees of the Lord, roast people on spits, and defile sacred sites through strategic placement of chunks of roasted meat — he decided to have his son killed.

He first ordered his palace guards to chop him to bits. But the guards found their blades went right through Prahlada with no effect. Hiranyakashipu then had him bitten by venomous cobras, trampled on by his biggest elephants, thrown into a furnace, attacked by his most terrible demon warrior, submerged in the ocean, and finally thrown off the highest peak in his empire, all to no avail. While

9 The Supreme Being in the form of the Lord Vishnu comes down to Earth in the form of eight *avataras*. Varaha is the Lord Vishnu's third *avatara*. The others are Matsya (fish), Kurma (turtle), Narasimha (man-lion), Parushurama (Rama with the axe), Lord Rama (from the *Ramayana* epos), Lord Krishna (from the *Mahabharata* epos), and Lord Kalki (yet to come). Lord Buddha is also sometimes listed as an *avatara* of Lord Vishnu; so is Dattatreya.

10 Do not mistake Lord Brahma, a finite being, with the *Brahman* of the *Upanishads*, which is thought to be infinite, eternal, unmanifest consciousness.

11 Lord Brahma, the present giver of the boon here, is the very same *deva* who, under the name of Prajapati, taught the demon king Vairochana that identification with the body is the true self. Since the demon accepted this corrupt teaching, it became henceforth known as the demonic teaching.

Prahlada remained in *samadhi*, the cobras' fangs fell out, the elephants' tusks broke off, the fire died down, the terrible demon warrior ran away, the ocean spat him out, and from his fall from the highest peak he landed lightly like a feather on a bed of lotus flowers.

Hiranyakashipu finally lost his temper and decided to finish off this unworthy son himself. He committed his final mistake on the stairs at the entrance to his palace when he dared Prahlada to invoke his mighty Lord on the spot and let him burst forth from one of the entrance pillars of the palace to prevent Hiranyakashipu from finally killing his son.

Prahlada only smiled and, closing his eyes, invoked the Lord. At that moment a huge cloud darkened the sky so much that there was hardly any daylight anymore; it was neither day nor night. With a clap of thunder, the huge pillar split apart and the Lord came forth in his terrifying Narasimha man-lion form, his fifth *avatara*. In this form he was neither man nor beast, but in between. He grabbed Hiranyakashipu on the stairs of the entrance to his palace, where he was neither inside nor outside of a dwelling. He lifted him up and placed him on his lap, where he was neither in the air nor on the ground. Without using any weapon at all — thus following the boon granted by Lord Brahma to the letter — the Lord in the form of the terrible Narasimha then tore Hiranyakashipu to shreds. (Here is a frequently occurring theme of Indian mythology: If we are in the position to ask a boon of a celestial, we should choose the wording of this boon very, very carefully.)

Whereas everybody else ran away in terror when Narasimha appeared, Prahlada just looked on, smiling, for he recognized the Lord Vishnu even in this terrifying form. The Lord then reverted to his benevolent four-armed form, placed Prahlada on the throne, and made him emperor of the demons.

Thus ends the story of Prahlada, the incarnation of the demon Shalabha. His father, the demon Hiranyakashipu, formerly Vijaya, the jealous doorkeeper of the Lord, had to go through two more demonic incarnations before becoming one with his master.

BHEKASANA (FROG POSTURE)

The term *bheka* denotes a frog. In Indian mythology, the frog is a metaphor for sweat and its inherent power of creation. We can see the basis for this metaphor in the following myths.

The *Katha Sarit Sagara* informs us how the frogs derived their strange voices and in so doing demonstrates the connection among frogs, water, and Agni, Lord of Fire.[12] Lord Shiva and his consort Uma were once engaged in love play. Since their activities were extremely long lasting and they were the most powerful beings in the universe, the entire world was excessively heated by the friction they created. The *devas*, lead by Lord Brahma, were concerned that the entire world would be destroyed as a result. So they singled out Lord Agni to interrupt Shiva and Uma's love play. Agni became very concerned, for he knew that when Kama (cupid) had dared to disturb the Lord's meditation with his flower arrows, he had been reduced to ashes by a mere glance from the mighty Lord's third eye. Agni therefore resolved to hide underwater in a lake rather than take up his task. But Agni's fire brought the water in the lake close to a boil. The frogs living in the water were in such unbearable pain that they revealed Agni's location to the *devas*. For this treason Agni cursed the frogs, and their voices turned into croaking.

The *Shatapatha Brahmana* also contains a passage that connects Agni to frogs.[13] It first describes the construction of the fire altar, and then the consecration and oblation thereof. A priest is advised to draw a frog on the central part of the altar. The story goes on to explain that in the beginning the *rishis* sprinkled Agni with water. When the water dripped off him, the drops became frogs. The drawing of the frog on the altar is used to appease Agni, who appears on the altar as fire to consume the oblations.

Agni represents the inner fire in yoga. Accordingly, the *sushumna*, visualized red, is called the fire *nadi*. Inner fire is created through ritualistic

12 C. H. Tawney, trans., *Somadeva's Katha Sarit Sagara,* vol. 2 (New Delhi: BRPC, 2001), p. 101.
13 *Shatapatha Brahmana,* ninth Kanda, first Adhyaya, second Brahmana.

practice (*tapas*) such as *asana*. The term *tapas* is derived from the verb root *tap*, to cook. Inner heat, produced by correct forms of exertion, is used to burn toxins and impurities. Any such activity brings about sweat, which is the water produced by the heated body.[14] Sweat has an important function in yoga. Shri B. N. S. Iyengar repeatedly instructed me that "sweat goes to the next life." This means, on one hand, that the fruit produced by right exertion is not lost when the mortal body is shed; and on the other hand, that creative power is ascribed to the sweat itself. In the *Puranas* there are several incidences of procreation happening when a drop of sweat falls off the brow of a celestial or *rishi*, and a new powerful being springs up from it. Procreation in the Golden Age (*Satya Yuga*) was thought to be possible without intercourse; the father merely wiped the sweat off his brow and rubbed it on the skin of his wife. Finally, the medieval Hatha texts inform us that the sweat produced by practice should not be wiped off but rubbed back into the skin. By this method, inner glow (*tejas*) is restored. *Tejas* is another form of Agni.

DHANURASANA (BOW-SHAPED POSTURE) AND *PARSHVA DHANURASANA* (SIDE BOW POSTURE)

Dhanu means "bow" and *dhanur* means "bow-shaped." The bow is highly significant in Indian culture and mythology because it was the chosen weapon of India's aristocracy. The following myths are just a few of the many in which a bow figures prominently.

The Rishi Bharadvaja had two students, Drona and Drupada. Both were very competitive, and hatred arose between them. At one point, Drona, who was a great warrior, humiliated Drupada. Drupada thought of revenge. He performed a ritual that gave him two divine children. The son was Drishtadyumna, who would eventually succeed in killing Drona, and the daughter was the beautiful Draupadi. Draupadi would become the wife of Arjuna and his four brothers and become the empress of India. At this early point, however, it

looked as if Arjuna had succumbed to attempts of his uncle and cousins to murder him. It was not known if he was in fact dead or simply in hiding.

Drupada had meanwhile become king of the Panchalas. He was worried how he could make Draupadi the wife of Arjuna, for it looked as if Arjuna were dead. Drupada's court priest suggested that he hold a tournament to determine who was the greatest archer, with Draupadi's hand as the prize. Draupadi was thought to be the most beautiful woman on Earth, so this tournament would surely get Arjuna out of hiding.

In his capital city, Kampilya, Drupada erected a huge palatial hall. Kings, great heroes, and the greatest archers from all over India and faraway countries were invited. They all came to try to win the hand of Draupadi. On the ceiling of the hall was mounted a rotating target in the form of a fish that could be felled only with five arrows. The celestial bow *Kindhira*, which possessed a bowstring of steel, was brought. Many kings tried to string the bow and failed. Others managed to string it but missed the target. Eventually Arjuna, disguised as a *brahmin* (a member of the priest caste), got up, strung the mighty bow *Kindhira* effortlessly and hit the rotating fish with all five arrows. Thus he won the hand of Draupadi.

Arjuna later used his bow *Gandiva* to vanquish his many enemies and win the Mahabharata war. The *Virata Parva* of the *Mahabharata* tells the story of Arjuna, who spent twelve years in exile in the forest and a thirteenth year in disguise, after which he reclaimed his hidden bow. When an onlooker asked him to explain the magic that the bow *Gandiva* exuded, Arjuna explained that it was famed throughout the entire world; it was the only one of its kind. Whoever possessed it would obtain eternal fame. Lord Brahma owned it for one thousand years, and after him Lord Indra for five thousand years. Lord Soma then held it for an eternity before he passed it on to Varuna, the Lord of the Ocean. From him Agni, Lord of Fire, obtained it, and he passed it on to Arjuna for the burning of the Khandava forest. Shortly thereafter, when Arjuna was attacked by the army of his enemies for the first time after the exile, the mere twanging of

14 Wendy Doniger O'Flaherty, *Shiva: The Erotic Ascetic* (London and New York: Oxford University Press, 1981), p. 41.

Gandiva's bowstring sent terror into the hearts of those in the opposing army.

Bows also feature prominently in the *Ramayana*.[15] The two biggest and most powerful bows in the world were said to be those of Lord Shiva and Lord Vishnu.

Lord Shiva was wedded to Sati, who was the daughter of Daksha. Daksha did not approve of the marriage, so he arranged a *yagna*, or ritualistic sacrifice, to humiliate Sati and mock Shiva. Although uninvited, Sati attended the sacrifice but could not bear her father's insults to Shiva, so she immolated herself on the spot. Shiva became enraged and manifested Virabhadra (of Virabhadrasana fame) to enact revenge on Daksha. Virabhadra killed all participants of the sacrifice, although Shiva later revived them in an act of grace. In the meantime, Lord Shiva gave his bow to the kings of Mithila to keep safe while he granted the penances. The bow came into King Janaka's possession when he ascended the throne. Nobody had ever been able to string this mighty bow or even lift it off the floor. King Janaka promised that whoever was able to string this bow would get the hand of his daughter Sita.

Rishi Vishvamitra then brought the two young princes Rama and Lakshmana to Mithila, after they had defeated some demons who had defiled the site of Vishvamitra's rituals by holding barbecues there. Vishvamitra introduced Rama to the king, who was happy that someone was trying to gain his daughter's hand, as many kings had failed. The bow was brought to the palace on an eight-wheeled cart and had to be unloaded by five thousand strong men. Meanwhile a huge audience congregated to watch the spectacle. Encouraged by Vishvamitra and King Janaka, the young Rama lifted the bow effortlessly, strung it, and under the eyes of the breathless crowd fixed an arrow and drew it back. He bent the bow to such an extent, however, that it snapped into two pieces, accompanied by an earthquake and tremendous thunder. After everybody had recovered, King Janaka happily gave his daughter Sita as wife to prince Rama.

15 Goldman, *Ramayana of Valmiki*, vol. 1, p. 251.

USHTRASANA (CAMEL POSTURE)

Ushtra means "camel." In this posture the back is arched, giving the body a rounded shape like the hump of a camel. The *Skanda Purana* uses the word *ushtra* metaphorically to suggest camel-like qualities.[16] It categorizes listeners of scripture according to the merit they derive from the activity. The listeners are first categorized as either superior or inferior; then those groups are divided into several subcategories. Among the inferior ones is a category called *Ushtra*. As the camel picks out bitter fruit and shuns the sweet varieties, so do listeners of the *Ushtra* type fail to take on the sweet and joyful aspects of scripture and instead focus on its bitter parts.

The *Harivamsha Purana* mentions an *asura* called Ushtra.[17] Ushtra participated in an epic battle between the celestials and demons. He was a follower of the one-hundred-headed king of the demons, Kalanemi, who fell only after his heads and arms were severed by the fiery *Sudarshana* disc of the Supreme Being in the form of the Lord Vishnu.

The following story is from the *Katha Sarit Sagara*.[18] On a hunting excursion, the King Pushkaraksha sees a camel that is about to swallow two snakes entwined in love play (entwined snakes are often a metaphor for the twin *nadis*, *ida* and *pingala*). Feeling grief for the snakes (similar to Rishi Valmiki's feelings for the *krouncha* birds), he shoots the camel with an arrow. Immediately the camel changes into the form of a *Vidyadhara* (a lower class of celestial being, often mentioned together with Gandharvas and Yakshas). Surprised, the king asks the *Vidyadhara* how he came to be entombed in the body of the camel. The *Vidyadhara* relates the story of how he had flown across the hermitage of a sage and spotted the beautiful Vinayavati, whom the sage had found in the forest as a little girl and had raised. The *Vidyadhara* was inflamed by lust and, descending, he attempted to drag Vinayavati away by force. The sage then appeared, attracted by his foster daughter's cries, and cursed the

16 *Skanda Purana* II.vi.4.19.
17 Bhumipati Dasa, trans., *The Harivamsha Purana*, vol. 1 (Vrindaban: Rasbihari Lal & Sons, 2005), p. 327.
18 Tawney, *Somadeva's Katha Sarit Sagara*, vol. 6, p. 15.

Vidyadhara to live in the body of an ugly camel until released by a king, who in turn would then marry Vinayavati. (The tale continues with numerous twists but does not involve any more camels.)

Laghu Vajrasana
(little thunderbolt posture),
Supta Vajrasana
(reclining thunderbolt posture),
and *Supta Urdhva Pada Vajrasana* (reclining thunderbolt posture with one foot upward)

Vajra means "hard, mighty, adamantine, impenetrable one." Patanjali lists *vajra* as a quality of the body of the yogi.[19] He suggests acquiring, through *samyama*, a form of objective *samadhi* that bequeaths adamantine stability of the body.

The mythological *vajra* is the thunderbolt, the weapon of Lord Indra. The following tale involving *vajra* is one of the oldest Indian tales and is mentioned in the *Rigveda*. Lord Indra had become very proud of being the king of heaven. He was sitting on his throne, attended to by thousands of dancers, musicians, celestial nymphs, and the other *devas*, when his preceptor Brhaspati entered the throne hall. Indra thought so greatly of himself that he did not deem it necessary to get up and bow to his preceptor. Brhaspati just looked at Indra, basking in his pride, and left. After Brhaspati had left, Indra realized that he was in trouble, for he would not be able to defeat the demon armies without his teacher's help. He looked for his teacher to apologize but could not find him, as Brhaspati had made himself invisible.

Indra, who now needed a new preceptor, then chose the service of Vishvarupa, son of Tvashtr. After initially staging rituals and sacrifices that helped Indra keep the demons (*asuras*) at bay, the two had a falling out, and Indra killed Vishvarupa. Vishvarupa's father, Tvashtr, decided to avenge the killing of his son and performed a powerful ritual. Out of the sacrificial fire an invincible demon was born, one that made the worlds tremble. His name was Vrtra. Vrtra, emitting a terrible cry and brandishing a trident, jumped out of the sacrificial

fire with the words, "What is your command?" to which Tvashtr said, "Go and kill Indra!"

Vrtra amassed a huge army of frightening demons, with whom he defeated the *devas* led by Indra. He humiliated Indra, who found that all his weapons bounced off Vrtra's body, unable to penetrate his skin. Indra then took refuge with Lord Brahma and from him learned that only a weapon formed from the adamantine bones of the Rishi Dadhicha could kill Vrtra, as Dadhicha's body was made from the essence of the world.

Dadhicha was a son of the Rishi Brighu and had an *ashrama* on the banks of the Sarasvati River. Dadhicha had been one of the few righteous ones who spoke out when Lord Shiva was insulted at Daksha's sacrifice. The *devas* went to Dadhicha's *ashrama* and found it to be a place where cats and mice, lions and elephants, mongooses and snakes were playing peacefully next to each other, having lost any intention to do harm in the vicinity of that great sage. (A peaceful coexistence such as this is described by Patanjali as a result of yoga practice.)[20] Dadhicha greeted the *devas* with the words, "Whatever you came here for shall be given to you." The *devas* described the situation and asked Dadhicha to surrender his body for the good of the world. Dadhicha, being a true saint, did not hesitate. He called those close to him and told them of his undertaking. Then in the presence of the *devas* he entered intense *samadhi*, cast aside his body, and attained the *Brahman* (infinite consciousness).

The *devas* then fabricated from his adamantine bones various weapons. The *vajra* was manufactured from Dadhicha's backbone; the extremely destructive celestial weapon the *Brahma shirsha astra*, or Brahma's head missile, was made from his skull;[21] other bones were made into other terrible weapons; his tendons formed nooses for Varuna, Lord of the Ocean, and Yama, Lord of Death.

The *devas*, led by Indra, then amassed a great army and challenged the *asuras*. The *asuras* appeared quickly, led by Vrtra, and hostilities intensified to such an extent that the three worlds were shaking.

19 *Yoga Sutra* III.46.

20 *Yoga Sutra* II.35.
21 *Skanda Purana* I.17.4–5. See more about *Brahma shirsha astra* under *Mukta Hasta Shirshasana*.

After the fight had claimed many casualties on both sides, the Lord of Heaven (Indra) met the leader of the *asuras*, the terrifying Vrtra, on the battlefield. Indra struck him with many weapons, which all seemed to bounce off the *asura*. Even the mighty *vajra* could not penetrate his skin. After the combat had gone on for a long time, Vrtra yawned. At this point, Indra hurled the *vajra*, which entered Vrtra's body through his open mouth and cut him in half.

KAPOTASANA (PIGEON POSTURE)

Kapota means "pigeon." The name *Kapota* in the *shastras* refers to three different figures. The *Mahabharata* tells of a Kapota who was a son of Garuda, the king of eagles.[22] The *Kalika Purana* informs us of the clandestine exploits of a sage named Kapota, to whom we return shortly. Most important, however, *Kapota* appears as one of the hundred names of Lord Shiva and as one of Lord Shiva's one thousand names. To chant the hundred or thousand names is itself a form of devotional practice (chanting the one thousand names is, of course, more time consuming and comprehensive).

The *Skanda Purana* informs us how Lord Shiva received the name Kapota.[23] He once undertook severe *tapas* (ascetic practices) in the form of living only on air and avoiding all pairs of opposites. Although he was the master of the eight forms (five elements, moon, sun, and Lord), he shrank to the size of a pigeon. Henceforth, he was known to his devotees by the name of Kapota.

Kapota is also the name of a sage who plays an important role in a tale described in the *Kalika Purana*.[24] Lord Shiva is at one point cursed to beget sons through intercourse with a mortal woman. He hatches a complicated plot so that he can fulfill this curse without violating the vows he made to his wife Parvati.

An old king, wishing for a son, asks Lord Shiva for the boon of progeny. Shiva grants the king his wish and makes himself be born as the king's son

under the name Chandrashekara (which means "he who wears the moon as a crown," another name of Shiva). At the same time, Parvati incarnates herself as the princess Taravati, who marries Chandrashekara once he succeeds his father to the throne.

One day Taravati bathes at a secluded spot on a river. She thinks herself well concealed, when in fact the sage Kapota observes her. Kapota, who is supposed to sit blissfully and beyond all earthly attachment in *samadhi*, is overcome with immense lust for Taravati as soon as he sees her. Kapota approaches her and tells her that she is so beautiful that she can only be Parvati or the queen of heaven. Taravati is actually both, but she is completely unaware of this fact. So she tells Kapota that she is the wife of King Chandrashekara (who is Lord Shiva in another form, again without being aware of it). Kapota then reveals to her how much he desires her and promises her that she will beget two strong and healthy sons if she yields to his advances. Taravati rebukes the sage for his illicit behavior, but Kapota then threatens to curse her if she does not consent.

Taravati manages to save herself by sending her younger sister Chidrangada, dressed as herself, to Kapota. After sage Kapota enjoys himself, he takes Chidrangada, posing as Taravati, to his *ashrama*, where later she bears the two promised sons. Not realizing that he has been cheated, Kapota resolves — now that he has had his way — to purify the queen from the sin of adultery through the power of his *tapas*.

After some months pass, Taravati makes the mistake of again bathing in the same spot at the river. At the same time, Kapota decides to get some fresh air and goes down to that lovely river spot. When he sees the beautiful Taravati, he realizes that he has been cheated. In anger he curses her to be raped by Lord Shiva in the form of a stinking, repulsive *Kapalika* (a fierce form of ascetic who bears the skull of Brahma as a begging bowl) and to give birth to two monkey-faced sons. To counter the curse, she swears by her marriage vows and the vows of her father (who begot her as a manifestation of Parvati) that she will never have intercourse with anybody but her husband, Chandrashekara (Shiva).

22 Kisari Mohan Ganguli, trans., *The Mahabharata*, vol. 4 (New Delhi: Munshiram Manoharlal, 2001), p. 208.
23 G. V. Tagare, trans., *The Skanda Purana*, vol. 5 (Delhi: Motilal Banarsidass, 1994), p. 83.
24 Quoted in O'Flaherty, *Shiva*, p. 56.

THE ORIGIN OF YOGA

The Supreme Being in the form of Lord Shiva is credited with the authorship of yoga (in the *Mahabharata*, Shiva is called *Yogeshvara*, Lord of Yoga) because many myths about the origin of yoga start with a dialogue between him and the mother of the universe, Uma Parvati, often called Shakti.[25] On one occasion when the Lord was teaching, the serpent of infinity, Ananta, was hiding close by and eavesdropped on the secret teaching. (Of course, Ananta is yet another aspect of the same Supreme Being, manifesting for the promulgation of the eternal teaching.) After he had heard enough, Ananta tried to slither away undetected, but Shiva apprehended him, having been aware of his presence all along. For his transgression, he sentenced Ananta to the task of relating this secret teaching (yoga) to the human beings. Ananta, the one-thousand-headed celestial cobra, then approached the next human village in his newfound role as ambassador of yoga. However, the Indian villagers — who didn't take too kindly to the appearance of normal, one-headed cobras, much less one-thousand-headed ones — pelted Ananta with stones. Ananta returned to Lord Shiva for advice, and the Lord suggested he take on a human form. After doing so, he succeeded in teaching yoga to human beings. This incident is still remembered today in the second *pada* of the opening prayer of the Ashtanga Vinyasa practice. It says, "*abahu purushakaram*," which means, "to him who is of human form from the arms upward." It also says, "*sahasrashirasam shvetam*," which means "one thousand white heads." This is to acknowledge the fact that Ananta, the one-thousand-headed serpent of infinity, took on a human form and was called Patanjali. To reflect this, Patanjali is depicted as a human torso placed on the coils of a serpent.

Kapota returns home and gets in some quality meditation time. In *samadhi*, he sees the true nature of Taravati and Chandrashekara as Parvati and Shiva, and from then on he honors Chidrangada as his wife.

When Taravati one day performs her worship of Lord Shiva, she becomes so engrossed that she no longer recognizes him as different from her husband, who is in fact only a manifestation of Shiva. Shiva then appears together with his wife Parvati. Shiva assumes the appearance of a horrible *Kapalika* and takes Taravati by force. Immediately afterward she gives birth to the two monkey-faced sons. Shiva and Parvati then reveal their identities to Taravati. When Chandrashekara returns, a mystical experience is bestowed on both Chandrashekara and Taravati, in which they see themselves as Shiva and Shakti, father and mother of the universe.

This tale has an important implication. The Lord Shiva does not hesitate to receive and fulfill a curse even though avoiding it would be within his power. Why does he take this course of action? He does it to achieve certain outcomes. Note that the unfolding of the curse's fulfillment results in the following: both Taravati's and Chandrashekara's fathers,

previously childless, are able to beget children by propitiating Shiva and Parvati, respectively; the sage Kapota, who veers from his path to violate a woman, learns to honor and respect each woman as the cosmic mother Parvati. Taravati learns that displacing her problem to her sister does not solve it; both Chandrashekara and Taravati learn that they are representations of the cosmic pair Shiva and Parvati. The listener of the tale comes to understand that the meeting of each human pair is nothing but a manifestation of the union of the cosmic father and mother, Shiva and Parvati (or Shakti).

BAKASANA (CRANE POSTURE)

Baka is the name of a demon who figures prominently in the *Mahabharata*. The *Mahabharata*, being seven times the length of Homer's *Iliad* and *Odyssey* together, is the largest piece of literature composed by humankind. It is a *dharma shastra*, meaning it inquires into what is right action, or *dharma*. Its main protagonists are the five Pandavas — the five sons of King Pandu — who find themselves coping with exceedingly difficult situations and thereby provide examples for right action.

The tale that revolves around the demon Baka begins after the still-juvenile princes and their

25 S. Sorensen, *An Index to the Names in the Mahabharata*, p. 777.

mother, Kunti, have escaped from a death trap. Enemies of the princes built a house that appeared to be soundly constructed but was in fact painted with layers and layers of highly flammable paint. Supporters of the princes warned them of the trap, and the princes escaped, while some of their assailants perished in the fire they set. The princes and their mother then hid in the Ekachakra forest.

While in hiding, Kunti hears of the terrible demon Baka who terrorizes the nearby villagers. To placate Baka, the villagers pay him tribute in the form of food and animals, but even this does not prevent the insatiable demon from swallowing the villagers who deliver the tribute to him. Kunti promises that her second son, Bhima, a son of the wind god, Vayu, will deliver the tribute for them and vanquish the demon. The villagers supply Bhima with the usual cartload of food for the demon, but Bhima happily shoulders it all without making use of the cart. While walking through the forest on the way to the demon's cave, he starts singing, pleased by the beautiful sunny day. It is a long distance to the cave, so he becomes hungry and starts to eat the food that was intended for the demon himself. He has just gulped down the last bite of his extensive meal when he arrives at the entrance to the demon's cave. Bhima yells into the cave and begins to taunt Baka with the news that he has eaten all of Baka's food. Baka does not remain idle for long. Eyes glowing red with anger, he emerges from the cave, tears out the nearest tree, and hurls it at Bhima. Bhima dodges the projectile and throws an even bigger tree back. This exchange goes on until all the trees in the vicinity of the cave are gone. The huge demon then charges at Bhima and starts to wrestle him. Bhima greatly enjoys this struggle. Finally, when he has had enough, he presses Baka down on the ground and crushes the life out of him.

We meet another demon with the name Baka in the *Bhagavata Purana*, a scripture consisting exclusively of the tales related to the Supreme Being in the form of the Lord Vishnu, particularly Vishnu's seventh *avatara*, Krishna.

In the tale that involves Baka, Krishna is a little boy who has been taken to the countryside to be protected from the wrath of his uncle, the demon king Kamsa. Kamsa has tried to kill Krishna many times, as it was prophesied that Krishna would one day kill Kamsa. After several thwarted attempts, Kamsa sends the demon Baka — who can take on the form of a giant crane — to kill Krishna.

At this time, Krishna is herding the cows with his brother Balarama (an incarnation, like Patanjali, of the serpent of infinity) on the banks of the Yamuna. They suddenly see a mountainous creature sleeping by the river. They inquisitively draw closer, at which point the creature, who is Baka in crane form pretending to be asleep, rises and swallows Krishna. Thinking that his job has been fulfilled, Baka suddenly feels a terrible burning pain in his throat and can do nothing but spit out Krishna. Outraged at the failure of his first attempt, he attacks Krishna, threatening to spear him with his huge beak.

Krishna waits calmly for Baka's approach, and just before Baka strikes him he grabs Baka by the two parts of his open beak, lifts him up into the air, and tears him into two pieces. When Krishna and Balarama return home, the villagers all marvel at the strength of the boy. Little do they know that he is no one else but the Supreme Lord. (Krishna takes great care not to display too much of his ability and to appear as human as everybody around him.)

Much later in the life of the grown-up Krishna it is revealed that the demon Baka was in truth a devotee who practiced Krodha Yoga, the yoga of hatred. By focusing on destroying the Lord, Baka had been drawn toward him and eventually found death at the hands of his master. In this way he became one with him.

BHARADVAJASANA
(POSTURE DEDICATED TO RISHI BHARADVAJA)

Bharadvajasana is the first of a two-part sequence of twisting postures. It is deeply symbolic that in previous postures the gaze is mainly directly ahead or backward, whereas these twists give the practitioner a lateral view and encourage "lateral thinking." It is also significant that both twisting postures are dedicated to human masters — and are in fact the only postures in the Intermediate Series or the Primary Series that represent human masters.

The two masters for whom these postures are named were very different. Bharadvaja was a Vedic *rishi*, while Matsyendranath — to whom the subsequent posture is dedicated — was a Tantric *siddha*. The juxtaposition of *Bharadvajasana* and *Ardha Matsyendrasana* is representative of the two roots of the Ashtanga Vinyasa system: Veda and Tantra. For a discussion of the difference between Veda and Tantra, see the sidebar "Veda and Tantra: The Twin Roots of the Ashtanga System."

Bharadvaja was one of the *Saptarishis* (seven *rishis*), the most prominent group of Vedic *rishis*. The *Ramayana* lists the *Saptarishis* as Vishvamitra, Jamadagni, Bharadvaja, Gotama, Atri, Vasishta, and Kashyappa.[26]

Bharadvaja was a son of the Rishi Atri and a disciple of the Rishi Valmiki, who authored the *Ramayana*. Bharadvaja is the author of large segments of the *Rigveda*, the oldest scripture of humankind. He is also the author of a *Dharma Sutra*, a *Shrauta Sutra*, and a Sanskrit grammar that is mentioned by the grammarian Panini but is no longer extant. Bharadvaja is also said to be one of the authors of the original Ayurveda. The *Brahma Purana* states that he taught this original Ayurveda to the king of Benares, but unfortunately this treatise also has been lost.[27]

According to the *Ayodhya Kanda* of the *Ramayana*,[28] Lord Rama went into exile and first visited the *ashrama* of Bharadvaja to seek his blessings. The *ashrama* is thought to have existed in what is now the Indian city of Allahabad, at the confluence of the Yamuna and Ganges rivers.

Bharadvaja was one of the fathers of Indian culture. His erudition represents in many ways the quintessence of Indic thought. As a young man, Bharadvaja set out to study the entire *Sanatana Dharma* (the eternal teaching of the Vedic sciences). Realizing that he was making slow progress, he commenced *tapas* (austere practices) to extend his life expectancy. As he continued to study, he came to learn about more and more areas of knowledge of which he was still completely ignorant. So he

intensified his *tapas* to buy himself more time. Each of the Vedic deities to whom Bharadvaja propitiated eventually appeared before him and, pleased with his *tapas*, granted him boons for a longer life span. At one point he asked Lord Indra for further extension of his lifetime. Lord Indra appeared before him and told him that what he had learned so far amounted to a handful of sand, whereas what still lay ahead equated to the huge mountain close by. Unperturbed, Bharadvaja took a further extension of his life and recommenced his study.

Bharadvaja's story exemplifies the determination and devotion of the founders of Indian culture and Vedic society. When we modern practitioners of yoga perform Bharadvajasana, we can ponder the path laid out by Bharadvaja and the other *rishis* as an inspiration for what is possible in this tradition. All of us who pursue any ancient *sadhana* (practice) — *asana*, *pranayama*, meditation, ritual, chanting of mantra, study of Sanskrit, and so on — are standing on the shoulders of the ancient sages of India.

ARDHA MATSYENDRASANA (POSTURE DEDICATED TO MATSYENDRANATH, HALF-VERSION)

Matsyendranath probably lived in Bengal or Assam. Legend has it that he was a fisherman who one day hooked a giant fish. The fish dragged him into the water and swallowed him. The fish subsequently traveled a long distance and came to rest exactly at the place in the ocean where Lord Shiva had chosen to impart the most secret teachings of yoga to his spouse, Shakti. By listening, Matsyendranath came into possession of the secret teachings, and then Lord Shiva ordered him to impart the teachings to suitable students. Matsyendranath practiced the Lord's teachings inside the fish; after many years another fisherman hooked the fish and Matsyendranath was freed.

He immediately set about to fulfill the Lord's order by founding the tradition of Hatha Yoga. This origin of Hatha Yoga is reflected in its most popular text, the *Hatha Yoga Pradipika*. It states that Adinatha (Lord Shiva) is the first *Siddha*, and Matsyendranath is the second.[29]

26 *Ramayana* 7.1.5.
27 *Brahma Purana* II.37.
28 The *Ayodhya Kanda* is the first of the seven books of the *Ramayana*.

29 Sinh, *Hatha Yoga Pradipika*, I.5, p. 1.

43

VEDA AND TANTRA

The Twin Roots of the Ashtanga System

During the times of the *Veda*, humans were able to stop their thinking process and listen, which allowed them to spontaneously realize the true nature of reality with their hearts ("heart" is a metaphor for consciousness). Listening to a simple sentence or a hymn from the *Vedas* could bring about a deep understanding. The time when Vedic *dharma* (teaching) was at its peak was India's golden age. Then as history and its various ages unfolded, entropy (disorder) increased, the knowledge of humankind dwindled and weakened, and people lost the ability to directly comprehend the knowledge of the *Vedas*. During each of those ages, new types of scriptures were revealed in an attempt to reconnect people with that original knowledge. The scriptures that are designed to fulfill this purpose in the current age (*Kali Yuga*) are the *Tantras*.

Tantra is a very generic term that means "scripture" or "teaching." The term *Tantra* is derived from the root *tan*, "to spread or stretch," and from the root *tra*, "to save or to protect." Since all *Tantras* accept the Vedas as their authority and reference point, the term *Tantra* refers to treatises that spread or propagate the "saving" knowledge, which is the knowledge of the *Vedas*. The *Tantras* do not introduce anything new; they simply present the ancient knowledge of the *Vedas* in a new way, designed for modern humanity.

The *Tantras* emphasize technique and precise method rather than intuitive wisdom, philosophical speculation, and direct insight. There are Shaivite, Vaishnavaite, Shaktaite, Buddhist, and Jaina *Tantras*. All these systems at some point in their history "went Tantric" so modern humans could understand them more easily.

The movement away from abstract philosophical teaching and intuitive metaphysical insight and toward simple "how-to" manuals has been most obvious in the yoga tradition. Whereas the former themes were covered in the ancient *Yoga Sutra* and *Upanishads*, Tantric yoga treatises such as the *Hatha Yoga Pradipika* and the *Gheranda Samhita* generally contain instructions on how to practice *asanas*, *bandhas*, *mudras*, and *kumbhakas* correctly. They also introduce the idea that if these methods are not practiced meticulously according to instruction, any higher realization will be impossible.

The Tantric approach differs from that of the *Vedas* in other respects as well. In particular, Tantric teaching's stance toward gender and sensuality is very different from that of Vedic teaching. While in the Vedic pantheon, female deities often play second fiddle, in Tantra they are considered at least as important as male deities and often more important. This reflects the Tantric view that the cosmic female principle (that is, the female energy that is in everything — not just women but also God and the universe in general) is essentially sacred. Whereas Vedic *rishis* are exclusively male, Tantric *siddhas* (those who have achieved the power of realization) can be of either gender.

To raise the awareness of their disciples, Tantric *siddhas* employ methods that are unorthodox compared to the methods of the Vedic tradition. For example, a liberated female *siddha* may use intercourse to initiate a suitable male student and thereby confer mental freedom on the student. Many of the great Tantric gurus were initiated in this way. The female adept is then seen not as a mortal woman but as a priestess representing the Cosmic Godmother, Shakti. The qualifications required of male students include many years of celibacy, the ability to be completely unwavering in concentration if encountering sensual thoughts, and a thorough training in *asana*, *pranayama*, and meditation. (These stringent requirements are usually cast aside in the commercialized version of Tantra that is popular in Western societies today.)

Tantric ritual follows the rationale that anything that can lead to your fall can also be used to lift you up. There is thus no wrong teaching in Tantra but rather teachings that may be unsuitable for some students but right for others. Methods in Tantra are judged not according to whether they hold up to a moral code but based on whether they produce results, namely *siddhi*, and awakening in the practitioner. Although Westerners welcome Tantra as importing sensuality into spirituality, the traditional Indian view is that Tantra introduces sensual people to spirituality.

Matsyendranath was a prolific and influential teacher. He is said to have authored the *Matsyendra Samhita*, the *Akula Vira Tantra*, the *Kaula Jnana Nirnaya*, and the *Kulananda Tantra*. Most of these are Shaktaite *Tantras* (dedicated to worship of the Goddess) written in Bengali rather than Sanskrit. According to the Sanskrit scholar Agehananda Bharati, Matsyendranath is also the author of *Gheranda Samhita*, which would make Gheranda another name for Matsyendranath.[30]

We know of Matsyendranath mainly through the fame of his student Gorakhnath. Gorakhnath made Hatha Yoga and the order of the Nathas popular. He authored many texts, such as the *Gorakshataka*, the *Goraksha Samhita*, *Siddha Siddhanta Paddhati*, *Yoga Martanda*, *Yoga Chintamani*, *Goraksha Sahasra Nama*, and many more. Swatmarama, the author of *Hatha Yoga Pradipika*, states that he learned Hatha Yoga through the grace of Matsyendranath and Gorakhnath.[31]

The Tantric scholar A. K. Banerjea argues that Matsyendra's and Goraksha's yoga techniques were later elevated to *Upanishadic* status — that is, viewed as official mystical doctrines of the upper echelons of Indian culture.[32] According to Banerjea, the group of *Upanishads* referred to as the *Yoga Upanishads* (the *Nadabindu Upanishad*, *Dhyana Bindu Upanishad*, *Tejo Bindu Upanishad*, *Yoga Tattva Upanishad*, *Yoga Chudamani Upanishad*, *Yoga Kundali Upanishad*, and so on) only repeat the teachings of Matsyendranath and Gorakhnath without referring to their compilers by name.

As the progenitors of some of Hatha Yoga's most quintessential texts, both Matsyendranath and Gorakhnath are of significance for modern Ashtanga practitioners. The *Hatha Yoga Pradipika*, which was authored by a student of Gorakhnath's, and the *Gheranda Samhita*, which was possibly authored by Matsyendranath himself, are the texts that place the most emphasis on the performance of the *bandhas*. The *bandhas* are a distinctly Tantric influence in the

Ashtanga system, and even though they may predate Matsyendranath, he is nevertheless remembered for them, especially in the performance of *Ardha Matsyendrasana*.

EKAPADA SHIRSHASANA (ONE-LEG-BEHIND-HEAD POSTURE) AND *DVIPADA SHIRSHASANA* (TWO-LEGS-BEHIND-HEAD POSTURE)

Leg-behind-head postures represent the destruction of the ego. It is easy to imagine the leg as a heavy sacrificial sword (*kadga*) ready to cut off the ego-containing head. The cutting off of the head as a symbol of reducing or destroying a bloated ego repeatedly occurs in Indian myth, such as in the beheading and subsequent resurrection of Daksha at the hands of Lord Shiva or the self-beheading of the goddess Chinamasta.

The symbolism of cutting off the head is powerfully displayed in the conflict between Lord Shiva and Lord Brahma. The *Kurma Purana* informs us that Brahma, the five-headed deity, once proclaimed that he was Ishvara, the Supreme Lord, and *Brahman*, the infinite consciousness, titles that more often than not refer to Lord Shiva or Lord Vishnu but not to Brahma.[33] When the four *Vedas* then materialized and informed him that Lord Shiva was the Supreme Being, Brahma argued that this could not be the case, since Shiva had a wife and was therefore displaying attachment, which he felt must surely disqualify Shiva. The sacred syllable *Om* then became audible, and out of it manifested the Supreme Being, the Lord Shiva. He informed Brahma that his wife, the goddess Uma, was nobody but himself, a manifestation of his ecstasy. Brahma refused to acknowledge this, and to make matters

30 Agehananda Bharati, *The Tantric Tradition* (New York: Anchor Books, 1970), p. 250.
31 Sinh, *Hatha Yoga Pradipika* I.4 , p. 1.
32 Akshaya Kumar Banerjea, *Philosophy of Goraknath* (Delhi: Motilal Banarsidass, 1983), p. 26.

33 G. V. Tagare, trans., *The Kurma Purana*, vol. 2 (Delhi: Motilal Banarsidass, 1982), p. 512. Lord Brahma is the name not of a deity but of an office. The first being that arises in each world age due to its past subconscious impressions becomes its Lord Brahma. Since this being is the first one, its subconscious impressions are not obstructed by those of others and it can create the universe according to its ideas. According to Indian tradition, the Lord Brahma of our world age is called Prajapati. He is thought to be almost omnipotent when compared to a human but mortal and of limited power when compared to the Supreme Being, who is usually identified with Lord Shiva, Lord Vishnu, or the goddess Uma.

worse, through his fifth head he ordered Shiva to bow down to him. At this point Lord Shiva raised his trident and cut off the fifth head of Brahma. As soon as the head was gone, Brahma could see that the Lord and the Great Goddess were in fact one and the same, the Supreme Being. Cured of his infatuation with himself and his obstinate ego, Brahma took refuge in the Lord.

By cutting off one of Lord Brahma's heads, however, Shiva had committed the sin of slaying a brahmin (brahmahatya). According to the law books, this was the worst of all sins, comparable to the murder of one's parents or one's spiritual teacher. The skull of Brahma's head attached itself to Lord Shiva's hand, and thus he became a Kapalin, a skull carrier. He would have to carry the skull until he had expiated himself from this sin.

To do this, Lord Shiva had to perform the mahavrata (great vow). The great vow includes living for twelve years in the forest, scantily clad and smeared in ashes, sustaining oneself only through roots and berries while carrying a skull. One is to use the skull not only as a begging bowl but also for consuming one's food and drink. The idea of the mahavrata is to make the sinner clearly visible as a slayer of a brahmin. This provokes the censorship and noncompassion of society, making the performer an outcast. Lord Shiva performed this penance symbolically. Since he is omnipotent, it was of course in his power to expiate himself from this sin. Nevertheless he undertook the penance willingly to show that nobody should deem himself above the law. He also showed that he did not have an ego since he did not hesitate to descend to the lowest social rung, that of a murderer.

Shiva's act of performing the mahavrata led to the formation of the order of the Kapalikas (skull bearers).[34] The Kapalikas emulate Shiva's penance by carrying human skulls, from which they eat and drink. They wear their hair matted, go naked, and smear themselves in ashes. They usually live alone in the forest, but if entering human habitations they act in a way that attracts the censorship of society;

by performing obscene gestures and making rude comments in the presence of women, they become outcasts and thus emulate Lord Shiva. They believe that the more society looks down on you, the closer you get to the Lord. They do this as an act of bhakti to Lord Shiva, spending their lives in exactly the same harsh conditions as he did during his mahavrata. The rationale behind the actions of the Kapalikas is that since Lord Shiva is omnipotent, liberation from conditioned existence can be had only through his grace. By emulating his mahavrata, the Kapalika seeks to attract the Lord's grace.

Because of their beheading symbolism, Ekapada Shirshasana and Dvipada Shirshasana remind us not to hold our heads too high and not to think too greatly of ourselves. Humility is one of the great qualities conveyed by leg-behind-head postures. If we think in terms of the penance Shiva performed for cutting off Lord Brahma's fifth head — and the order of the Kapalikas that arose from it — these two postures teach us not to judge too quickly those who stand outside society, because they could be in that position for valid reasons that are outside our understanding.

YOGANIDRASANA (YOGIC SLEEP POSTURE)

Patanjali lists nidra as one of the five fluctuations of mind. He calls nidra the state in which both the dreaming and waking states are negated, which makes it a third state of mind.[35] This third state and the fourth state, turiya (consciousness), are similar in the sense that in both the flame of the mind is not fanned by the wind of prana, meaning the mind is steady. Nidra and turiya are different from each other, however, because awareness is present in turiya but not in nidra. In yogic sleep (yoga nidra) one combines the awareness of turiya with the mind-steadiness of nidra. There is absolutely no movement of the mind, yet awareness of this stillness is present. According to Monier-Williams, yoga nidra, or yogic sleep, is a state halfway between meditation and sleep.[36]

The tale that gave rise to the name of this posture is related to Lord Vishnu, who assumes the state of yoga nidra at the end of each Mahayuga. A

34 The Kapalika order has been immortalized in the Ashtanga system through Krakachasana, a posture in the Advanced C series. Krakacha was one of the leaders of the Kapalika order and at home in the Mysore state.

35 Yoga Sutras I.6 and I.10.
36 Monier-Williams, A Sanskrit-English Dictionary, p. 857.

Mahayuga, or great *yuga*, is the period the world takes to go through one whole cycle of the four ages.

Mrkandu, a grandson of the Rishi Bhrigu, remained childless for a long time. Eventually he started to perform *tapas* dedicated to Lord Shiva. When Shiva was pleased with him, he gave him the choice of having either a long-lived but evil and dim-witted son or a noble, erudite, and virtuous son who would die when completing his sixteenth year. Mrkandu chose the latter. When Mrkandu's son, Markandeya, was approaching the age of sixteen Mrkandu informed him of his fate. Markandeya sat down in front of an image of Lord Shiva and fell into deep contemplation. When in due time Yama, the Lord of Death, appeared, he had to cast his noose around both the divine image and Markandeya to catch his victim. This enraged Shiva who, manifesting from the image, killed Yama and blessed his devotee, Markandeya, so that he would remain eternally at the age of sixteen years and thus continue to elude death.

Markandeya then spent several world ages in deep meditation without having any awareness of the change of ages that happened outside him. One day while he was meditating, a strong wind started to blow and soon turned into a hurricane. Torrential rain commenced, and quickly the rivers left their beds and submerged everything. Markandeya was thrown around by mountainous waves, when suddenly he saw a huge banyan tree on top of a king wave. He was attracted to the tree by the great effulgence that seemed to exude from it. Drawing closer he noticed a light stemming only from one branch. Coming even closer, he could see that this light came from only one leaf of the tree. On this leaf he saw a shining infant lying on its back, sucking on its big toes.

Markandeya was sucked by an inhalation into the body of the infant. There he could see, to his great amazement, the entire universe with its galaxies, suns, planets, oceans, continents, mountains, rivers, trees, and so on. He saw the whole creation passing before his eyes, powered by time. As he watched, ages drew past in fast succession. Then, suddenly, an exhalation of the infant threw him out. When he saw the infant lying there in its golden light on the leaf of the banyan

tree with the entire creation suspended in its body, he realized that this was the Lord Vishnu and that this was the time of the great deluge Mahapralaya, when the entire creation was drowned in water at the end of the *Mahayuga*.

Lord Vishnu, the sustainer of the universe, inhales the creation at the end of each world age and enters the state of yogic sleep. In this state the universe and time remain suspended in the infant body of the Lord until Vishnu breathes it forth at the beginning of the next new world age.

The posture *Yoganidrasana* symbolizes the posture of the infant form of the Lord Vishnu on a leaf of the world tree on the king wave in the primordial ocean during the grand dissolution at the end of time.

TITTIBHASANA (INSECT POSTURE)

Tittibha means "insect." In assuming this posture, one resembles the shape of an insect with its wings raised.

In the *Katha Sarit Sagara* we learn the story of a pair of *tittibhas* living by the sea.[37] It is time to lay eggs, so the female *tittibha* suggests that they move to a different location, as the sea could carry away the eggs at any time. The male *tittibha* refuses to budge, however, and assures the female that whatever happens, he can take care of it. The sea listens to this boastful talk and decides to teach the *tittibha* a lesson by washing the eggs away. Hurled into action by the wailing of the female, the male *tittibha* calls a meeting of his relatives and relates the insult meted out against him at the hands of the sea. The clan of *tittibhas* decides to take the issue further and send a petition to Garuda, the king of all airborne beings. Garuda takes up their cause and approaches his master, the Lord Vishnu, who resides in the ocean. Lord Vishnu, always inclined toward his vehicle Garuda, threatens to burn up the sea, and the sea has to return the eggs to the shore.

In this same text we also learn of an encounter between the louse Mandavisarpini and a flea named Tittibha.[38] Mandavisarpini leads a luxurious life in the bed of a king, and since she bites the king only

37 Tawney, *Somadeva's Katha Sarit Sagara*, vol. 5, pp. 56–57.
38 Ibid., p. 52.

at night and in a clandestine way, she is not discovered. Then Tittibha appears, wanting to share Mandavisarpini's royal host. Although initially ill disposed to the new arrival, Mandavisarpini assents to Tittibha's moving in because Tittibha has never drunk the blood of a king. Mandavisarpini allows Tittibha to stay, on the condition that he never bite the king in a way that wakes him up. Tittibha, however, cannot help himself, and as soon as the king enters the bed, he starts to gorge himself on the king's blood. In the morning, the king orders his servants to search the bed. Sure enough, they find the louse Mandavisarpini and she is killed, whereas Tittibha escapes.

PINCHA MAYURASANA
(FEATHERS OF THE PEACOCK POSTURE) AND
MAYURASANA (PEACOCK POSTURE)

Mayura means "peacock." Peacocks are thought to be immune to snakebite venom and other poisons, a quality that connects them — through the following myth — to Lord Shiva.

When the *devas* and demons churned the primordial ocean to obtain the elixir of immortality, the great world poison *Kalakuta* appeared. As it threatened to destroy the entire world, the *devas* asked Lord Shiva to swallow it, knowing that he would never refuse a request. When he put the poison into his mouth, his spouse, Uma, stepped up from behind and wrung his neck to prevent him from swallowing it and being killed. The poison thus remained in his throat and colored it blue, earning him the name Nilakantha, the blue-throated Lord. As the peacock is also blue throated, the *Skanda Purana* assigns to the Lord Shiva epithets such as *Mayuresha* and *Mayureshvara*, both meaning "Lord of the Peacock."[39]

Appropriately, *Mayurasana* and *Pincha Mayurasana* are both believed to expel toxins from the abdominal organs and cure abdominal diseases such as duodenal and stomach ulcers.

Peacocks have further significance in Indian mythology. The peacock Mayura is thought to be the son of the mythical eagle Garuda, who created him

from his feathers. The *Skanda Purana* tells us that Garuda gave Mayura to Lord Skanda to use as his vehicle upon his installation as commander-in-chief of the celestial army.[40] One of Skanda's names is thus Mayuraketu, which means "having a peacock as one's banner." The peacock is also the vehicle (*vahana*) of Devi Sarasvati, the goddess of learning, art, and speech.

KARANDAVASANA (WATERFOWL POSTURE)

Descriptions of celestial lakes in the *shastras* are usually replete with three waterbirds: *chakravaka* (ruddy sheldrake), *hamsa* (swan), and the bird for which this posture is named, *karandava* (goosander or merganser).[41] (The other two birds have lent their names to *asanas* as well, although they are not practiced in Ashtanga Vinyasa Yoga.) This posture was named after the *karandava* because in the final version of the posture, the practitioner's forearms resemble this bird's large feet.

There are several passages in the *Ramayana* that mention *karandavas*. One concerns Sita, King Janaka's daughter, who was wedded to Prince Rama of Ayodhya, the sixth *avatara* of Lord Vishnu. Rama was forced into forest exile by his ill-disposed stepmother, Kakeyi. Along with Rama's brother, Lakshmana, Sita followed Rama into exile. The demon king Ravana then abducted Sita and brought her to the island fortress Lanka. Rama enlisted the help of Hanuman to search for Sita. When scanning Lanka in search of Sita, Hanuman saw *karandavas*.[42]

In another passage of the *Ramayana*, the sky is likened to a large lake or ocean, with the sun resembling a lake full of *karandavas*.[43] A third passage likens the beauty of the women in the demon king Ravana's harem to rivers covered by *hamsas* and *karandavas*.

Karandavas are also mentioned several times in the *Skanda Purana*.[44] In all three passages they are mentioned together with swans, a metaphor for the

39 Tagare, *Skanda Purana*, vol. 11, p. 25.

40 Tagare, *Skanda Purana*, vol. 2, p. 257.
41 Robert P. Goldman and Sally J. Sutherland Goldman, trans., *The Ramayana of Valmiki*, vol. 5 (Delhi: Motilal Banarsidass, 2007), p. 363.
42 *Ramayana, Sundara Kanda*, Sarga 2, Shloka 9–13.
43 *Ramayana* V.55.1–3.
44 Tagare, *Skanda Purana*, vol. 15, pp. 7, 97, 110. (V.III.2, 26 and 28).

soul. In the first and second passages, the presence of swans and *karandavas* is used to enhance the natural beauty of two sacred sites. The third passage describes the destruction of the three demonic cities (Tripura) by the Lord Shiva. As the cities are engulfed in fire, their usually calm and clear lotus ponds are stirred up by the swans and *karandavas*, adding to the destructiveness of the image.

NAKRASANA (CROCODILE POSTURE)

The crocodile, or *nakra*, is frequently employed as a metaphor in Indian mythology and scripture. The *Skanda Purana*, for example, likens our present age, the dark age of *Kali Yuga*, to a crocodile.[45] It gives instructions to those "who are in the fangs of the crocodile of Kali." This metaphor is used because the *Kali Yuga* has the tendency to drag us down into the lower recesses of our animalistic and demonic nature, much as a crocodile gets hold of its prey and drags it under water to drown it.

Despite its aggressive nature, the crocodile is accorded a protected status in scripture. The *Devi Bhagavata Purana* contains a passage that describes the various hells that await those who transgress divine law; *Nakra Kunda* (crocodile hell) is reserved for killers of sharks and crocodiles.[46] After having roasted in that hell for some time, says the *Purana*, the assailants of crocodiles will then have to be born in the form of their victims for some time — possibly several lifetimes — until purification is complete.

In the *Mahabharata*, we hear of Arjuna in a close encounter with crocodiles.[47] While on a *tirtha yatra* (pilgrimage to sacred sites) to expiate a sin, Arjuna travels through South India. Here he learns of a group of five famous *tirthas* (sacred bathing sites) that are considered very sacred and powerful but cannot be used because anyone who tries to bathe in them is taken by crocodiles. Arjuna decides to put himself to some good use and rid the sacred sites of the crocodiles. He proceeds to the first lake and

takes his ritual bath, only to be grabbed by a huge crocodile and dragged under water. However, being Arjuna, he is able to lift the crocodile out of the water and drag it ashore. At this moment the crocodile disappears in a puff of smoke, and Arjuna finds himself embracing a beautiful *apsaras* (celestial nymph).

Dumbfounded, Arjuna asks this most beautiful of all *apsarases* how she came to be hiding in the lake in the form of a crocodile. The *apsaras* replies that from their heavenly abode, she and four friends had once spotted a young, handsome sage in deep contemplation in the forest. Through the power of his mantras and *samadhi*, the young sage shone more brilliantly than the sun. As it is in the nature of an *apsaras* to distract sages from their austerity through erotic exploits and thereby restore the balance of the cosmos, the five celestial nymphs descended into the forest and started singing, dancing, and cavorting in front of the saint, all the while being covered only by the most skimpy of attires, revealing their shapely forms at their every move. However, this sage did not react at all to their advances. After they had danced before him for some time, he turned toward them and cursed them to live as crocodiles under water. They were to sustain themselves by eating visitors to the sacred sites until a man came along who was strong enough to drag them out of the water, at which point they were to regain their original forms.

After Arjuna learns all this, he goes on to the other four lakes in the vicinity and drags the other four crocodiles out of the water. After he thus rids the *tirthas* of their plague and reinstates the celestial nymphs to their respective forms, he continues his *tirtha yatra*.

VATAYANASANA (WINDOW POSTURE)

Vata means "wind" and *yana* means "path," so *vatayana* means "wind path." As such, the word commonly refers to a window, which provides the path for the wind in a house. *Vatayanasana*, then, simply means "window posture." The original sense of *vatayana* as an opening through which the wind blows is still present in the modern English word *window*.

45 Tagare, *Skanda Purana*, vol. 6, p. 287.
46 *Devi Bhagavata Purana* XXXIII.86–103.
47 Kisari Mohan Ganguli, trans., *The Mahabharata, Adi Parva*, sec. 215, vol. 1 (New Delhi: Munshiram Manoharlal, 2001), pp. 416ff. The same episode is retold in Tagare, *Skanda Purana*, vol. 2, p. 2.

The window in *Vatayanasana* is the space between the knee of the leg in half-lotus and the foot of the supporting leg. The goal in the posture is to bring both close together. When the foot and the knee are touching, the window is considered closed.

PARIGHASANA (IRON CAGE POSTURE)

Parigha means "iron bar" and can refer to the bar used to shut a gate or door. The Sanskrit prefix *pari*, however, means "around," and for this reason I translate *Parighasana* as "iron cage posture." The torso in this posture is firmly enclosed by the "cage" formed by the arms and the straight front leg.

The term *parigha* features prominently in the *Ramayana*. After Lord Hanuman finds Sita, who had been held captive in the demon fortress Lanka, he decides to destroy the pleasure grove of the demon king Ravana and thus challenge the demons to a fight. Outraged, Ravana sends the Kimkara demons to kill Hanuman. Hanuman, who has not brought any weapons to Lanka, simply tears a huge iron beam (*parigha*) from a gateway and uses it to bludgeon the demons to death.[48] Next, Ravana dispatches one hundred palace guards, whom Hanuman defeats by means of a column that he rips out of a palace. Ravana then sends the demon Jambumalin into battle. Jambumalin attacks by hitting Hanuman with many arrows. Hanuman then hurls a huge rock at the demon, which Jambumalin manages to destroy in midair by hitting it with his arrows. Hanuman then uproots an enormous tree and throws it at the demon, but again Jambumalin destroys it with his arrows. Hanuman finally wields the same *parigha* he used previously to kill the Kimkara demons. He hits Jambumalin on the chest, at which point the demon's body crumbles to dust.[49]

GAUMUKHASANA (COW FACE POSTURE)

Go means "cow" and *mukha* means "face." The term *gaumukha* can be used for anything odd or randomly shaped, such as an unevenly built house. Even an odd-shaped hole that thieves would create to enter a house can be called a cow face.[50] The posture's name is derived from these connotations of *gaumukha*. Also, *Gaumukh* is the name of the source of the Ganges, a place said to resemble a cow's mouth.

In the symbolic realm, the cow in India is rich with significance. For example, it is a symbol for motherhood and all those who freely give much and take little. Kamadhenu, the cow of plenty, is a metaphor for abundance. Govinda, which means "cowherd," is a name of the Lord Krishna, reminding us of the fact that he spent the first part of his life in Brindavan, tending the cows. The cow is regarded as sacred in India and is not to be killed. The *Shatapatha Brahmana* states that the flesh of the cow and the ox should not be eaten, as they support everything on Earth.[51]

The following myth demonstrates the importance of the cow. After a long time of lawlessness and famine, Prithu became emperor. His subjects complained that the herbs, grains, and vegetables had all been withdrawn into the Earth and there was nothing to eat. Prithu took his bow and arrows and went in pursuit of the Earth Goddess. The Earth Goddess took the form of a cow and ran away. After a long pursuit, the cow/Earth eventually consented to be milked by Prithu, and through this act all the Earth's fertility and abundance returned. The cow is thus a symbol of the abundance the planet provides us with.

Nowhere is the importance of the Earth's abundance clearer than in the conflict between the Rishi Vasishta and the great king Kaushika.[52] As was common with Vedic kings, Kaushika visited the *ashrama* of the Rishi Vasishta when he was passing by with his army on the way to battling his foes. The king and the sage exchanged pleasantries and grew fond of each other, so that eventually Vasishta invited Kaushika, together with his entire army, to be his guests for the night. Kaushika tried to prevent this, as he did not want to be a strain to the *ashrama* kitchen, but Vasishta insisted. Vasishta then instructed his wish-fulfilling cow, Kamadhenu, to provide everything that was needed. The cow (again

---

48 *Ramayana* V.4.31.
49 *Ramayana* V.42.14–17.

50 Monier-Williams, *Sanskrit-English Dictionary,* p. 366.
51 Max Mueller, ed., *The Shatapatha Brahmana* III. I 2.21, pt. II (Delhi: Motilal Banarsidass, 1963), p. 11.
52 Goldman, *Ramayana of* vol. 1, p. 224.

symbolizing the abundance of the Earth) manifested mountains of steamed rice, rivers of curd, and uncountable delicacies of all varieties.

At the end of the meal, Kaushika pointed out to the sage that the cow was truly a jewel, and since by law all jewels belonged to the king, Vasishta should hand her over. When the sage refused, Kaushika offered him first a hundred thousand cows, then fourteen thousand elephants, and then additionally eight hundred golden chariots. But Vasishta remained steadfast and refused. Eventually the king told his soldiers to drag the cow away by force. Kamadhenu, however, managed to tear herself away. She ran to Vasishta and asked him to protect her. Vasishta pointed out to her that as a *brahmin* he had no power over the king who was a member of the warrior caste (*kshatriya*) and commanded a huge army. Kamadhenu then told Vasishta that no *kshatriya* in the whole world could withstand the power of a *brahmin*. She offered to take care of the situation if only Vasishta would order her to manifest destructive forces instead of benevolent ones.

Vasishta ordered the cow to manifest an army to destroy Kaushika's army. After Kaushika's men withstood the first onslaught, the cow manifested a bigger army consisting of more bloodthirsty and demonic warriors. Eventually, all of Kaushika's men and also his hundred sons lay slain on the battlefield. At this point, Kaushika realized that the military might of a *kshatriya* could not face up to the spiritual power of a *brahmin*. He abdicated as king and retired to the forest in the hope of acquiring by means of asceticism the spiritual power of a *brahmin*.

MUKTA HASTA SHIRSHASANA (FREE HANDS HEADSTAND) AND BADDHA HASTA SHIRSHASANA (BOUND HANDS HEADSTAND)

One challenge of a headstand posture is that once you begin falling out of it, you cannot reverse the fall. Thus it is recommended that you not go into a headstand unless you can sustain it. In the broader world, this translates into an important principle: Never unleash a force unless you can withdraw it.

This lesson is taught in a tale from the *Mahabharata* that involves, quite appropriately, the

head of Lord Brahma.[53] In the days of the *Mahabharata*, the main weapon of the great warriors was the *astra*. An *astra* was an arrow released with a magical incantation that turned it into a destructive missile. There were many types of *astras*, the destructive power of which could be released only by those warriors who had mastered their incantations through *tapas* and initiation. The most terrible of these *astras* was the *Brahma shirsha astra*[54] or "missile of Brahma's head," which contained the destructive power of Lord Shiva tearing off Lord Brahma's fifth head. The *Skanda Purana* states that this *astra* was manufactured from the adamantine skull of the Rishi Dadhicha, who also gave his backbone for forming Lord Indra's Vajra. The *Brahma shirsha astra* was never meant to be used against humans but only against demons.

Lord Shiva gave the *Brahma shirsha astra* to the Rishi Agastya. After a long time Agastya passed it on to Drona, Arjuna's martial arts guru. Drona passed it on to Arjuna, since he knew of Arjuna's strong *tapas* and self-mastery. Drona's son, Ashvatthama, grew jealous of Arjuna's achievement and coaxed his father, against Drona's better knowledge, to reveal to him the incantation for this terrible weapon. Drona finally assented but not without obtaining from his son the promise that he would never use this weapon against human beings.[55]

Later, during the Mahabharata war, Ashvatthama was an opponent of Krishna and Arjuna. Bhima, Arjuna's older brother, challenged Ashvatthama to a fight. Since Bhima was a great warrior, Ashvatthama decided to take no risks and released the *Brahma shirsha astra* at Bhima, with the words, "May the world be Pandava-less." Arjuna then entered the battlefield. He realized that to protect himself and his brother he had to counteract

---

53 Ganguli, *Mahabharata, Sauptika Parva*, sec. 14, vol. 7, pp. 34ff.
54 An alternative spelling is *Brahma-shiras*, which has the same meaning, according to Monier-Williams (p. 740).
55 The use of the *Brahma shirsha astra* was permitted against powerful foes such as *rakshsasas* and *asuras* (classes of demons). In ancient days, warriors had to adhere to a code of conduct according to which certain weapons were not to be unleashed against one's own kind even if they were one's foes. Modern humanity unfortunately has lost all such restraint.

ASHTANGA YOGA — THE INTERMEDIATE SERIES

Ashvatthama's *astra* by releasing the *Brahma shirsha astra* himself.

As the two *astras* raced toward each other, mountains started to shake and oceans began to boil. It became apparent that the combined force of the *astras* would destroy the whole world. The two celestial *rishis* Vyasa and Narada appeared between the two *astras* to prevent them from colliding. They each raised their hands, and with the power of their accumulated *tapas*, stopped the *astras* in midair. The *rishis* called upon Arjuna and Ashvatthama to recall their *astras*, explaining that a weapon of this magnitude should not be used at all on the fragile planet Earth nor against fellow humans. Arjuna obeyed, and with great concentration and under great strain, he recalled his *astra* by the power of his accumulated *tapas*.

Ashvatthama, however, could not recall his *astra*. He had never learned to recall it, and he never showed any interest in recalling any destructive force that he sent out. He was interested only in destroying and reaching his goals. Since Arjuna and his brothers were protected by the *rishis*, Ashvatthama directed the *astra* against all the unborn children of the Pandavas, to fulfill his curse of making the world Pandava-less. By the power of Lord Krishna, one of the unborn children, Parikshit, was saved. After Emperor Yudhishthira's death, Parikshit ascended the throne and ruled for sixty years. Lord Krishna cursed Ashvatthama to wander the world alone, stinking, infested by diseases, and without friends or love for thousands of years.

Chapter 5
The Antiquity of Ashtanga Vinyasa Yoga

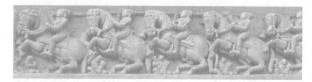

Frequently I have been approached by students who were disturbed by modern scholars' claims that Ashtanga Yoga is a modern invention. This brief chapter asserts that Ashtanga Vinyasa Yoga is in fact an ancient practice and offers evidence supporting this conclusion. I consider this a vital point because to realize that your *sadhana* (practice) is handed down by a living ancient tradition and to energetically connect with this tradition will elevate the quality of your practice to a completely different level; that is, it will transform you not just physically but spiritually.

Ashtanga Vinyasa Yoga has grown out of the fertile ground of the *Vedas*, which form a vast body of ancient knowledge. As noted in chapter 1, there are four main Vedic texts, the *Rigveda, Samaveda, Yajurveda,* and *Atharvaveda*. There are also four *Upavedas* (ancillary *Vedas*) addressing the subjects of medicine (*Ayurveda*), economy (*Arthaveda*), military science (*Dhanurveda*), and art (*Gandharvaveda*). The *Vedas* have six limbs called *Vedangas*, namely Sanskrit grammar (*Vyakarana*), astrology (*Jyotisha*), etymology (*Nirukta*), phonetics (*Shiksha*), meter (*Chandas*), and ritual duty (*Kalpa*). The Vedic teaching is divided into six systems of philosophy, called *darshanas*: logic (*Nyaya*), cosmology (*Vaisheshika*), creation (*Samkhya*), psychology (*Yoga*), Vedic ritual (*Mimamsa*), and ultimate reality (*Vedanta*).

Yoga, the ancient Vedic branch of psychology, does not compete with the other five *darshanas* but rather works in conjunction with them. Accordingly, Yoga uses the findings of the *Samkhya darshana* as its philosophy;[1] in this regard Yoga may be seen as the psychological branch of *Samkhya*. Yoga also uses the findings of the *Nyaya darshana* in regard to logic. All the other *darshanas*, however, look to the Yoga *darshana* as the authority on meditation.

Patanjali, the author of the *Yoga Sutra*, contributed to the Yoga *darshana*; he also contributed to the Vedic limb of *Vyakarana* (Sanskrit grammar) by writing his Great Commentary (*Maha Bhashya*) on Panini's grammar. Furthermore, he compiled a treatise on one of the *Upavedas*, namely, the *Ayurvedic* text *Charaka Samhita*. Vyasa, the compiler of the *Brahma Sutras*, the authoritative text on Vedanta, also authored the most important commentary on Patanjali's *Yoga Sutra*. Patanjali's *Yoga Sutra* is the basic text accepted by all forms of Ashtanga Yoga. We thus find a thorough interweaving of yoga in general and Ashtanga Yoga in particular with the other branches of Vedic science.

What, however, is the origin of Ashtanga Vinyasa Yoga? The *vinyasa* method is only one of the schools that come under the general name of Patanjali's Ashtanga Yoga, and strictly speaking, the terms *Ashtanga Yoga* and *Ashtanga Vinyasa Yoga* are not identical. Some modern Western scholars have argued that Ashtanga Vinyasa Yoga must be a recent invention because it has a multitude of *asanas* and because there appears to be no scriptural evidence indicating that it has ancient origins. Both of these arguments are invalid, as I explain below.

---

1   The findings of the *Samkhya* consist of its analysis that the phenomena of the world can be grouped into twenty-five categories. This has led to the term *Samkhya* often being translated as "categorization." Patanjali subscribed to *Samkhya*'s twenty-five categories but added a twenty-sixth: Ishvara — God.

The Dwindling Number of Asanas

Some scholars who argue that Ashtanga Vinyasa Yoga is a modern invention claim that *asanas* have accumulated over time. They base this claim on the fact that medieval texts such as the *Gheranda Samhita* or the *Hatha Yoga Pradipika* mention relatively few postures, while our system today includes many. They argue that Ashtanga Yoga must therefore be a nineteenth-century invention, as it contains too many *asanas* to be truly ancient. This argument is flawed. From the number of postures given in particular scriptures, it is not possible to gauge the antiquity of its system or lack thereof. The *Hatha Yoga Pradipika*, for example, does not give an exhaustive list of postures, and it was never its intention to do so. The *Pradipika* does not list all the *asanas* explicitly because they were to be learned through personal instruction from a teacher and not from merely reading a text.

In fact, the older the yoga system is, the more *asanas* you will find. Under the influence of entropy (disorder), over time we have lost not only more and more Sanskrit treatises and knowledge but also more and more *asanas*. The *shastras* state that originally there were 8,400,000 *asanas*, equaling the number of living species in the universe, which were known in their entirety only by the Supreme Being in the form of Lord Shiva.[2] This passage states that at the outset of time, we began with a virtually infinite number of asanas. The nineteenth- to twentieth-century yogi Ramamohan Brahmachary reportedly knew seven thousand *asanas* and taught three thousand of them to Shri T. Krishnamacharya.[3] Most modern *asana* systems contain only a few dozen or in some cases in excess of one hundred postures. Over time, therefore, the numbers of *asanas* has decreased, not increased.

The Lack of Scriptural Evidence

Unfortunately, most yogic schools did not leave any scriptural evidence behind. Even the *Vedas* weren't committed to paper until the nineteenth century. The traditional view was that a body of knowledge could be read and sullied if it was written down. Most yogic schools kept their teachings secret and confined to memory. *Asanas* were learned only through personal instruction from someone who had mastered them. Some Western scholars discount all aspects of Indian spirituality that were not recorded in books. This is often due to the fact that they see themselves merely as observers and do not want to get their feet dirty on the ground. But Indian spiritual traditions are mainly oral traditions. If you wanted to learn something, you needed to get the trust and acceptance of somebody who knew what you wanted to learn. Most knowledge that was confined to texts was considered so general that it was hardly usable. The mere absence of scriptural evidence, therefore, does not prove that Ashtanga Vinyasa Yoga is not ancient or that a large number of postures came into existence only recently.

Ashtanga Vinyasa Yoga as a Vedic Adjunct

The Ashtanga Vinyasa system, authored by the Vedic seer Vamana, is not a modern creation but follows the most ancient of Vedic designs. It is in fact a Vedic adjunct. The oldest of the systems of philosophy (*darshanas*) is probably the *Mimamsa darshana*. *Mimamsa* describes and analyzes Vedic rituals. The elaborate Vedic rituals are not senseless jumbles, as some Westerners have stated, but symbolic representations of the entire cosmos.

Although the practice of yoga does not include any traditional Vedic rituals, it is nevertheless closely connected to and influenced by them, as we can see from the following dialogue recorded in the *Brhad Aranyaka Upanishad*, the oldest of the philosophical portions of the *Veda*:[4]

Yajnavalkya, the foremost of the Upanishadic *rishis*, finds himself invited to a dialogue with the emperor Janaka. First, however, he has to undergo a cross-examination by nine learned court priests. The priests are hostile to this outsider from the forest, as they are worried that he might gain influence over

2   The *Gheranda Samhita* II.1, trans. R. Chandra Vasu (Delhi: Sri Satguru Publications), p. 12.
3   T. K. V. Desikachar, *Health, Healing and Beyond* (New York: Aperture Foundation, 1998), p. 43.

4   *Brhad Aranyaka Upanishad* III.1. 3–6.

the emperor, so they try to keep the upper hand in the dispute.

Yajnavalkya's first opponent, Ashvala, erroneously assumes that Yajnavalkya has no deep understanding of ritual and asks him how a performer of the Vedic ritual attains *mukti* (emancipation, freedom). Yajnavalkya answers by noting what the four priests who officiate the ritual represent: fire and speech for the *Hotr* priest, the eye and the sun for the *Adhvaryu* priest, the wind and breath for the *Udgatr* priest, and mind and the moon for the *Brahmana* priest. Fire, sun, wind, and moon are represented by the Vedic deities Agni, Savitri, Vayu, and Soma, which partake of the ritual. Wind (*vayu*) is symbolic for the life force (*prana*), and the various forms of *prana* are called *vayus*. Yoga holds that the location of the sun in the body is the stomach and the location of the moon is the so-called *soma* chakra, located at the soft palate in the head. But fire, moon, and sun represent together the three main energy channels: *ida* (moon), *pingala* (sun), and *sushumna* (fire). Fire, moon, and sun also represent the six chakras: fire, the *muladhara* and *svadhishthana* chakras; sun, the *manipuraka* and *anahata* chakras; and moon, the *vishuddha* and *ajna* chakras.

In this way, Yajnavalkya interprets the offices of the four priests as having the functions of speech/sound, sight, breath, and mind. Through those four powers, the performer of the Vedic ritual attains freedom, he says. Significantly, sound, sight, breath, and mind are the defining factors in Ashtanga Vinyasa Yoga.

Producing the *Ujjayi* sound and listening to it represents sound. Keeping one's focus on *drishti* (focal points) represents sight. Breath, anatomical and *pranic*, is the permanent core focus of the practice (correct practice is to let movement follow breath rather than vice versa). When all these are bound together through *bandha* (*bandh* means "to bind"), then the mind is stilled. The stilling of the mind eventually reveals consciousness, since the mind is what veils consciousness in the first place because of its clouded, opaque nature. As the *Brahmana* is the chief priest of the four in the Vedic ritual, so is the mind the chief ingredient in Ashtanga Vinyasa Yoga. We can thus see from Yajnavalkya's ancient discourse that Ashtanga Vinyasa Yoga is an exact application of the esoteric principles of the Vedic ritual. Even today we can perform our daily Vedic ritual by means of the Ashtanga Vinyasa method, giving us the opportunity to invoke the wisdom and might of the ancient Vedic sages, who lived as long ago as ten millennia before our time.

While practicing Ashtanga Vinyasa Yoga, many of us have intuitively felt that we were partaking in a truly ancient practice, but we never knew its exact origins. The Yajnavalkya discourse shows that its principles were conceived at the dawn of time.

For modern practitioners it is important to realize that Ashtanga Yoga is not just the latest exercise craze, newly developed just to get your body into shape. When you practice this yoga, you become part of an ancient tradition that has weathered many a storm. Connect with this age-old wisdom and honor its founders and many contributors. Know that when this practice was conceived, many concepts and ideas that make up our life and society today did not exist. And this tradition will still exist when many of these ideas are gone. In the meantime, continue your practice mindfully and respectfully of the ancients and don't worry too much what modern scholars, who barely dip their toes into the ocean of yoga, have to say about it.

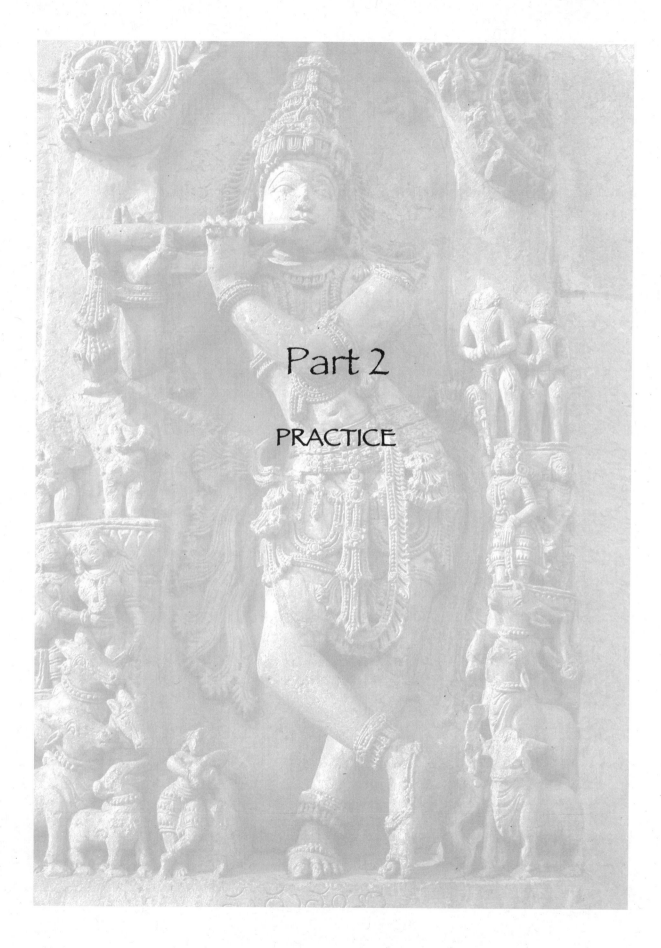

Part 2

PRACTICE

Chapter 6
Anatomy: Understanding the Capabilities and Limitations of Your Body

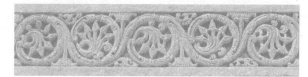

In bygone times, yogis could easily perform postures properly, as people's minds (*chitta*) were habitually suspended (*nirodha*) or single-pointed (*ekagra*).[1] The *nirodha* mind was predominant during the time when the *Vedas* were composed. Ancient people generally had the ability to reabsorb the mind into the heart and could therefore "see" the divine matrix that gave rise to an *asana* and its respective alignment. The *ekagra* mind was predominant during the time of the *Upanishads*. Although the tendency toward habitual suspension (*nirodha*) was lost by then, people generally could still concentrate their minds to such an extent and for such a time span that they could "download" the matrix behind the *asana*, its essence (*dharmin*). Both of these states of mind are nowadays exceedingly rare.

In the current age (*Kali Yuga*), our minds are habitually infatuated (*mudha*) with our bodies, wallets, and gene pools or families.[2] The infatuated, or *mudha*, mind has neither the ability of the *nirodha* mind to look right into the heart of things nor the capacity of the *ekagra* mind to slice like a laser through mere appearances to arrive at their deepest layer. The *mudha* mind tends to superimpose past conditioning

onto present sensory input. In other words, it usually lives in the past, relating to its fear and guilt, or in the future, projecting its desires onto the present. The scriptures say that those who live in the *Kali Yuga* need clear instructions to perform all actions, such as *asanas*, correctly. The *Shiva Purana*, for example, says that during the *Kali Yuga* one's actions can be crowned by success only when they are performed with utmost precision.[3] There is a special class of scriptures, called the *Tantras*, in which every single act performed by humans is described in detail.

India's Tantric phase was characterized by the analysis and deconstruction of accepted beliefs and systems of thought.[4] Interestingly enough, the same tendency surfaced, albeit much later, in the West in the form of Western science. Since Western anatomical inquiry allows us to fulfill the directive of the *Shiva Purana* and other texts — that is, to perform our actions (in this case, *asana*) with utmost precision — it should be one of the tools of modern yogis. For most of us, anatomical inquiry into *asana* provides the best way to practice postures precisely, without pain or injury.

This chapter will provide you with the tools you need to use anatomical inquiry to illuminate your *asana* practice. It identifies the various forms of pain and explains why pain during *asana* practice needs to be avoided. It then explores the relationship between the postures of the Intermediate Series and the parts of the body on which these postures focus. This sets the stage for the remainder of the chapter, which goes into the anatomical details of these parts of the body and discusses the various issues that may arise during *asana* practice, including injuries and the limitations imposed by anatomical abnormalities. You

---

1 For a detailed discussion of the relationship of the historical phases to stages of mind see *Ashtanga Yoga: Practice and Philosophy*, pp. 133ff.
2 The Indian traditional view is that the *Kali Yuga*, which has the Tantra as its scriptures, started five thousand years ago.

3 *Shiva Purana, Vidyeshvara Samhita* XI. 66.
4 Western scholars say India entered its Tantric phase in the eighth century CE. They do, however, admit that as a grassroots movement, Tantra is much older. For example, the Harappa-Mohenjodaro culture (more than four thousand years old) appears to have been Tantric.

will find many tips for performing the most challenging postures in the series as well as suggestions for rehabilitation. I deem this chapter one of the most important and practical in the book and recommend that you revisit it often.

Do Postures Have to Be Painful?

There is a widespread misconception that postures should be painful. As a rule of thumb, postures should *not* be painful, which is something that even the ancient masters pointed out. Patanjali states in *Yoga Sutra*, "heyam duhkham anagatam," which means that new suffering needs to be avoided.[5] The reasoning behind this injunction is simple. Every experience you have forms a subconscious imprint (*samskara*). Every subconscious imprint, whatever its content, calls for its own repetition.

This means that if you frequently practice postures in a way that causes pain, you will create more pain in your postures in the future. The adage "No pain, no gain" may work in some areas of life, but applied to *asana* it becomes destructive. Apart from damaging bodily tissues, you may become more and more preoccupied with pain and with the body if you imprint pain into your subconscious again and again. All intense physical sensations call for more identification with the body. The goal of yoga, however, is not to increase this identification. It is to perfect the body so as to transform it into a capable and reliable vehicle on the road to freedom. Think of your body as akin to your car: the better you treat it, the better it will run. You need to service it regularly, maintain fluid levels, and correct tire pressure. Treating the body respectfully does not mean identifying with it. If you identify with your body, it becomes an obstacle to spiritual evolution, not a vehicle for it. This is nowhere clearer than at the moment of death, one of the key moments in terms of spiritual evolution. If you have not learned detachment from the body, dying will not elevate you. This potentially most powerful moment then becomes a painful experience.

Another scriptural injunction against pain appears in the *Bhagavad Gita*. The Supreme Being in the form of the Lord Krishna criticizes those who torture the body.[6] He, as the true self of the world, lives as the self in our hearts and thus lives in every body. Those who cause pain to the body desecrate his abode. This has led to the notion of the body as the temple of God. We need to treat our bodies as we would the home of the Supreme Being.

There are three types of unpleasant physical sensations that can occur in postures. I call them (1) creative discomfort, (2) unnecessary pain, and (3) necessary, karmic pain.

CREATIVE DISCOMFORT

In *asana* it is important to recognize the difference between pain and discomfort. When you stretch a muscle or hold a demanding strength posture, there is necessarily a certain amount of discomfort involved. This discomfort comes from stretching the muscle or making it stronger, both of which are among the goals of the practice. In regard to *asana*, therefore, we may say, "No discomfort, no gain." (Postures that are to be held for a long time for the purpose of *pranayama* and meditation are an exception; they need to be completely comfortable.) If the discomfort crosses the line into pain, on the other hand, injuries can happen. This is particularly true if the pain is felt in a joint, ligament, or tendon. If you feel pain, you need to back off or adjust the posture and work more precisely so that you can return to the zone of discomfort. Anatomical knowledge guides this process.

Practitioners should analyze the postures and continually correct their performance of them until awareness is spread all over the body. When that happens, the body is hardly felt anymore. This sounds paradoxical, but you feel the body mainly when something is wrong. The absence of negative feedback means that everything is okay. When the body is correctly aligned, a feeling of stillness and firmness yet vibrant lightness arises. The mind becomes luminous, still, and free from ambition and egoic tendencies. This is the state that you are looking for. It is conducive to meditation. When this quality is achieved in a posture, that posture is fit as a platform for the higher limbs of yoga.

5 *Yoga Sutra* II.16.

6 *Bhagavad Gita* XVII.5–6.

There is no point in waiting for this state to suddenly and miraculously appear by performing the same faulty postures again and again. From a faulty action, no correct result can be achieved. Faulty postures cause more faulty postures in the future.

UNNECESSARY PAIN

Any pain experienced in joints, ligaments, tendons, and at the origins and insertions of muscles is likely to be unnecessary pain. This type of pain accounts for the vast majority of pain experienced in *asana*. It is completely avoidable and almost always due to faulty technique. This may sound like a steep claim, but this type of pain can easily be recognized because it disappears in due time when postural alignment is analyzed and corrected. For this reason, you should always assume that the pain you experience when executing a posture is in the category of unnecessary pain. All such pain can be avoided by applying the tool of anatomical inquiry into posture. If unnecessarily painful practice is continued, an already existing negative tendency — toward self-torture, perfectionism, or egotism, for example — may be increased instead of reduced.

NECESSARY, KARMIC PAIN

This form of pain is more difficult for Westerners to understand, as it involves the concept of karma. Through our past actions, words, and thoughts, we have created who we are today, including, according to Patanjali, the type of body, span of life, and form of death we will experience. When Patanjali stated that future pain is to be avoided, he did not elaborate about past pain. Past pain in this context is the pain that we have created through our past actions. It may be experienced now or in the future. We cannot change our past actions. Once the seeds of our actions have sprouted, the karma associated with those actions cannot be intercepted, and the pain resulting from them needs to be endured — not grudgingly endured but willingly accepted as ordained. If it is willingly accepted, it will lead to a karmic purification, to a burning of the old karma associated with that pain.

Occasionally in life we have to go through letting-go processes, and they are not complete without painful sensations. Grief is an example of such a process. Nobody will doubt that a possibly lengthy grieving process, during which we learn or come to terms with letting go, follows the death of a loved one. These processes can come to a conclusion only if we willingly and consciously enter into them.

Karmic pain in *asana* is that pain that cannot be removed by anatomical inquiry and attention to detail. If you have done everything in your power to correct the posture and the pain still persists, it may be necessary, karmic pain, something you may have to go through. It is very challenging for a yogini to know that she has done everything in her power and yet continues to suffer. Many people at this point will stop practicing because they feel unfairly treated. If you manage to continue your practice, you are fostering *tapas*, the ability to sustain your practice in the face of adversity. If you refuse to work through karmic pain and simply endure it, your yogic progress may stagnate.

Yoga in this regard is similar to a marriage. When you get married, you commit to sticking with your partner through good and bad times. The same unwavering commitment is necessary in your *asana* practice. However, it needs to be an intelligent commitment. You need to be able to clearly identify whether the pain is the avoidable result of faulty technique or whether it is caused by demerit accumulated in the past. You can achieve this by doing everything in your power to make sure that you perform *asana* correctly and are therefore sure beyond doubt that avoiding the pain that you experience is not possible.

A word of caution: If you do not correctly identify your pain, you may make matters worse. Again, the overwhelming majority of pain experienced during *asana* is unnecessary and due to faulty technique. Never accept that your pain is karmic until you have ruled out beyond doubt that it is caused by poor alignment. This point shows the importance of anatomical inquiry. If your understanding of the anatomical principles of the body and the posture under discussion are sound, you will know whether you have done everything to avoid the pain. Anatomical knowledge must be used to determine whether pain is karmic or not.

The instruction given in the previous paragraphs may easily lend itself to abuse. Often students are only too happy to believe that their pain is necessary, as this way they don't have to take responsibility for changing their approach to *asana*. For the correct identification of pain, consult a qualified yoga instructor steeped in the study of anatomy and alignment. This section in no way constitutes medical advice. If you experience any ongoing pain, consult your physician.

Anatomical Foci of the Intermediate Series Postures

On an anatomical level, the Primary Series focuses on lengthening the hamstrings, opening the hip joints, and establishing the *bandhas*. The Intermediate Series expands this focus to the spine, the sacroiliac joints, and the shoulder joints, while giving intensified attention to the hip joints.

Recall the outline of the Intermediate Series given in the Introduction. There I noted that of the seven distinct sequences making up the Intermediate Series, three form the core of the series, while the remainder serve as "connective tissue" linking these core parts together. These three core parts are the backbending sequence (eight postures), the leg-behind-head sequence (three postures), and the arm-balancing sequence (four postures). The backbends are the postures that work primarily on the spine and the sacroiliac joints; the leg-behind-head postures are those that further open the hip joints (while also working on the sacroiliac joints); and the arm balances are the postures that give attention to the shoulder joints.

These three core sequences, or posture themes, are primarily what produce the defining effect of the Intermediate Series of postures — the purification of the *nadi* system. If you can become proficient at the postures making up these three themes, you will enjoy the benefits of this series of postures. None of the three themes is easy, and sometimes students are so eager to progress that they attempt them while yet ill prepared. Apart from listening to the advice of your teacher, understanding the information in the remainder of this chapter will be a helpful aid in learning to practice these postures correctly.

In the rest of the chapter, I look sequentially at the four major parts of the body — the spine (particularly the thoracic spine), the sacroiliac joint, the hip joint, and the shoulder joint — on which the core sequences of the Intermediate Series focus. I explain the structure of each of these body parts and how it functions, focusing in particular on information useful in practicing the postures correctly, avoiding injury, and healing existing injuries. Table 3 on the next page indicates which Intermediate Series postures focus on each of these body parts.

The Spine

Knowledge of the spine's various movements and restrictions is important in backbending, and it is also applicable in forward bending and twisting. Let's look first at the thoracic spine, which is inherently less flexible in extension than the cervical and lumbar spines.

Anatomically, the vertebrae of the thoracic spine are wedge shaped, thereby forming its kyphotic (bent forward) curve. Here, long, overlapping spinous processes add stability and prevent extensive backward arching. Additionally, the almost vertical plane of the facet joints is specifically designed for rotation versus extension, as this facilitates the varied activities we perform with our upper limbs. Finally, the attachment of the ribs to the vertebral bodies and the sternum form a stable cage to house our most vital organs.

Since the armor of the heart prevents the thoracic spine from arching, you need to consciously distribute part of your effort in backbending toward your rib cage and thoracic spine. If you do not make a conscious effort to do so, your backbend will translate into your lumbar spine, which is weak and unsupported and thus prone to overstretching.

The thoracic spine is especially designed for flexing forward and for actions that require twisting. The ability to rotate or twist our thoracic spines gives us a much greater range of motion in the use of our upper limbs and hands. The wedge-shaped vertebral bodies forming a kyphotic curve, the long overlapping spinous processes, and the attachment of ribs make the chest much less suited for extension (20–25 degrees extension compared to 30–40 degrees

TABLE 3. RELATIONSHIPS BETWEEN BODY PARTS
AND THE INTERMEDIATE SERIES POSTURES THAT FOCUS ON THOSE PARTS

Posture Theme	Primary Body Parts	Relevant Postures
Twisting	Spine Sacroiliac Joints	*Pashasana* (noose posture) *Bharadvajasana* (posture dedicated to Rishi Bharadvaja) *Ardha Matsyendrasana* (posture dedicated to Matsyendranath, half-version) *Supta Urdhva Pada Vajrasana* (reclining thunderbolt posture with one foot upward)
Forward Bending	Legs Spine	*Krounchasana* (heron posture) *Parighasana* (iron cage posture) *Tittibhasana* (insect posture)
Backbending*	Spine Sacroiliac Joints	*Shalabhasana* (locust posture) *Bhekasana* (frog posture) *Dhanurasana* (bow-shaped posture) *Parshva Dhanurasana* (side bow posture) *Ushtrasana* (camel posture) *Laghu Vajrasana* (little thunderbolt posture) *Kapotasana* (pigeon posture) *Supta Vajrasana* (reclining thunderbolt posture)
Leg-Behind-Head*	Hip Joints Sacroiliac Joints Spine	*Ekapada Shirshasana* (one-leg-behind-the-head posture) *Dvipada Shirshasana* (two-legs-behind-the-head posture) *Yoganidrasana* (yogic sleep posture)
Arm Balancing*	Shoulder Joints Spine	*Pincha Mayurasana* (feathers of the peacock posture) *Karandavasana* (waterfowl posture) *Mayurasana* (peacock posture) *Nakrasana* (crocodile posture)

* Theme constituting the core of the Intermediate Series

flexion). Additionally, the angle of the facet joints (nearly vertical with a front-to-back orientation) provides an uninterrupted surface for these articulations to glide and for rotation to occur easily. In comparison, the lumbar facet joints have a side-to-side orientation, which prevents rotation and promotes flexion and extension.

In general, the magnitude of rotation in the thoracic spine decreases in a head-to-tail direction. The lowermost thoracic vertebrae, T12, has its superior facet joints at the angle of a thoracic vertebra and its inferior facets at that of a lumbar vertebra. This transitional segment also takes the brunt of many opposing muscular forces that attach into this area and is thereby prone to dysfunction and/or instability. Additionally, the diaphragm

SCOLIOSIS

If you find twisting to one side much harder than twisting to the other, you may have scoliosis. Scoliosis is a deformity of the spine that involves lateral or rotational curvatures. Whether you experience discomfort or dysfunction from your scoliosis depends on the severity of the angle of the curve(s) and whether or not your body has compensated successfully.

If you have scoliosis, do not follow your tendency to go deeper on your flexible side; instead, follow the general rule to balance the extremes and work on your weaknesses. Also, find out whether the scoliosis is structural or functional. A *structural scoliosis* is one caused by the underlying structure, meaning the bones. In a structural scoliosis the sacrum is not level. Eighty percent of structural scolioses are idiopathic — that is, the cause is unknown. The remainder are usually caused by congenital abnormalities (present at birth) or are secondary to another condition, such as cerebral palsy. A small minority of structural scolioses are due to anatomical leg length discrepancies (LLD). If one leg is longer than the other, the pelvis and the sacrum will be raised on that side. The L5 vertebra will be slightly tilted toward the side of the shorter leg. Depending on the severity of the leg length discrepancy, the entire lumbar spine may curve toward the side of the shorter leg, with the thoracic spine balancing into the opposing direction as a compensatory mechanism to keep the spine upright and the head level. The compensating vertebrae are also usually rotated. A structural scoliosis can also be caused by an asymmetry or deformity of the pelvic bones.

A *functional scoliosis* is one in which an imbalance of the pelvic or spinal musculature is responsible for the lateral spinal curve. A tilt of the pelvis can, for example, be caused by the left adductor muscles and the right abductors being tight and chronically in spasm. This will result in the pelvis being lifted on the left side, especially if the opposing muscle groups (the right adductors and the left abductors) lack tone and strength.

Yoga practice cannot change the underlying cause of a structural scoliosis, but it can alleviate symptoms, reduce discomfort, and prevent degeneration. If you have a structural scoliosis, practice asymmetrical postures to strengthen weak areas.[7] When you are performing symmetrical postures, your stronger side will always perform the bulk of the work, and thus the imbalance will be exacerbated. When you perform asymmetrical postures, you can target each side separately, exercise your weak side more, and so work toward a state of balance. You are likely to need a program of therapeutic exercise that can be done as a warm-up before your *vinyasa* practice.

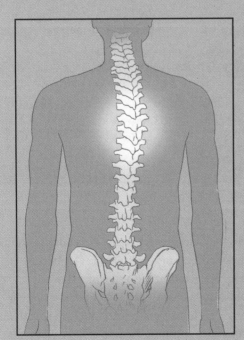

A functional scoliosis can be corrected by resetting the muscles to their proper tone. Yoga can help you to stretch tight muscles and strengthen weak ones. If you suffer from a functional scoliosis, analyze all forms of physical labor and recreational activity that you engage in for imbalance. Change sides for some time and see what influence that has. If you are a gardener, start using the shovel with the other hand. Change the side on which you carry your bag or, if possible, abandon handbags altogether and switch to backpacks. If you have young children, change the side on which you carry your baby. It is very common for a mother to twist her pelvis by carrying her baby exclusively on one side.

If you are an Ashtanga Mysore–style teacher, change the leg that you place in front when adjusting *Supta Kurmasana* and drop-backs. Inevitably you will twist your pelvis when you always use the same leg. I used to place my left foot in front when adjusting, and consequently suffered from pelvic obliquity, colloquially referred to as a twisted pelvis, for a long time. I had to place my right foot in front for one year to become balanced. Since then I have frequently changed sides.

FIGURE 1: Example of scoliosis

7   This approach was taught to me by Shri A. G. Mohan.

muscle influences one's ability to twist freely because of its horizontal plane and position in the floor of the thoracic cage. Practically speaking, all of the above means that when performing twists you need to carry as much of the action out of your lumbar spine, which is unsuited to twisting, and up into the thoracic spine.

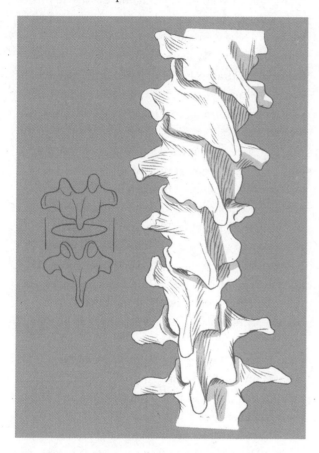

FIGURE 2: The role of facet joints in twisting

Compared to the thoracic spine, the lumbar spine is much more unstable. Injuries of the intervertebral discs are far more common in the lumbar spine. This is due to the absence of the protective corset of the rib cage. The yogi has to train the abdominal muscles to the extent that they give the lumbar spine all the necessary support it needs to avoid damage. Such training is given through application of *Uddiyana Bandha*; the *vinyasa* movement of jumping back and through; leg-behind-head postures; and arm balances. Most important, the yogini needs to use abdominal bracing during backbending. Through abdominal bracing, backbending is distributed from the lumbar

spine to the thoracic spine. Abdominal bracing is different from tucking in the abdomen. Tucking in the abdomen does not support the low back. The main difference between the two is that during abdominal bracing you bear down with the diaphragm, thus increasing intro-abdominal pressure. Tucking in the abdomen requires sucking up the diaphragm into the thoracic cavity. Bearing down with the diaphragm not only stabilizes the low back but also (through increase of intra-abdominal pressure) draws the lumbar vertebrae away from each other and thus takes pressure off the lumbar intervertebral discs during backbending.[8]

The Sacroiliac Joints

The sacroiliac (SI) joints are essential for backbending. They also play a major role during leg-behind-head postures and twisting. If forward bending is not executed properly, it can lead to strain of the sacroiliac joints. A proper understanding of the movements and function of these joints is therefore necessary for all yogis.

The sacroiliac joints form an integral part of the pelvic girdle. The pelvic girdle is connected to the spine via the sacrum and to the lower extremities via the hip joint. The upper part of the pelvic bone is called the ilium, and its articulation with the sacrum forms the sacroiliac joint. The sacrum is actually an extension of the spine, being composed of the fusion of five vertebrae. It is wedged in between the two pelvic bones. The coccyx, or tailbone, attaches to the end of the sacrum and is usually made of three small vertebrae.

We will look at the pelvic bone first. Before skeletal maturity the pelvic bone consists of three un-united bones, which eventually fuse to form the pelvis. This is reflected in the three names given to the different parts of the pelvic bone: the ilium, ischium, and pubis. The acetabulum, with which the head of the femur articulates, sits in the lower, lateral aspect of the ilium. The four spines of the ilium provide points of origin for many muscles.

The ischium (sit bone) is the lower (inferior),

---

8   This is described in detail in *Ashtanga Yoga: Practice and Philosophy*, pp. 113–14.

rear (posterior) part of the pelvic bone. The adductor magnus and the hamstring muscles originate here. The pubic bone is the inferior, anterior part of the pelvic bone. Here the two halves of the pelvis join via a cartilaginous pad. The adductor muscles insert at the pubis along with the muscles that form the pelvic diaphragm.

The wedge-shaped sacrum connects to the lumbar spine via the L5 intervertebral disc and to the coccyx, which Western scientists allege to be a rudimentary leftover of a tail.[9] The sacrum has a kyphotic shape. It is part of the primary curvature that the infant acquires in the womb, where the entire spine is curved in this direction. The thoracic spine is the other area of the spine that has retained its primary curvature. Two areas of the spine adapt to a lordotic (bent backward) curvature during the maturation process to produce the double-S curve of the spine of the upright walking hominid. The lordotic curve of the cervical spine begins to form during infancy with the constant effort of lifting the head while lying on the belly; it is necessary to

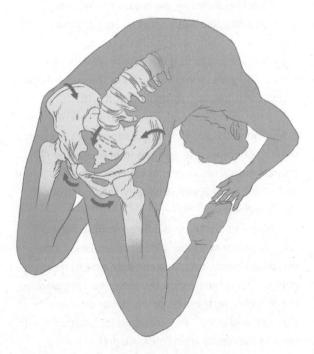

FIGURE 3: Sacroiliac joints showing joint movement

9 The lumbar spine consists of five vertebrae, which are numbered from the top. The L1 vertebra borders the thoracic spine, and the L5 vertebrae is located above the sacrum.

support our heads in an upright position. The lordotic curvature of the lumbar spine begins to form when we stand upright and start to bear weight in an upright position.

The sacroiliac joint is composed of two auricular (ear-shaped) articulations, which form a relatively rigid joint between the sacrum and the two ilia. The open sides of the semicircular, boomerang-shaped joints face backward, in the opposite direction of the kyphotic sacrum. When we look at the sacrum from the side and draw a horizontal line through both joints, we can understand that the joints enable the sacrum to perform up to 10 degrees of rotation around this axis.

The SI joint is unusual because the lower third of the joint is a synovial type of joint (consisting of a joint capsule containing fluid), while the upper portion resembles a fibrous joint (consisting of connective fibers). In childhood it has all the characteristics of a synovial joint. This changes between puberty and young adulthood, and with age the SI joints develop intra-articular grooves and interdigitating bony growths (osteophytes), and become increasingly fibrosed and less pliable. The resultant reduction of mobility develops as an adaptive, stability-promoting response to the stresses of weight bearing. Anthropologists use the condition of the SI joint as a reliable indicator of the approximate age of a specimen.

The SI joint provides two functions: stress relief within the pelvic ring, and (along with the pubic symphysis) shock absorbance between the lower limbs and the spine. It is principally a ligamentous joint, supported and stabilized by strong ligaments. Some are primary stabilizers that cross the joint, while others act as guy-wires to surrounding structures. The stabilizing action of the muscles surrounding the SI joints is based on their attachments to the fascia and ligaments. The only muscle that spans the joint itself is the piriformis, which originates on the anterior aspect of the second to fourth sacral tubercle and inserts onto the greater trochanter of the femur.

Some describe the SI joint as a friction joint. The forces that act on the joint, associated with weight bearing and the stresses placed on ligaments and muscles that attach to surrounding structures, tend to force the joint closed. Thus, the SI joint is stabilized by its form (angle, grooves, and later osteophytes) and the force of the ligaments and muscles that increase the friction between the joint surfaces when weight bearing is added.

It is important to understand the movement of the sacrum in relation to the ilia (hip bones) on either side. When the spine flexes, as in forward bending, the ilia move in the opposite direction — that is, backward. The opposite occurs with backbending: the ilia roll forward. For this reason, "jutting out" the pubic bone in backbends is contraindicated. Doing so causes the ilia to move in the same direction as the sacrum, preventing normal function of the SI joint. This reciprocal flexion–extension pattern causes each side of the pelvis to rotate slightly out of phase with the other while we are walking. Some musculoskeletal specialists describe the kinesthetic action of the sacrum with its articulating ilia as "floating." This is a wonderful image to keep in mind when practicing both forward and backward spinal movements, because it helps to keep a harmonious relationship of movement between the sacrum and ilia at the SI joints.

Another important concept of sacral movement is nutation. When the pelvic bone is stationary and the top edge of the sacrum moves forward and down around this axis, this movement is called nutation (bowing, nodding).[10] If the top of the sacrum returns from nutation and moves backward, the movement is defined as counter-nutation. Nutation is a flexion-like movement, and counter-nutation an extension-like movement. The differing terms were chosen because the range of the movements involved are too insignificant for them to be called flexion and extension.

When we look at the sacrum from above and draw lines through the SI joints, we notice that the lines meet at an angle of roughly 45 degrees. This means that a movement of the sacrum around the

horizontal axis will change the position of the two sides of the pelvic bones relative to each other.

If the sacrum nutates (bows forward), it will pull the ilia toward each other. Since the ilia and the ischia are fused as one unit, the drawing together of the ilia will pull the ischia apart from each other, a movement that in yoga is dubbed as the "broadening of the sit bones."

This movement occurs during childbirth (parturition), and examining how it works enables one to more clearly understand the reciprocal movement of the ilia and the sacrum. In the early stages of parturition, when the head of the baby enters the pelvic bowl, the sacrum counter-nutates (bows backward). This counter-nutation draws the ilia apart and thus opens the top of the pelvic bowl to give more space for the baby's head. When in the final phase of the birth the head passes through the birth canal, the sacrum nutates. This nutation has two effects. The moving together of the ilia squeezes the baby down from above, aiding its passage, while the broadening or moving out to the side of the ischia provides a wider opening for the passing of the head of the baby.

We have observed during our yoga teaching that those females who are very proficient in backbending and nutation of the sacrum (all else being within normal limits) tend to give birth easily, whereas those who have difficulties in sacral nutation tend to find giving birth more challenging. Perhaps it would be wise to establish a high culture of backbending in females as a preparation for giving birth.

There are other important functions of nutation and counter-nutation of the sacrum. One of these is that this movement enables the sacrum to act as a pump for cerebrospinal fluid (CSF). The brain floats in cerebrospinal fluid, which nourishes, removes toxins from, and protects the brain with its shock-absorbing qualities. The pulse of the cerebrospinal fluid, which occurs about eight times per minute, also has a massaging or stimulating quality. It is important for the sacroiliac joints to be mobile to perform the oscillation of the cerebrospinal fluid. In this way the sacrum acts as a CSF pump.

10 The term *nutation* is also used to describe the third movement of the planet Earth. The first movement is its rotation around the sun; the second, its rotation around itself; and the third is a minute wobble in this second movement, which is strong enough to make us change the position of the pole star about every five hundred years.

When the cerebrospinal fluid does not properly pulse, the individual will have more adverse reactions to stress, tire more quickly, and be more susceptible to aggressive behavior or depression. We believe that the health of the sacroiliac joints contributes to the overall well-being of the individual. It is important to mention that aggressive backbending, like other forms of aggressive exercise, can have a detrimental effect on the sacroiliac joints and thus on the entire organism.

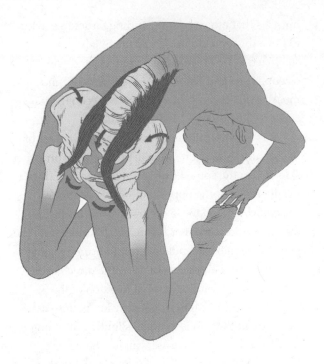

FIGURE 5: The psoas in relation to sacroiliac-joint movement

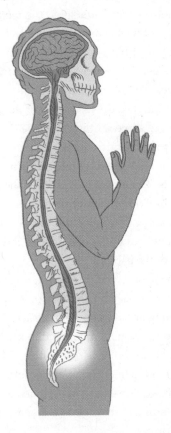

FIGURE 4: Sacrum orientation and the channel of cerebrospinal fluid

Although contraction of the erector spinae pulls the sacrum forward, contributing to a nutational force, there is no muscle that directly performs this action. Such a muscle would need a position that would impinge on the integrity of the female reproductive system. The muscle that can strongly affect the action of nutation, therefore, originates higher up on the lumbar vertebrae and, circumnavigating the uterus, travels through the pelvis and attaches at the lesser trochanters of the femurs. It is the psoas.

The lower fibers of the psoas in particular are in an ideal position to pull the upper part of the sacrum in the anterior direction (forward). However, a muscle that also inserts at the lesser trochanter of the femur, the iliacus, and is usually used together with the psoas, will pull the entire pelvic bone and thus the ilium forward. This will make our attempts to nutate the sacrum futile. The iliacus therefore must be released, while the psoas is engaged. This is possible because different nerves innervate the two muscles. The psoas is innervated by the branches of the lumbar plexus, a group of nerves that exit the spinal cord at the levels of the first to fourth lumbar vertebrae. The iliacus is innervated by the femoral nerve, which shares the same nerve roots at L2 to L4.

When you engage the psoas separately from the iliacus, the ilium has a tendency to follow the sacrum forward. If you are initially unable to isolate the iliacus and release it, allowing the sacrum to "float" in the SI joints and the natural reciprocal movement of the ilium to take its natural course, try gently drawing the pelvis down in the back. I suggest performing this action by ever so slightly engaging the hamstrings, rather than the gluteus maximus, because the gluteus externally rotates the femurs.

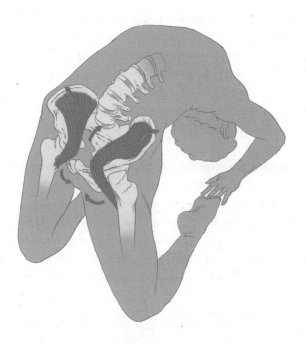

FIGURE 6: The iliacus in relation to sacroiliac-joint movement

The Hip Joint

The hip joint performs the essential function during leg-behind-head postures. If the hip joints are opened properly, there is no or very little pressure on the various segments of the spine. If the movements and limitations of the hip joints are not properly understood, execution of leg-behind-head postures can lead to subluxated vertebrae and damage to the intervertebral discs.[11]

The hip joint consists of the femur, which is articulated by its large, spherical head with the acetabulum (socket of the hip joint) of the pelvis. The right and left halves of the pelvic bone are each divided into three parts. The upper part is the ilium, the lower anterior part is the pubis or pubic bone, and the lower posterior part is called the ischium. All three bones of the pelvis intersect and form part of the acetabulum. The deep socket of the acetabulum stabilizes the femoral head and is

11 A subluxated vertebra is somewhere between its ideal position and the dislocated state. The ideal anatomical position of a vertebra or in fact any joint of the body will give us 100 percent function, whereas a dislocated joint provides 0 percent function. In between these extremes are the many shades of subluxation in which some function of varying degrees exists, albeit often accompanied by discomfort.

RELATIONSHIP OF *UDDIYANA BANDHA* TO SACRUM NUTATION

In *Ashtanga Yoga: Practice and Philosophy*, *Uddiyana Bandha* was defined as the engaging of the lower part of the transverse abdominis muscle. For novices it is essential to isolate this part of the muscle not only from the upper part but, more important, from the rectus abdominis (six-pack muscle, or "abs"). The rectus abdominis will lift the pubic bone up toward the chest and flatten out the lower back, which means it counteracts nutation of the sacrum. The lower part of the transverse abdominis, however, attaches mainly over fascia at the anterior superior and anterior inferior iliac spines (ASIS and AIIS, respectively). The ASIS especially move toward each other during nutation of the sacrum. *Uddiyana Bandha*, if correctly implemented, will encourage and support nutation, whereas to mistake *Uddiyana Bandha* with the indiscriminate contracting of all abdominal muscles will oppose it! A sophisticated understanding and performance of *Uddiyana Bandha* rather than a "tucking in" of the entire abdomen is necessary to foster nutation of the sacrum.

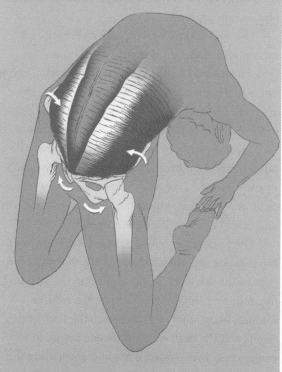

FIGURE 7: The lower transverse abdominis in relation to sacroiliac-joint movement

69

surrounded by an extensive set of capsular ligaments. Many forceful muscles insert onto the pelvis and around the hip joint. These provide the necessary torques needed to propel the body forward and upward. Weakness in any of these muscles has profound impact on the mobility of the body as a whole.

The femur is the longest and strongest bone in the human body. The head of the femur is connected to the shaft via the femoral neck. The neck serves to displace the femur laterally away from the hip joint to reduce the likelihood of any bony impingement against the hip joint. Anatomically, leg-behind-head flexibility may be limited by a short, less concave femoral neck, as it will come in contact with the hipbone earlier and thus limit further movement. This needs to be understood especially by teachers giving leg-behind-head adjustments to their students and also by students who are practicing forcefully. The sensation of encountering a bony obstacle to movement is completely different from that of movement being limited by ligaments, muscles, adipose tissue, or even lack of support strength. A teacher needs to be able to determine, by the quality of the barrier, the type of tissue that is obstructing progress.

The angle between neck and shaft (angle of inclination) is about 125 degrees and causes the femoral shaft to be angled inward (medially), giving optimal alignment for the hip joint surfaces. The angle of inclination places the knees and feet closer to the midline of the body, which allows humans to walk upright without leaning from one side to the other as apes do. An angle markedly less than 125 degrees, termed *coxa varus*, causes the knees to bow out. An angle markedly greater is called *coxa valgus* and causes a knock-kneed condition.

The neck of the femur points not exactly out to the side but slightly backward if we choose the hip joint as the reference point. Viewed in the standing (anatomical position) from above, the relative rotation (twist) that exists between the neck of the femur and the shaft is called torsion angle. In conjunction with a normal angle of inclination this affords optimal alignment and congruence of the hip joint. The degree of torsion is normally approximately 12 to 15 degrees and is called normal anteversion.[12] A torsion angle significantly greater than 15 degrees is called excessive anteversion and often produces a compensatory toe-in posture and gait. Excessive anteversion hampers the ability to place one's leg behind the head. In contrast, an angle significantly less than 15 degrees is in retroversion and may produce an externally rotated leg posture with a toe-out gait. This angle complements leg-behind-head postures. This torsion angle allows a person to place her leg not only behind the head but way down the back if she radically combines three of the movements of the hip joint (flexion, abduction, and external rotation). Through this movement, the hip joint is taken through its entire range of more than 180 degrees.

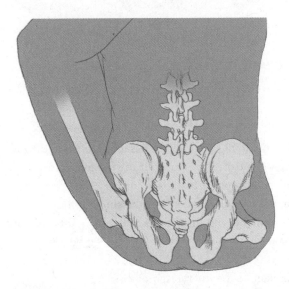

FIGURE 8: The hip joint during leg-behind-head postures

The opening of the hip joint is an important goal in Ashtanga Vinyasa Yoga. If, however, the force of an adjustment is obstructed by the shape of the participating bones, this force may be diverted. Typical locations that receive the stress of the force during leg-behind-head adjustments are the lateral longitudinal (collateral) ligament of the knee, the lateral semilunar cartilage (meniscus), the sacroiliac

12 Since the torsion angle describes the twist between shaft and neck of femur, the reference point used here is the shaft of the femur and not, as it is in yoga, the hip joint. The normal angle of the neck of the femur is therefore called anteverted, which means it points forward of the plane of the femur.

joints, and the lumbar intervertebral discs. All of these are potentially vulnerable and sensitive structures. If damaged, their repair requires considerable time, as ligaments and cartilage have limited circulation, which is of course necessary in the healing process. A ligament or sacroiliac joint sprain, for example, may take six weeks to stabilize or heal. Additionally, scar tissue is never as strong as original healthy tissue. It is therefore wise to proceed with caution in leg-behind-head postures. Needless to say, this is also valid for backbending and other areas of yogic *asana* practice.

The axis of pelvic movement is the hip joint. An unlevel or oblique pelvis is another issue that may cause asymmetry in flexibility in leg-behind-head postures. This may be due to a sprain, instability, or fixation of the sacroiliac joint. Additionally, symptoms of knee, sacroiliac joint, groin, or low-back pain may arise if the pelvis is torqued or twisted. A malpositioning of the sacrum in relation to the pelvis can also be a source of problems. The sacrum is the axis of spinal movement. Its correct position in the pelvis is therefore paramount to full and optimal function of both the spine and the pelvis.

As described previously, the pelvis is made of two separate bones (innominates) that articulate with the sacrum in the back and are joined in the front by a fibrocartilage pad, forming the pubic symphysis. This allows substantial scope for the innominates to move. Because of their attachments, these composite parts act as one unit and therefore, the position of one part will affect the motion and/or position of the other. Additionally, all of the muscles that attach to the pelvis act as guy wires in providing support and stability. Any change in position of either innominate will cause particular muscles to be lengthened or shortened. If the ilium (upper part of the pelvis) moves backward, it is referred to as a posterior tilt of the pelvis, which is accompanied by a forward movement of the pubic bone. If, for example, one ilium is positioned posterior and therefore inferior to its counterpart, the muscles that attach to the front of the ilium will be drawn taut, while the muscles on the posterior side will be shortened and contracted. Because of the angle of the femur in the hip joint, a posterior inferior ilium will draw the leg on that side upward,

causing a functional leg-length discrepancy. The psoas and/or quadratus lumborum muscles may also go into spasm. An innominate may also flare out to one side, which will cause the groin muscles to be stretched and taut with the external hip rotators shortened and contracted.

The Shoulder Joint

The shoulder joint carries most of the workload during arm balances. Arm balances are very important and beneficial; unfortunately, however, long-term Ashtanga practitioners frequently give up performing them due to shoulder problems. These problems can be avoided or, if incurred already, the shoulders can be rehabilitated through proper anatomical understanding and ensuing action.

The shoulder joint is described as a ball-and-socket joint, similar to the hip joint. The difference between these joints is the vast range of movement in all directions that the shoulder joint has compared to the hip joint. Since range of movement is always a trade-off against stability, this also means that the shoulder joint is much less stable than the hip joint due to its minimal osseous support.

The socket of the shoulder joint is formed by the glenoid fossa of the scapula, in which the head of the humerus (arm bone) is located. To enable the arm's enormous range of movement, the glenoid fossa of the shoulder joint is much more shallow than the glenoid cavity of the hip joint, the acetabulum. The actual shoulder socket cannot prevent the dislocation of the head of the humerus as the hip socket can do for the head of the femur. Therefore, the labrum, joint capsule, ligaments, and a complex of tendons take on the function of keeping the head of the humerus in position. The labrum of the glenoid fossa is a fibrocartilaginous pad, analogous to the meniscus of the knee. It lines the glenoid fossa, deepening the concavity for the humeral head and thereby stabilizing the joint. The biceps tendon inserts into the labrum and serves as a crucial anterior support for the shoulder joint. Additionally, active support is provided directly through the capsular integration of the rotator cuff muscles. The rotator cuff muscles insert into the joint capsule. These are the supraspinatus, infraspinatus, teres minor, and subscapularis muscles. Contraction of these muscles tightens the capsule, which has a stabilizing effect. Besides having a stabilizing role, the rotator cuff muscles also perform dynamic movements. The supraspinatus mainly performs abduction; the infraspinatus and teres minor both perform external rotation; and the subscapularis performs internal rotation of the humerus.

The shoulder joint is only indirectly connected to the axial skeleton (spine, thorax, and pelvis) through the clavicle (collarbone), which is joined distally to the acromion process of the scapula and proximally via the sternoclavicular (SC) joint to the sternum. There are in fact three joints and one "articulation" that make up the shoulder girdle. These are the glenohumeral joint, the acromioclavicular (AC) joint, the sternoclavicular joint, and the scapulothoracic articulation — that is, where the scapula glides over the thoracic cage. These four work together to permit the full range of motion appreciated at the shoulder joint. Function of the shoulder joint is dependent on coordinated integration of this complex of joints as well as an integrated, position-dependent system of ligaments, muscles, and tendons that provide stability.

also enables us to raise our arms above our heads. For the first 30 degrees of abduction, the scapula seeks a stable position on the rib cage via contraction of the trapezius, rhomboid, and serratus anterior muscles. Beyond 30 degrees, for every two degrees of abduction of the humerus, the scapula moves one degree laterally and superiorly on the back of the chest. Abduction is performed by the supraspinatus and deltoid muscles. The fact that the scapula "swims" on the posterior aspect of the thorax with almost no limitation to its movement poses the main problem in prevention and rehabilitation of shoulder joint injuries. It led the American orthopedic surgeon Dr. Stephen Michael Levin to develop the model of the scapula as a sesamoid, a floating bone.[13]

Sesamoid bones are bones that are not directly attached to other bones, their movements being solely guided by the attached bones and ligaments. Examples of sesamoid bones are the patella (kneecap) and the hyoid bone in the neck. Levin compared the scapula to the hub of a bicycle wheel, which is placed in position by a network of spokes. The spokes can be tightened or released, and thus the position of the hub changed. Similarly, the scapula is held in position only by the tension or tone of its stabilizing muscles. When the prime mover muscles of the shoulder girdle exert their pull on the humerus, the stabilizers maintain the optimal position of the glenoid fossa (the most lateral aspect of the scapula) as it articulates with the head of the humerus. Maintaining the proper position of the scapula allows the instant center of rotation to be maintained. These muscles are of utmost importance because, ultimately, they determine the position and thereby function of the entire shoulder girdle.

The correct functional position of the scapula influences the tone of

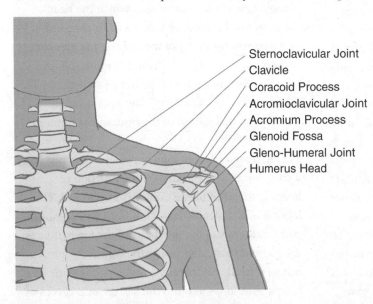

Sternoclavicular Joint
Clavicle
Coracoid Process
Acromioclavicular Joint
Acromium Process
Glenoid Fossa
Gleno-Humeral Joint
Humerus Head

FIGURE 9: The shoulder joint

Besides permitting the actions of protraction and retraction of our arms, movement of the scapula

13 Stephen Michael Levin, "The Scapula Is a Sesamoid Bone," *Journal of Biomechanics* 38, no. 8 (August 2005): 1733–34.

all the muscles of the shoulder girdle. Just as the abdominal muscles anchor the anterior chest wall to enable the diaphragm to function optimally, so the rhomboids, the lower trapezius, and the serratus anterior muscles stabilize the scapula to enable the other prime mover muscles of the shoulder-girdle to perform their actions. The tone of the stabilizer muscles can be lost or become aberrant through trauma, imbalanced use, or poor posture. Once this has happened, the scapula is no longer anchored properly when the other shoulder-girdle muscles are engaged. This may result in inflammation or dysfunction of any of the structures of the shoulder (muscles, tendons, ligaments, or bursa). The action of the stabilizing muscles is unconscious, so one can correct dysfunction only by isolating and targeting the individual muscles through specific strengthening exercises. Attempting to strengthen the stabilizing muscles through general shoulder exercises alone will only exacerbate the problem.

The rhomboids are a pair of muscles of prime importance for balancing the strong muscles on the posterior surface of the rib cage. The majority of the population and especially those with desk jobs have rounded shoulders. Those with this posture will automatically have weak, underdeveloped rhomboid muscles, as rounding the shoulders places the rhomboids in a lengthened position. Additionally, many Ashtanga practitioners do not bring the rhomboids into play enough; they often perform the *vinyasa* movement of jumping through and jumping back without enough awareness of the importance of engaging these scapular stabilizing muscles. Concurrently, this movement encourages the use of serratus anterior and pectoralis minor together with the deltoid. These muscles become stronger and stronger while their antagonists (the rhomboids) recede more and more into the background. If such an imbalance exists, the rhomboids need to be targeted through isolated strengthening exercises.

The rhomboids originate at the spinous processes of the lowest cervical (C7) to upper thoracic (T1–T5) vertebrae and insert along the entire length of the medial border of the scapula. When contracting they adduct the scapula (draw the shoulder blades in toward the spine); they are fixed in adduction especially when the humerus (arm bone) is extended or adducted under load, such as when doing chin-ups. As this movement does not occur in Ashtanga Yoga, the rhomboids may become underdeveloped if the practitioner does not focus on the action of "sucking the heart through" or "leading with the heart" in various postures, including jumping through to a sitting posture. If the practitioner has a shoulder injury and the rhomboids are weak, he must enhance their functioning. The jump-through to sitting, however, contains too much serratus anterior activation to bring the rhomboids sufficiently into play (the serratus anterior is an antagonist of the rhomboids). Chin-ups, on the other hand, require you to suddenly lift your entire body weight without any preparation. Such intense exercises are unfortunately often performed without developing sufficient awareness. For this reason they are unsuitable for the correction of faulty motor patterns. It is more effective to exercise the rhomboids with very small weights, such as resistance bands, slowly and with maximum awareness.

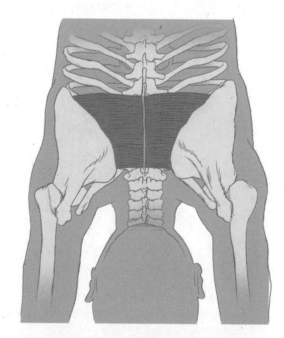

FIGURE 10: The rhomboid muscles

Since the rhomboids slightly elevate the shoulder girdle, an action that in *asana* can lead to "hunching of the shoulders around the ears," their action needs to be combined with that of the lower trapezius and latissimus dorsi, which depress the shoulder girdle, to have a major stabilizing impact on the scapula and thus the entire shoulder joint.

Another important muscle in the stabilization of the shoulder joint is the subscapularis. This rotator cuff muscle originates on the anterior surface of the scapula and surfaces to attach on the inside of the humoral head (the lesser tubercle). Apart from being a strong internal rotator of the humerus, the subscapularis, through its origin on the front of the scapula, is in the unique position to suck the shoulderblades (scapulae) into the back of the chest. If the shoulderblades have a winged appearance — that is, if the medial borders of the scapulae lift off the posterior surface of the thorax under load — the shoulder joint complex is not properly stabilized and shoulder injury and strain are more likely. Engagement of the subscapularis, along with the serratus anterior muscle, can correct this problem.[14] Their use is crucially important during all arm balances and weight-bearing exercises.

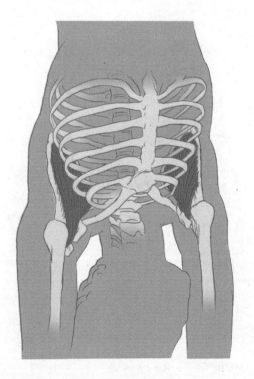

FIGURE 11: The subscapularis muscle

14 For a detailed description of the action of the serratus anterior muscle, see *Ashtanga Yoga: Practice and Philosophy*, p. 48.

The subscapularis muscle, however, should not be contracted indiscriminately, as it vigorously internally rotates the humerus. In yogic forearm balances (for example, those in the Intermediate Series), this would lead to the elbows sliding out to the sides and the hands moving together. To prevent this, the subscapularis needs to be used in unison with the infraspinatus muscle and its "little helper," teres minor. The infraspinatus and teres minor muscles originate on the posterior surface of the scapulae and insert on the outer surface of the humeral heads (the greater tubercles). The action of these other two rotator-cuff muscles balances the inward rotation of the subscapularis and, in concert with the action of the subscapularis, stabilizes the humeri. When the insertion of the subscapularis muscle is thus fixed in space, its contraction leads to the movement of its origin, the anterior surface of the scapula. In other words, as long as the infraspinatus accompanies the action of the subscapularis, the subscapularis will suck the shoulderblades into the back, thereby functioning as an essential stabilizer of the shoulder joint.

SHOULDER INJURIES

Most shoulder injuries are caused by performing rapid movements under load. Tears of the glenoid labrum, the cartilage lining of the glenoid fossa, are often produced in the attempt to catch a heavy falling object. This object can be your own body if, for example, you fall off a chair, a ladder, or a bicycle and try to brace your fall with your arm.

Many people have decreased space between the humerus and the acromiocoracoid ceiling. This condition increases the likelihood of the joint becoming inflamed due to constant friction from exercise or repetitive movement. In all exercises where the arms are raised the supraspinatus tendon may rub against the acromion process and coracoacromial ligament and become inflamed. The insertion of the supraspinatus tendon onto the greater trochanter of the humerus has a relatively poor blood supply, making it susceptible to injury and delayed repair. Inflammation may also spread to the infraspinatus and long head of the biceps tendon. Once a tendon is inflamed it can no longer glide properly in its sheath and becomes susceptible to tear during fast movements. The body's chemical reaction to a chronically inflamed tendon is to either lay down scar tissue in an attempt to repair the damage or to eventually calcify the tendon. These processes make future tears more likely, especially during dynamic movements that involve a humerus flexed to its maximum. These movements rarely occur in yoga, but handstand drop-backs and so-called backflips are examples.

Shoulder injuries are more common in practitioners over forty years of age. The incidence of injury is more frequent, and recovery is usually slower due to a loss of elasticity and reduced cellular activity. If you injure your shoulder, it is important that you avoid reinjuring it. If you do reinjure your shoulder while it is healing, you may set yourself back for many months. After repeated episodes, the shoulder injury will be chronic and less likely to respond to any sort of treatment.

A drawn-out shoulder injury often comes with dysfunction of the lower cervical spine. The arm and shoulder are common sites for referred pain from the cervical spine. The nerves that supply the muscles of the shoulder, arm, and hand exit the spinal cord between the lowermost cervical vertebrae. If there is any disruption to the nerve supply to the muscles, causing over- or underactivity of the muscles, the shoulder joint will be susceptible to injury and its ability to heal will be impeded. For optimal functioning of the spine, the muscles, and the nervous system, it is important that the cervical vertebrae move freely in all directions. As the shoulder-girdle muscles attach to the thorax, it is additionally important for the thoracic spine and rib cage to function optimally. The single most important way to avoid rigidity of the rib cage is to apply the three stages of breathing, drawing the inhalation all the way up into the manubrium (the uppermost part of the sternum, right under the collarbones), avoiding exclusive abdominal breathing. The important word here is *exclusive*. Exclusive chest breathing is of course equally detrimental. In the case of shoulder injuries any therapy must involve breathing exercises that draw the breath into the upper thorax, thus directing a wavelike healing motion of breath all the way up to the topmost thoracic vertebrae.

Another underlying cause of shoulder injury is the inability to use the abdomen as a support structure to lift weight. When we are lifting heavy weights during standing, or in fact during all strenuous actions, the abdomen forms a hydraulic system.[15] Supported from underneath with *Mula Bandha* and by bracing in front with *Uddiyana Bandha*, the descending of the diaphragm during the inhalation leads to increased intra-abdominal pressure. With the glottis then partially closed to create the *Ujjayi* sound, the pneumatic pressure in the chest will rise at the same time and the thorax and abdomen will form one solid support structure, enabling us to lift heavy weights. This is all the more necessary in the case of yogic arm balances. The more the abdominal wall is firmed during the lifting of the body, the more the shoulders are supported and kept in an anatomically sound position during yogic arm balances.

Another common cause of inflammation of the shoulder joint is an imbalance between the muscles on the anterior surface of the rib cage (the pectoralis major and minor, and often the serratus anterior) and the muscles on the posterior surface of the rib cage (typically the latissimus dorsi, teres major, lower trapezius, and rhomboids). People often acquire this imbalance slowly through poor posture or faulty technique. One cause can be the failure to shorten one's stance in *Chaturanga Dandasana* as one increases in strength.[16] If the hands are kept under the shoulders, the pectoralis muscles and serratus anterior will continue to build through the constant push-up motion. Since the latissimus dorsi, teres major, and rhomboids are not getting a comparable amount of exercise, they do not grow stronger. The result will be that the anterior muscles will pull the shoulder forward and rotate the head of the humerus internally, all of which can in due time lead to inflammation.

Imbalance of the shoulder girdle may be due to trauma, such as from catching a heavy falling object,

15 *Hydraulic* refers to a system containing a liquid under pressure in a confined space.
16 See *Ashtanga Yoga: Practice and Philosophy*, p. 28.

jolting the shoulder in an anterior direction, or even repeating smaller stressful movements, such as carrying a growing child. Such trauma can decrease the proprioceptive awareness of the shoulder joint.[17] This simply means that you will perform *asanas* and believe your shoulders to be in the proper position when in fact they are not. It will be difficult to rectify your problem since you have no awareness of it. You can only deduce the problem from the presence of its symptoms, such as pain and/or eventually dysfunction. Often this pain results from the biceps tendon being pulled out of its groove by the fascia attached to the pectoralis major. It is unlikely that you can fix this problem in the practice itself. You will often need to add therapeutic exercises in which the muscles in question are isolated so that you can restore proprioceptive awareness.

As mentioned earlier, the rotator cuff muscles both stabilize the shoulder joint and produce torque forces for larger movements. An imbalance between these muscles is a common cause of shoulder problems. Inflamed shoulder joints can be due to excessive inward or outward rotation. Either can be preexisting as a postural imbalance and then lead to inflammation or can be acquired through faulty exercise technique.

Most beginners start Downward Dog with their shoulders hunched around their ears, which usually accompanies internally rotated humeri (arm bones). The problem usually starts with an overworked upper trapezius muscle (which elevates the shoulders) and the subscapularis muscles rotating the arm bones inward. If the practitioner does not correct this imbalance, the trapezius and the other muscles build up even more, increasing the already existing dysfunction. Especially during strenuous arm balances or dynamic backbends, an already existing imbalance in the shoulders can be exaggerated to the point of inflammation.

In the other extreme are avid students who analyze their imbalances and correct them excessively. There is a natural imbalance of strength in the shoulder, with the internal rotator muscles of the shoulder girdle being stronger than the external

rotators. Most students will, at some point, need to externally rotate their arm bones in Downward Dog, arm balances, and backbends. The problem is knowing when this action is performed to satisfaction and then allowing one's shoulders to settle in the neutral or balanced state. If you go beyond that point through overuse of the infraspinatus muscle (which externally rotates), friction will occur, often involving the biceps tendon. The body will now communicate its predicament through inflammation, which leads to pain and loss of range of motion.

The neutral position of the humerus in the respective postures needs to be assessed by a qualified teacher. Do not expect the practice to miraculously fix everything, a belief that would permit you to continue practicing without using inquisitive intelligence. Experience shows that in unmindful practice the exact opposite usually happens; that is, students increase their already existing tendencies and conditioning rather than counteracting them to find a state of balance.

The following points summarize what's important to keep in mind in healing shoulder injuries:

- Avoid reinjury. The healing of shoulder injuries, especially in practitioners over forty years of age, can be very drawn out. Every time you reinjure your shoulder, you set yourself back for several more months and greatly increase the chance that your injury will become chronic.
- Shoulder injuries often have dysfunctional lower cervical vertebrae as a precipitating factor. If such a cervical joint dysfunction persists, chances of healing are reduced. See a musculoskeletal specialist.
- Shoulder injuries are often associated with the inability to draw the inhalation all the way up to the upper part of the thorax. The upper rib cage should enlarge, meaning it should increase its volume to the front and back during the inhalation. Failure to do so will lead to a lack of energy supply to the shoulder girdle.

17 *Proprioceptive* refers to an awareness of the placement of one's limbs in space that does not rely on visual clues.

- Make sure you use a short stance in *Chaturanga Dandasana*, with your hands beside your waist. This will encourage you to bring your latissimus dorsi, rhomboids, and lower trapezius more into play. Consciously focus on engaging these three muscles whenever you bear weight into the hands.
- If you have a shoulder problem, consider not lowering down into *Chaturanga Dandasana* but rather performing it with straight arms until your condition improves. Remove any postures and movements from your practice that aggravate your condition. Examine critically all fast dynamic movements, such as drop-backs.
- Train the weak and underused muscles by using exercises that isolate these muscles.

Start with isometric exercise (where the muscle stays the same length) and progress into the use of very low weights such as graded resistance bands or tubing. Perform these exercises slowly and with maximum awareness.
- Massage and release the overworked and tight muscles daily. Include "trigger point therapy" in your daily massage. Trigger points are tender spots in the muscles that when pressed may radiate pain into areas other than that point.

In this chapter, I hope that I have created some openness toward Western anatomical inquiry. My stance is that if we can improve the effectiveness of our yoga by reducing pain and increasing precision, then we should do so, whether the tools we use are old or new.

Chapter 7
Respiratory Movements and the Breath

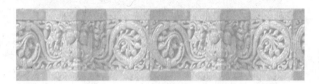

Breathing and the breath have central roles in Indian spirituality. *[A]ta eva pranah* — "the breath verily is the *Brahman* (infinite consciousness)" — sound the immortal words of the *Brahma Sutra*.[1] The ancient Vedic seers saw the universe as performing a pulsating movement of expansion and contraction very much like breathing. The *Upanishads* say the universe was "breathed forth" by the *Brahman*.[2] Similarly, the respiratory rhythm of the individual was seen as linked to a cosmic rhythm.

The inhalation is thought to emit the sound *sa* and the exhalation, the sound *ham*.[3] Together they form *soham*, "I am that (the *Brahman*)," one of the four *mahvakyas* (great formulas) of the *Upanishads* (the mystical portion of the *Vedas*). If you exhale first and then inhale, the sound becomes *hamsa*, "swan." The swan is the metaphorical emblem of the soul or spirit of the individual that is held to be one with the *Brahman*. By breathing, therefore, throughout life each individual emits the two great mantras of creation, *soham* and *hamsa*.

But the spiritual significance of breathing goes far beyond the symbolic. Of all the body's many unconscious activities, breathing is the one with the most important consequences for the gross body, the subtle body, and the mind. Western thought has created a great dichotomy between body and mind, a separation that Indian thought does not recognize. Yoga holds that body and mind are intricately connected; in fact, they are expressions of each other, and their link is nothing other than the breath.

Patanjali, the ancient codifier of yoga, said that every thought, word, or action leaves a subconscious imprint[4] that is accumulated[5] in what's called the "karmic deposit."[6] This karmic deposit eventually forms the subtle body with its energy channels (*nadis*) and centers (chakras) and from that the gross body with its various tissues. The important connection here is that encrusted thought patterns (called *subconscious imprints* and *conditioning*) determine the flow of *pranic* currents, which in turn determine creation of tissue. It also works in the opposite direction: once established, bodily tissue determines *pranic* flow, which determines movement of thought patterns. Whereas tissue and mental structures are slow to change and difficult to influence by one's will, *pranic* flow can be altered — and this is done by consciously manipulating the breath, which is nothing but the gross expression of *prana*. By directing the breath, you direct *prana*, and wherever *prana* goes, so goes the mind.

Properly understanding the gross or Western anatomy of breathing and incorporating this understanding in one's practice results in correctly supplying all tissues with oxygen and thus ensuring their health. Knowing and applying the subtle energetic anatomy of *prana* means harmonizing the *pranic* flow in the subtle body, focusing the mind inward (*pratyahara*), and concentrating the mind's focus (*dharana*). In this way the yogic science of breath leads to a balanced, healthy body and

---

1   *Brahma Sutra* I.1.23.
2   *Brhad Aranyaka Upanishad* II.4.10.
3   Some traditions assign it the other way round but the point is still the same.

4   *Yoga Sutra* I.50.
5   *Yoga Sutra* II.12.
6   Sanskrit: *karmashaya*. In modern language we would call this the subconscious.

prepares the mind for the higher meditation techniques and ultimately for the realization of consciousness.

Anatomy of the Outer, or Gross, Breath

Of all movement patterns in the body, respiration is perhaps the most important. The diaphragm muscle is the initiator and prime mover of respiration, so it deserves our attention first. The diaphragm is a dome-shaped muscle that separates the thoracic cavity from the abdominal cavity. It attaches to the inside of the sternum, the lower (seventh through twelfth) ribs, and the upper (first through fourth) lumbar vertebrae — and is usually divided into these areas functionally. Some claim that there are sixteen functional areas of the diaphragm. It has apertures for the oesophagus, the aorta (the major artery that transports oxygenated blood away from the heart), and the vena cava (the largest vein in the body that returns blood to the heart). When fully functional, the diaphragm works in coordination with the intercostal muscles (between the ribs); the abdominal wall, especially the transverse abdominis muscle; the pelvic floor; and the deep stabilizing muscles of the low back. Its insertions interdigitate with those of the transverse abdominis on the rib cartilages, which signifies their close working relationship.

During an exhalation, the diaphragm relaxes, expands, and rises up into the rib cage. During an inhalation, it contracts and descends, increasing intra-abdominal pressure. This pressure creates a resistant force in the abdomen, which tonifies the pelvic floor, the abdominal wall, and the deep stabilizing muscles of the low back. Upon inhalation there is a concentric (or shortening) contraction of the diaphragm and an eccentric (or lengthening) contraction of the transverse abdominis; conversely, with a concentric contraction of the transverse abdominis, the diaphragm must work eccentrically, tonifying the transverse abdominis as it works against resistance. Additionally, the pressure exerted by the movement of the diaphragm massages all the other abdominal organs, and its pressure on the

stomach reduces the likelihood of developing a hiatal hernia.

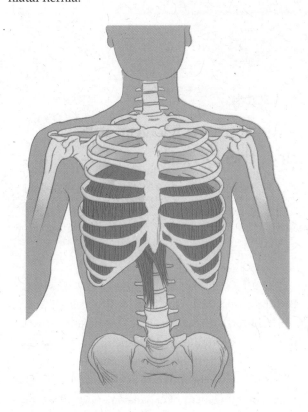

FIGURE 10: The diaphragm

Normal, healthy breathing involves both the chest (thoracic cavity and rib cage) and the abdomen. When we are anxious, we tend to adopt a form of breathing called chest breathing, in which the abdomen does not move, and breathing happens only in the chest. During chest breathing, the thorax moves up and down with the breath, and the low back is destabilized. Since it is associated with an anxious state, chest breathing tends to support anxiety and an agitated mind, even when it arises for other reasons. Chest breathing can be mild, moderate, or severe — mild if it occurs only with a deep inhalation, moderate if it occurs when seated or standing but not when lying down, and severe if it also occurs when lying down.

At the other end of the spectrum is exclusive abdominal breathing. This occurs when the abdominal muscles are completely relaxed and the entire abdomen, upper and lower, protrudes and the thorax does not participate in the breathing. This kind of breathing may occur in individuals with a weak abdominal wall. If that's not the underlying cause, continuing to breathe in this way will certainly *lead to* weakness in the abdominal wall. In the long run, exclusive abdominal breathing is as detrimental as exclusive chest breathing.

Upon inhalation, the thoracic spine should flex, while the cervical and lumbar spines extend. The opposite happens on exhalation, which has a mobilizing effect on thoracic extension. If the thorax does not move with the breath, the cervical and lumbar spines will compensate, and increased movement will occur in these areas. This has several detrimental effects. For example, if upon inhalation there is no movement in the thorax (no flexion), the cervical and lumbar spines incur a greater amount of extension. Over time the muscles in these areas will become hypertonic, and/or the vertebral segments may become hypermobile, incurring greater wear and tear, which ultimately leads to degeneration of the spine.

Ideally, a thorax that is anchored down by the abdominal muscles in the front and sides and the quadratus lumborum in the back will cause the upper belly to expand slightly as the diaphragm descends and presses against the stomach and abdominal cavity. This is the first stage of breathing. In the second stage the rib cage expands horizontally. Last, if the breath is full and deep, the chest will expand. In this type of breathing, both the abdomen and the thorax participate. We may therefore call it thoraco-abdominal or diaphragmatic breathing. This is the form of breathing used during yoga *asanas*.

There is a natural tendency for the abdominal wall to protrude upon inhalation as the diaphragm descends. Breathing that instead contracts the abdominal wall (sucks it inward) upon inhalation and relaxes (expands it) upon exhalation is referred to as paradoxical breathing.[7] This form of breathing may occur under stress or during moments of fear or danger, but it can also result from a misunderstanding of the function of *Uddiyana*

Bandha. If the upper abdominal muscles are vigorously included in *Uddiyana Bandha*, they press the abdominal contents upward against the thoracic cavity. This means that the diaphragm has to work harder. Only by lifting the thorax even higher can we produce a full inhalation. These added tensions may cause the diaphragm to go into spasm or become chronically tight and thereby dysfunctional. This denies the low-back stabilizing muscles and the surrounding organs the tonifying qualities of the action of the diaphragm. It also prevents deep back-bending, as the ribs cannot fan open. Paradoxical breathing can easily happen in Ashtanga Yoga during backbends such as *Kapotasana* (see p. 118), especially when students perform them in a class situation or when the teacher asks the student to perform to a certain specification or level of achievement, putting the student under stress.

Pranayama and the Anatomy of the Inner, or Subtle, Breath

The anatomy of the subtle breath is the anatomy of *prana* — its flow in the *nadi* system and its relationship to breathing. *Pranayama*, in turn, is the science of manipulating the flow of *prana*. It consists of an extensive set of breathing exercises.

We encounter the term *prana* in several contexts, and in each context the meaning is somewhat different. Some yogic scriptures instruct you to draw the *prana* in through the right nostril and expel it through the left. Here, *prana* simply refers to breath. We also come across passages that advise us to draw the *prana* into the elusive *sushumna*, the central channel. Here, *prana* means "the subtle life force"; this is the word's most common meaning. We also find textual passages saying that *prana* and *apana* need to be mingled at the navel. In such contexts, *prana* (as well as *apana*) refers to only one of the ten vital airs (*vayus*), which in themselves are subdivisions of the broader life force, *prana*. Keep these various meanings in mind when you encounter the term *prana*.

The term *prana* is inextricably linked to *pranayama*. The practice of *pranayama* has three important effects on the subtle breath, and through

7 David Coulter, *Anatomy of Hatha Yoga* (Honesdale, PA: Body and Breath, 2001), p. 135.

it the mind and the gross body. *Pranayama* draws *prana* back into the body, balances the flow of *prana* in the *nadi* system, and allows *prana* to enter the central energy channel. We look at each of these effects in turn.

The *Yoga Yajnavalkya* states that in an untrained person *prana* is scattered and therefore extends twelve angulas (finger widths) above the surface of the gross body.[8] When your *prana* is in this state you are likely to be uncentered, ungrounded, and scattered. You will find it difficult to concentrate, you will tend to waste your energy in useless pursuits, and your mind will not be able to focus long enough on a particular problem to come to the right solution. When this is the case, the practice of *pranayama* will draw the *prana* back into the body. You can recognize this first effect of *pranayama* easily: a person who was scattered and "out there" now rests in themselves and is calm and confident.

The second result of *pranayama* is the harmonizing of *prana* between the lunar and solar *nadi* systems.[9] In the average person, the prana oscillates between the two; prana may also be mostly stuck in one *nadi*. If you have a preponderance of *prana* in the solar *nadi*, your mind will tend to attach itself to one position and declare all others wrong. You may then appear to be very ignorant and walk through life with tunnel vision. If you have a preponderance of *prana* in the lunar *nadi*, your mind will tend to see the truth in all positions and, lacking critical judgment, you will become incapable of taking responsible action. You will be without direction, like a nutshell tossed about in a stormy ocean.

Both conditions lead to the manifestation of the many obstacles to yoga that Patanjali lists, such as rigidity, doubt, false views, and the inability to attain and retain a desired state.[10] Rigidity is caused by too much *prana* in the solar *nadi*. Doubt is produced by too much *prana* in the lunar *nadi*. False views may be produced by too much *prana* in the solar *nadi*, which may lead one to stubbornly hold on to a senseless position; however, it can also be produced by excess *prana* in the lunar *nadi*, which leads to the inability to reject a wrong position. The inabilities to attain or retain a desired state are both caused by a reduced amount of *prana* in the solar *nadi*.

Pranayama leads to an even distribution of *prana* between the two aspects of the *nadi* system. This in turn leads to freedom from the extremes of the mind and the removal of many of the obstacles on the path of yoga. The balancing of the *nadis* also prepares for the third and most important effect of *pranayama*, the suspending of the mind.

The yogic texts state that where *prana* (breath or life force) goes, there goes *vrtti* (oscillation of mind). Similarly, the *Hatha Yoga Pradipika* says that mind and breath are united together, and that both of them are equal in their activities. The *Pradipika* goes on to explain that the mind starts to think only when a thought is powered by *prana*, and that *prana* begins to flow only when there is mental involvement.[11]

Oscillation of the mind — its constant rummaging and mulling — obstructs the view of our inherent natural state, which is divine ecstasy (*ananda*). According to the yogic texts this happens through the following mechanism: Before the gross body (*sthula sharira*) is manifested, the life force is established in the central energy channel (*sushumna*). Through the process of manifestation, also called evolution, the energy centers of the subtle body develop one by one, starting from the top (*sahasrara* chakra) and ending with the lowest, the earth chakra (*muladhara*). Once the earth chakra manifests, the lower opening of the central energy channel, which is located within the earth chakra, closes. Through this closure, the *prana* is prevented from entering the central channel and is thus diverted into the two adjacent channels, similar to what happens when a blood clot suddenly blocks an artery and the body attempts to solve the problem

8 *Yoga Yajnavalkya* IV.6–10. A.G. Mohan, trans., *Yoga Yajnavalkya* (Chennai: Ganesh), p. 57.

9 The lunar and solar *nadis* can be likened somewhat to the parasympathetic and sympathetic nervous systems. If we draw such parallels, however, we always need to keep in mind that the minute *nadis* are part of the subtle body, whereas the nerves, being discernible by the naked eye, are part of the gross body. Similarity exists here only in function, not in structure.

10 *Yoga Sutra* I.30.

11 Pancham Sinh, trans., *Hatha Yoga Pradipika* IV.24 (Delhi: Sri Satguru, 1915), p. 50.

by diverting the blood into collateral arteries. The *shastras* (scriptures) say that in this moment, knowledge of our divinity is lost, while knowledge of the world is gained. The knowledge of the world is gained by the fact that the closure of the central energy channel causes the production of the gross (anatomical) body. The loss of knowing oneself as the infinite consciousness causes not only the machine of the mind to switch on but also the body to manifest. (This makes the phrase "enlightened body, enlightened mind" somewhat problematic.) The presence of mind and body together means that the individual needs to order occurrences in a time sequence (meaning some earlier, some later) because he cannot process them simultaneously. In contrast, when one is established in consciousness, one is aware of everything simultaneously, whether it happens in past, present, or future. The presence of the body is thus generally an indicator of one's limitation and not of one's evolution.

This needs to be deeply contemplated and understood. It is for this very reason that sages such as Jnaneshvar did not hesitate to shed their bodies at a very young age, since they thought that holding on to their bodies would not contribute to their experience of divine ecstasy. Also, modern sages such as Shri Nisargadatta Maharaj or Ramana Maharshi weren't at all concerned by the breakdown of their aging bodies. Nisargadatta's worried audience could barely convince him to take his medicine when he was terminally ill.

To recap: The blocking of the central energy channel in the *Muladhara* (base) chakra causes the life force to be diverted into the two adjacent channels, which are the solar (*pingala*) channel, relating to the right nostril, and the lunar (*ida*) channel, relating to the left nostril. The oscillation of life force between *ida* and *pingala* and the analogous oscillation of breath between left and right nostrils drives the oscillation of the mind between the extremes of relativism on one hand and fundamentalism on the other.

Pranayama practice restores the balance between the extremes of the mind and thus keeps the mind from oscillating between its extremes; more important, *pranayama* draws *prana* back into the central channel, which enables us to recognize the world as it really is (*sat*), return to abiding in infinite consciousness (*chit*), and finally reenter our natural state of divine ecstasy (*ananda*). *Pranayama*, then, is the training that utilizes the power source of the mind (*prana*) to return the mind to its original purpose and function.[12]

Essential for the opening of the central channel, which is blocked within the *muladhara* chakra (*mula* = root, *adhara* = support), is *Mula Bandha*. By the practice of *Mula Bandha* the *prana* is made to enter *sushumna* "like a snake disappears into its hole."[13] *Mula Bandha*, however, can have this effect only when it has become very subtle and refined. Through years of practice, *Mula Bandha* is transformed from a gross muscular contraction into a subtle energetic seal.

The various forms of alternate nostril breathing balance the solar and lunar channels, whereas the different forms of breath retention (*kumbhaka*) guide *prana* back into the central channel. *Kumbhaka* is *pranayama* proper.[14] *Kumbhaka*'s highest expression is the spontaneous breath retention that accompanies *samadhi*, called *kevala kumbhaka* (or the fourth *pranayama*) by Patanjali.[15]

However, the *nadis* must be cleansed before this balancing of *ida* and *pingala* can occur and the subsequent breath retentions can be practiced. The cleansing of the *nadis* is done in Ashtanga Vinyasa Yoga by practicing the Intermediate Series of

12 The purpose of the mind initially is to gain knowledge of the outer world. When self-knowledge — that is, knowledge of the inner world — is desired, the mind needs to be reabsorbed into the heart. Indian authors often describe *pranayama* or yoga as "mind control." Although this term is usable in the Indian cultural context, which is mystical and devotional, it is not helpful if translated into a Western context. This is due to the fact that Western culture is built on the concept of controlling the mind to get control of the outer world. The state of ecstasy, however, cannot be "conquered" by what Westerners understand as mind control.

13 *Hatha Yoga Pradipika* III.68.

14 There is the somewhat naïve belief among Ashtanga practitioners that just because they are practicing *Ujjayi* during their *asana* practice they have therefore comprehensively covered *pranayama* (expressed in the saying, "It's all happening on the mat"). However, the *Hatha Yoga Pradipika* talks only about *kumbhakas* (and not *pranayama*), thus suggesting that *pranayama* exercises that do not contain breath retention are preliminary.

15 *Yoga Sutra* II.51.

postures in conjunction with *Ujjayi pranayama, Mula Bandha,* and *Uddiyana Bandha.*

AN ALTERNATIVE METHOD FOR PURIFYING THE *NADIS*

Although it is not impossible for students who commence yoga in their fifties to complete the Intermediate Series, it will be difficult. The progress of a student may also be impeded by an ailment or a handicap. For cases like these, traditional teachers such as Shri T. Krishnamacharya have taught a preparatory *pranayama* method that has an effect similar to that of the Intermediate Series of postures and therefore has the same name, *Nadi Shodhana.* As a preparatory method, *Nadi Shodhana Pranayama* is done without any breath retentions, and the inhalations and exhalations are practiced to a breath count that does not strain the practitioner at all.[16] To cleanse the *nadis*, it must be practiced daily for a minimum of fifteen minutes for three months. It does not bestow the benefits on the gross body that performing the Intermediate Series of postures offers.

Similarly, the *dosha*-harmonizing and detoxifying effect of the Primary Series of Ashtanga Yoga can, to a certain extent, be simulated by practicing the six actions (*shat karmas*) described in the *Hatha Yoga Pradipika*: the *Dhauti, Basti, Neti, Trataka, Nauli,* and *Kapalabhati.*[17]

These options are further examples of the principle that there is not one practice fit for all, but that the form of practice needs to be consistent with the practitioner's fitness (*adhikara*) or the stage (*bhumika*) he or she has attained.

Breathing during Performance of Intermediate Series Postures

When performing the Intermediate postures, the breathing method to employ is *Ujjayi pranayama*, meaning "the victorious extending of the breath." *Ujjayi* requires a slight constriction of the glottis — the upper opening of the larynx — which is

achieved by partially closing it with the epiglottis. With the glottis slightly constricted, we stretch the breath and create a gentle hissing sound, which we listen to throughout the entire practice.[18]

When breathing in this way, make sure not to restrict the movement of the diaphragm. Instead of "tucking in" the abdomen, use abdominal bracing. "Tucking in" consists of partially sucking the abdominal contents up into the thoracic cavity, an action that when performed in combination with movement leads to a tightening of the diaphragm, with its various health concerns. Abdominal bracing, in contrast, is accomplished by engaging only the lower part of the transverse abdominis muscle and keeping the diaphragm relaxed. The upper part of the transverse abdominis needs to be isolated from the lower part because the upper part interdigitates with the diaphragm and engaging it, as done by many nonrefined Ashtanga Yogis, leads to a tightening of the diaphragm as well. Keep the abdominal wall soft above the navel and firm below the navel, so that the lower abdominal wall functions as does the belt of a weight lifter.

When practicing the Intermediate postures, draw the inhalation all the way to the manubrium (the top of the sternum) to move more *prana* into the upper areas of the body. If you neglect to do this, your practice of the Intermediate *asanas* will be less effective. At the end of the inhalation, the upper lobes of the lungs should be completely filled. To achieve this, start the inhalation literally at the pelvic floor. Let the breath fill your entire torso from the bottom up. This should feel like a wave starting at the lower abdominal wall and running all the way up along the front of the torso, terminating at the manubrium.

On the exhalation, the wavelike motion flows back downward, toward the lower abdominal wall. When sitting in meditation, you can visualize this sensation by imagining that your torso is hollow and that you are breathing in water. As the inhalation proceeds, your torso slowly fills with water. At the end of the inhalation, the water level reaches the base of your neck. Try to feel this

16 The full version of this *pranayama* (that is, not the preparatory version) is described in *Hatha Yoga Pradipika* II.7–10 and *Shiva Samhita* III.22–26.
17 *Hatha Yoga Pradipika* II.22.

18 For a more exhaustive discussion of *Ujjayi pranayama*, see *Ashtanga Yoga: Practice and Philosophy*, p. 9.

wavelike motion during every breath that you take in your practice. This is difficult, of course, as there are many other things you will need to focus on. One approach is to devote one day of practice per week to focus mainly on breathing.

Let every movement into a posture be borne from the inhalation, and every movement out associated with exhalation. Do not let the breath follow the movement; rather, let the breath *initiate* the movement. Distribute the breath evenly over the entire movement as you enter and exit each posture. All too often, practitioners inhale to 80 percent of their capacity in the early phases of a movement and are then surprised to find their lungs full before they get deeply into the posture. In particular, while jumping through to sitting, if you suck the air in all at once and blow your chest up like a balloon, you will likely find that you cannot transit through without touching down. Instead, start the inhalation as your feet leave the floor, inhale rather sparsely during the first 30 percent of the movement, and only once you feel that the momentum of your jump has worn off, open up your epiglottis more and start to suck in the air more powerfully. This should feel as if you are creating a vacuum in your thoracic and abdominal cavity that makes you float through; indeed, this — and not the build-up of copious muscle bulk — is the *pranic* mechanism that makes floating through effortless. Let the inhalation

conclude just as your momentum fades out. The same approach applies to jumping back.

The vital link between breath and movement is *Mula Bandha*. *Mula Bandha* is the contraction of the pubococcygeal muscle used to reverse the downward flow of *prana* that invites death and decay. Initially, at a learning stage, *Mula Bandha* is done exclusively on a gross, muscular level and mainly benefits the gross body. More experienced yogis and yoginis practice it on a more subtle level, where it aims more at the *pranic* body. Masterly practice of *Mula Bandha* is done on a mental level, when hardly a muscular contraction is noticeable. It then influences *karana sharira*, the causal body. The *karana sharira* consists of knowledge and only the longest-lasting *vasanas* (conditionings) and *samskaras* (subconscious imprints).

Let the inhalation reach all the way down to the pelvic floor and rebound off it, at which point the exhalation commences. Imagine your inhalation to create an energetic suction from the pelvic floor — the center of which is formed by the pubococcygeus — all the way up to the crown of the head. Especially during a lifting movement such as jumping through to sitting, hook the inhalation into *Mula Bandha* and be carried through and lifted by the force of the breath. For a more detailed discussion of *Mula Bandha* see *Ashtanga Yoga: Practice and Philosophy*, pages 11–14.

Chapter 8
Reaping the Benefits
of the Intermediate Series

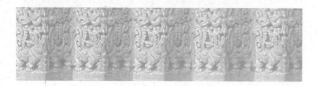

A large amount of information has been presented in this book to help create for the practitioner a broad context in which to place his or her practice of the Intermediate Series of postures. All the many elements of this context, from appreciation of the ancient roots of Ashtanga Vinyasa Yoga to the specifics of the gross anatomy of the sacroiliac joint, are, I believe, essential — not only for enriching one's practice but also for getting the most out of what the Intermediate Series has to offer. As these elements are both numerous and diverse, I offer in this chapter an easily digestible summary of what in my opinion are the most important points presented in the foregoing chapters, couched in terms of practical guidelines.

General Guidelines

REMEMBER THE ULTIMATE GOAL OF YOGA

While practicing postures, remain aware of the fact that yoga was created to support you in the process of realizing that you are the infinite consciousness (sometimes called the soul or the spirit) and not the body. Although you are practicing the methods of one of the many schools of Karma Yoga, you are working toward the same objective as that of the ancient Jnana Yoga. Follow "instant enlightenment" approaches if you are attracted to them. If they do not prove successful, you can always return to structured Karma/Ashtanga Yoga practice.

Practice the postures with a devotional and respectful attitude. Do not look at the Intermediate Series as a whimsical combination of stretches. Look at it as a sacred dance that existed in its eternal perfection long before the ancient seer Vamana saw it in *samadhi*. Practice it with what Patanjali called a "good attitude," an attitude of devotion.[1] This means expressing gratitude to the Supreme Being for having taught yoga; it means practicing with an attitude of giving and of service rather than of personal gain. Move your body in a way that extols the glory of the aspect of the Divine that you worship. To practice Ashtanga Vinyasa Yoga is to pray in movement.

If you do not have a form of worship but are open to the idea, then use the mythological descriptions of the posture names combined with further study of *shastras* (scriptures) to find your *ishtadevata*, your own private communication frequency to the Supreme Being (see chapter 2). Remember that the Indian scriptures agree on this point: There is only one God. Different cultures and individuals have described the One in various ways due to different constitutions. All ways to the Divine are equally valid.

To find your *ishtadevata* and deepen your practice, study *shastra*. If you have a mystical constitution, study the *Upanishads*. If yours is an intellectual-philosophical mind-set, the *Sutras* are the most appropriate set of scriptures. If you have a devotional-emotional tendency, the *Puranas* will best fit your constitution. If you have more of a physical-athletic attitude, study the *Tantras*. If you are a teacher of yoga, study all these scriptures so that you can cater to the various dispositions of your students.

Do not feel superior because you believe the mode of Karma Yoga that you practice is better than

1 *Yoga Sutra* I.14.

the others. Each form of yoga is suited to a different group of practitioners. Further, different stages (*bhumika*) of practice accommodate different levels of fitness (*adhikara*) in practitioners.

If you practice with devotion and dedication, be open to and ready for the descent of grace.

EMBRACE THE EIGHT LIMBS

Always be aware that *asana* is but one limb of eight. Integrate your practice of *asana* with the fourth, fifth, and sixth limbs, and think of this as preparation for limb seven (meditation) and, ultimately, limb eight (*samadhi*). The integrated practice of limbs 3 through 6 begins with proper execution of *Ujjayi pranayama* (a technique of the fourth limb; see chapter 7) during *asana* practice. It continues with withdrawal of the senses (*pratyahara*, the fifth limb). Withdraw the visual sense by following the prescribed *drishtis* (focal points). Withdraw the aural sense by listening to the sound of your own breath. Withdraw the tactile and kinesthetic senses by focusing on proprioception, your intuitive awareness of the proper placement of your limbs. Withdraw the olfactory sense by engaging *Mula Bandha*,[2] and the gustatory sense by engaging *Uddiyana Bandha*.[3]

When you willfully engage your mind in all of these without letting it escape into the future or the past, your mind becomes concentrated, and you achieve *dharana* (the sixth limb). When, after due practice, all takes place uninterruptedly and spontaneously, you reach the stage of *dhyana* (meditation, the seventh limb).

Remember that *samadhi*, the eighth limb, is of two kinds. If the mind is so pure, powerful, and concentrated that the meditation object becomes identical with the mind's representation thereof, the state is called objective *samadhi*. It is in this state that Patanjali conceived the *Yoga Sutra* and Rishi

Vamana, the *Yoga Korunta*. When, through all of the above, one recognizes oneself in a moment of grace as eternally abiding in the true self, the infinite consciousness, the state is called objectless *samadhi*.

OPEN YOURSELF TO SANSKRIT

Whatever your native language is, remember that it is *vaikharic* (based on the gross, fourth phase of sound). Give Sanskrit the respect it deserves as a *madhyamic* (based on the subtle, third phase of sound) and mantric language. Try not to balk at the idea of learning Sanskrit, but rather assemble, ever so slowly if necessary, a toolbox of Sanskrit terms. Meditate on the sacred syllable *Om*, the origin of all mantras, the only *pashyantic* (manifest, second phase of sound) syllable, the sound into which all sounds return.

Learn to properly pronounce the names of the postures and all Sanskrit terms directly related to yoga. Remember that all matter, all knowledge, and all sound are in essence vibrational patterns (*shabda*). Proper intonation in speaking the posture names and Sanskrit words will alter your brain and produce knowledge (see chapter 3).

STUDY ANATOMY

Know and understand in detail the applied yogic anatomy and kinesiology of the human body and how they relate to each posture that you are performing. It is helpful to know which muscle ends where and what it does. When you are about to perform a posture, ask yourself, What main actions make up the posture? Which muscles do I need to use concentrically or eccentrically and isotonically or isometrically when performing it? What is the range of movement of the joints and ligaments involved?

Most of the postures are counterintuitive (based on what's left of intuition in modern humankind). This means that if you do not use refined method and analysis, you will probably perform them incorrectly. The human mind has the tendency to simplify things and will likely tell you to do such things as contract your back during backbending when in fact the opposite needs to be done. Keep in mind the two constitutional laws of posture practice:

---

2 According to *Samkhya*, the philosophy on which yoga is based, the sense of smell is located in *muladhara* chakra, the earth chakra. Looking toward the tip of the nose activates *Mula Bandha* and *Mula Bandha* withdraws the olfactory sense.
3 *Uddiyana Bandha*, the lower abdominal lock, is related to *svadhishthana* chakra, the lower abdominal chakra. According to *Samkhya*, the sense of taste is located in *svadhishthana*, the water chakra.

(1) Expand simultaneously into all opposing directions; and (2) after entering a posture, annul or negate each action that moved you into the posture by performing its opposite. Following these two rules constitutes the way of moving through the world without causing disharmony.

BREATHE MINDFULLY

Stay conscious of the fact that your respiration is nothing but a manifestation of the mantra *Soham*, meaning, "I am verily nothing but the infinite consciousness." Create a solid foundation for your breathing during *asana* practice by using *Uddiyana Bandha* correctly: contract only the lower abdominal wall but stay soft above the navel. This allows the diaphragm to move up and down freely. Restricting the movement of the diaphragm may lead to aggressive, egotistical, ambitious, and anxious character traits.[4] Breathe neither in the chest alone nor exclusively in the abdomen; use the correct method of thoraco-diaphragmatic breathing.

Use the waves of the breath to move deeper into the postures; that is, utilize thoracic flexion and lumbar extension on the inhalation and thoracic extension and lumbar flexion on the exhalation. Breathe through your entire torso, as if your breath was a liquid, filling even the most hidden recesses of an empty cavern. Let all movement be borne from the waves of the breath rather than allowing the movement to precede, dictate, or arrest the breath.

As you practice, remain aware that the purpose of applying *Ujjayi pranayama* in conjunction with the Intermediate postures is twofold: to calm the mind and become deeply centered by drawing *prana* from the surface of the body to its core; and to become balanced and harmonious by evenly distributing *prana* between the lunar (*ida*) and solar (*pingala*) parts of the *nadi* system.

Remember that the ultimate purpose of all breathing exercises is to move the *prana* into the central channel (*sushumna*). If *prana* is made to rise through the chakras up to *sahasrara* (crown chakra), then Deep Reality (*Brahman*) and Ishvara (Supreme Being) will automatically be realized and "seen." If

4   The first three are usually a result of deep-seated anxiety.

you cannot master the Intermediate Series, then alternative methods are available.

Let each posture grow out of the root of *Mula Bandha* (root lock). As you become proficient in contracting the pubococcygeus during practice, make *Mula Bandha* more subtle; that is, shift from a muscular contraction to an energetic and eventually mental contraction.

Specific Guidelines
ADD THE POSTURES ONE BY ONE

The safest and most effective way to begin practicing the Intermediate Series is to slowly add Intermediate Series postures one by one while you continue practicing the Primary Series every day. The postures of the Intermediate Series are very powerful, especially when done in the traditional sequence. You should practice each posture individually until you gain proficiency in that posture. Only then should you undertake the next posture. Practicing in this way enables you to allocate enough energy to working on each new posture. Only when you add on the postures in this traditional method can you harvest the many benefits of the Intermediate Series. If you were to switch one day to practicing a full Intermediate Series, you would not be able to focus and allocate enough energy to the individual postures to perform them proficiently. I have seen many students who abruptly switched from Primary to Intermediate in a follow-the-leader or talk-through type of class. Their practices remained insipid despite all my attempts to change them.

The Primary Series acts as your foundation, your launching pad for progress, and as such you shouldn't abandon it prematurely. During the adding-on process (or even once you have completed the Intermediate Series) you may be confronted by certain issues that force you to go back to practicing the Primary Series. This will be much less disruptive if you have continued practicing the Primary Series all along.

Once you begin practicing the Intermediate Series in its entirety, practice it on days one through five of your practice week, and then practice the

Primary Series on the sixth day. Devoting the last day of your practice week (the sixth day) exclusively to the Primary Series energetically seals the body before rest is taken on the seventh day. If you ever reach a point when nothing feels right in your Intermediate practice, then return to practicing the Primary Series for a few weeks. In that situation, your body may be like an electronic device that has lost its default settings; returning to the Primary Series for a while is like pressing the button that restores those settings.

CONSULT OR WORK WITH A QUALIFIED TEACHER

You should let a qualified teacher decide when you are ready to take on the next posture. It is difficult to judge your own progress, and ambition can easily cloud your judgment. An impartial and knowledgeable teacher is in a better position to make the right decision. Undertaking a new posture before you have mastered the previous one may lead to injury or exhaustion. In most cases, mastering the series and reaping its full benefits will end up taking longer (or never occur at all!) if you take on new postures too early. As with those who try to learn a language without a teacher, most people who teach themselves the Intermediate Series will not realize their full potential. Likewise, those who limit their input to dead media such as books (including this one) and DVDs usually end up with a shallow, superficial practice.

MAINTAIN A STEADY PACE AND STAY WITH THE FLOW

When beginning to practice the Intermediate Series, some students tend to slow down, as the postures have more dimensions than do most of the Primary Series postures. You may warm up to do the postures, become too analytical, and generally fidget and fiddle while attempting the postures. Although it may be good to do this once a week as an experimental tool, it is detrimental to let this approach creep in permanently.

The Intermediate Series is still Ashtanga Vinyasa Yoga, which means there needs to be flow rather than stop-and-go. Once the postures have become familiar, try to practice them in the same rhythm as you do the Primary Series postures. If you slow down too much, you will not build up enough heat and you won't tax yourself enough cardiovascularly. Even a technically refined practice won't be as beneficial if it is too slow. Also, slow practice allows your mind to control you too much. Keep surrendering to the rhythm of the practice and make sure that you do not succumb to any extremes of the mind, such as an obsession with performing postures perfectly.

Of course, you shouldn't practice at too quick a pace either. At a fast pace, you cannot give enough attention to detail, and the quality of the postures suffers as a result; the postures can even become dangerous. Practicing too fast will also drain the life force out of the body, especially when it is hot and humid. If you practice these more difficult postures while cultivating a medium pace — not too fast, not too slow — you will find that you are mobilizing much more energy, which you can use creatively in your practice. To learn the right pace you will need a teacher. Only a teacher can see from the outside whether your practice is too slow or too fast.

The Intermediate Series of postures is difficult to master. However, if you combine the advice given in this and the preceding chapters with dedication to your practice and the guidance of an experienced teacher, your journey through the Intermediate Series will be highly rewarding.

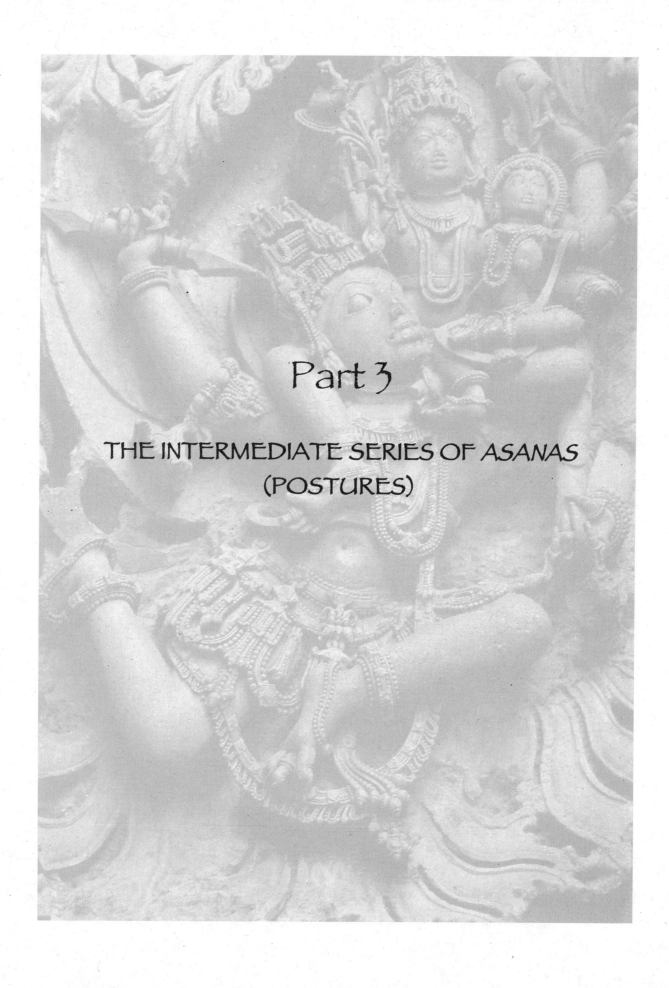

Part 3

THE INTERMEDIATE SERIES OF ASANAS
(POSTURES)

INTRODUCTION

The Intermediate Series described here is to be taken up once proficiency in the Primary Series, covered in *Ashtanga Yoga: Practice and Philosophy*, is gained. The Intermediate Series is made up of twenty-seven *asanas*, many of which comprise A, B, C, and even D versions, and each version is broken down further into a multitude of *vinyasas* (sequential movements).

When analyzing the structure of this series of *asanas*, we discern two different elements: one element, the active one, consists of the three *essential sequences* that produce the effect of the series; the second element, the passive one, consists of the four *connective sections*, which function as fascia, or connective tissue, surrounding the essential sequences. Let's have a closer look first at the essential sequences and then at the connecting sections.

The Three Essential Sequences

The three essential sequences of the active element are the sequences of backbending, leg-behind-head postures, and arm balances.

The first sequence of the Intermediate Series, the backbending postures, consists of the eight postures from *Shalabhasana* to *Supta Vajrasana*. Backbending is a theme that may be new to the practitioner, as it was not treated in the Primary Series.[1]

The second essential sequence is the leg-behind-head sequence, consisting of three postures from *Ekapada Shirshasana* to *Yoganidrasana*. The theme of leg-behind-head was alluded to in the Primary Series through *Supta Kurmasana*, but the Intermediate Series presents its first serious treatment.

The third essential sequence is the arm-balance sequence, consisting of four postures from *Pincha Mayurasana* to *Nakrasana*. Again, this theme was alluded to in the Primary Series through *Bhujapidasana*.

The Connective Sections

Each of the three essential sequences is preceded and followed by one of the four connective sections of the Intermediate Series. The first connective section, to be performed before the backbending sequence, consists of two postures (*Pashasana* and *Krounchasana*). The second connective section, performed between the backbending sequence and the leg-behind-head sequence, consists of three postures (*Bakasana*, *Bharadvajasana*, and *Ardha Matsyendrasana*). The third connective section, which separates the leg-behind-head sequence from the arm-balance sequence, consists of one posture only (*Tittibhasana*); the fourth and final connective section is made up of six postures (from *Vatayanasana* to *Baddha Hasta Shirshasana*).

Function of the Essential Sequences and Connective Sections

The purpose of the active element of the three essential sequences is to purify the *nadi* system and prepare the so-called royal pathway (*sushumna*), the gross manifestation of which is the spine.[2] This purpose is achieved by combining backbending and leg-behind-head postures with arm balances.

Except for the last two postures of the fourth connective section (*Mukta Hasta Shirshasana* and *Baddha Hasta Shirshasana*), which fulfill several functions at the same time,[3] all four connective sections are made up of forward bends

---

1 Up to this point, the yogini would have performed only *Urdhva Dhanurasana* as a backbend. *Urdhva Dhanurasana*, however, is done at the end of each sequence and thus is not an integral part of the Primary Series.

2 The central channel plays the role in the subtle body that the spine plays in the gross body. The subtle body, according to yoga, appears first, then the gross body. *Sushumna* manifests itself as the spine on a gross level.

3 The functions are setting and positioning the shoulder joints for the third (Advanced) series, preventing the burning of *amrita* (nectar) by the gastric fire (this is a function that these headstands share with all other inversions), and drawing *prana* into the core, thus energetically sealing the series and linking it with the upcoming finishing/cooldown postures.

(*Krounchasana, Tittibhasana, Parighasana*), twists (*Pashasana, Bharadvajasana, Ardha Matsyendrasana*), hip openers (*Vatayanasana, Gaumukhasana, Supta Urdhva Pada Vajrasana*), and postures that are kyphotic and *apanic* in nature, such as *Bakasana* and *Tittibhasana*. Many postures fit into more than one of these groups. The postures of the connective sections are identical in structure to the postures of the Primary Series. Their function is to calm and ground the yogi after and in between the exhilaration of the three essential sequences and thus, so to speak, "take the edge off" the practice.

Relationship of Intermediate Series with Other Series

There is conflicting information about the total number of series of postures, but it appears that Shri T. Krishnamacharya taught four: Primary, Intermediate, Advanced A, and Advanced B.

The four connective sections discussed here are an important element of the Intermediate Series. The Advanced Series (not described in this book) stands out because of its lack of connective postures. During advanced practice, the yogi goes from one extreme direction to the opposite extreme. The defining themes of the Advanced Series (except for the extreme hip rotations) are present in the Intermediate Series; however, they are buffered by connective tissue that makes them less blunt in their impact and lessens their effect.

The Intermediate Series is similar to the Advanced A Series in that both contain back-bending, leg-behind-head, and arm-balance sequences. The Intermediate Series is also similar to the Primary Series in that it contains the buffering and mollifying connective sections. The Intermediate Series thus forms a bridge from the Primary to the Advanced A Series.

You will find among the posture descriptions references to *pranayama* (fourth limb of yoga), *pratyahara* (fifth limb of yoga), and so on. This is to remind you that the integral purpose of the postures is to climb the ladder to higher yoga and not just to achieve fitness, health, and good looks.

WARM-UP POSTURES

The warm-up to the Intermediate Series consists of the same sequences as the warm-up to the Primary Series. The warm-up is not an integral part of the series itself; hence it is not described in this book. Perform as a warm-up the following postures as described in detail in *Ashtanga Yoga: Practice and Philosophy* (pp. 22–52) and pictured below:

> *Surya Namaskara* A — 5 repetitions
> *Surya Namaskara* B — 5 repetitions
> *Padangushtasana*

Pada Hastasana
Utthita Trikonasana
Parivrtta Trikonasana
Utthita Parshvakonasana
Parivrtta Parshvakonasana
Prasarita Padottanasana A, B, C, D
Parshvottanasana

Do not include the extended warm-up from *Utthita Hasta Padangushtasana* to *Virabhadrasana* B, as this is done only in combination with the Primary Series.

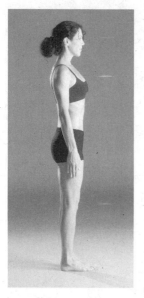

Samasthiti

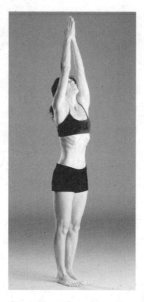

Surya Namaskara A,
vinyasa one

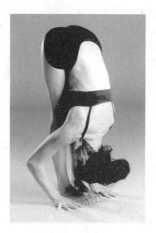

Surya Namaskara A,
vinyasa two

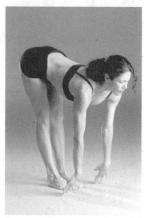

Surya Namaskara A,
vinyasa three

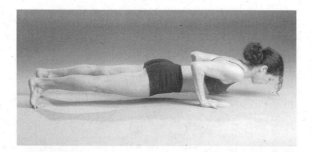

Surya Namaskara A,
vinyasa four (*Chaturanga Dandasana*)

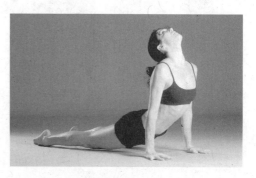

Surya Namaskara A,
vinyasa five (Upward Dog)

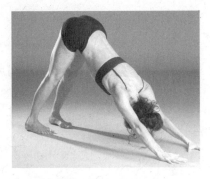

Surya Namaskara A,
vinyasa six (Downward Dog)

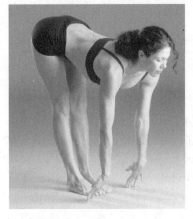

Surya Namaskara A,
vinyasa seven

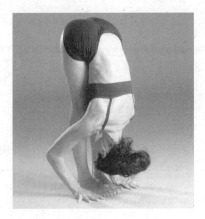

Surya Namaskara A,
vinyasa eight

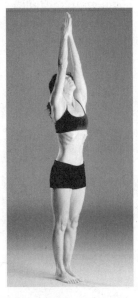

Surya Namaskara A,
vinyasa one

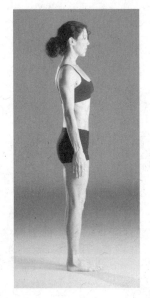

Samasthiti

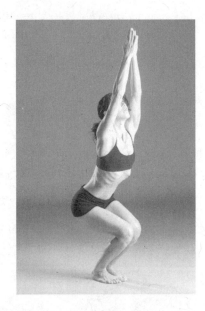

Surya Namaskara B,
vinyasa one (*Utkatasana*)

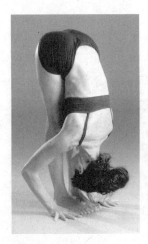

Surya Namaskara B,
vinyasa two

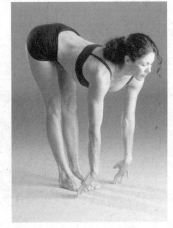

Surya Namaskara B,
vinyasa three

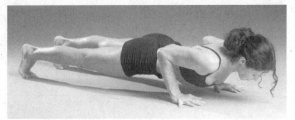

Surya Namaskara B,
vinyasa four (*Chaturanga Dandasana*)

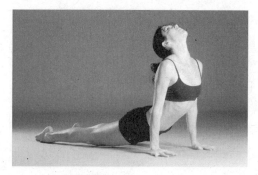

Surya Namaskara B,
vinyasa five (Upward Dog)

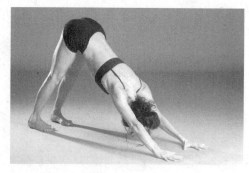

Surya Namaskara B,
vinyasa six (Downward Dog)

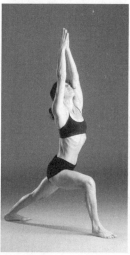

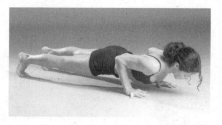

Surya Namaskara B, *vinyasa* eight
(*Chaturanga Dandasana*)

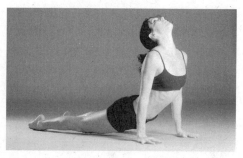

Surya Namaskara B,
vinyasa nine (Upward Dog)

Surya Namaskara B,
vinyasa seven
(*Virabhadrasana* A, right side)

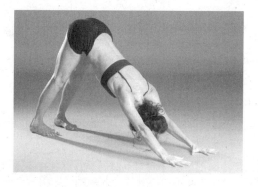

Surya Namaskara B,
vinyasa ten (Downward Dog)

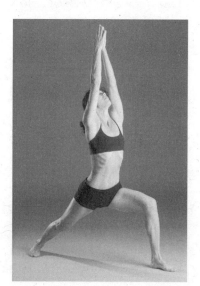

Surya Namaskara B, *vinyasa* eleven
(*Virabhadrasana* A, left side)

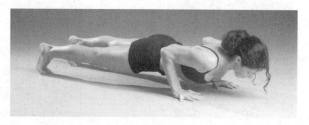

Surya Namaskara B, *vinyasa* twelve
(*Chaturanga Dandasana*)

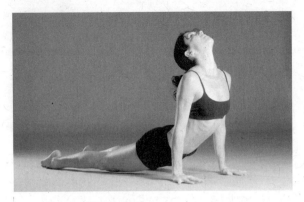

Surya Namaskara B,
vinyasa thirteen (Upward Dog)

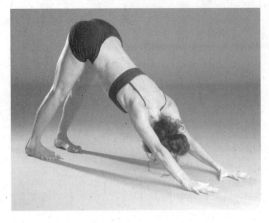

Surya Namaskara B,
vinyasa fourteen (Downward Dog)

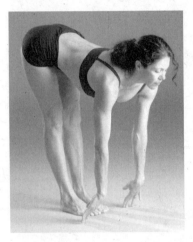

Surya Namaskara B, *vinyasa* fifteen

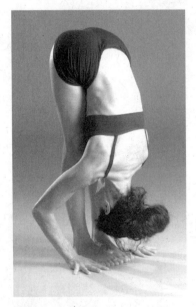

Surya Namaskara B, *vinyasa* sixteen

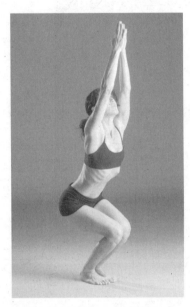

Surya Namaskara B, *vinyasa* seventeen

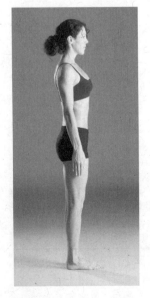

Samasthiti

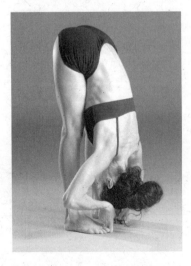

Padangushtasana

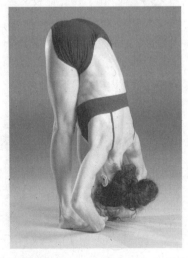

Pada Hastasana

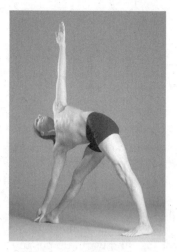

Utthita Trikonasana

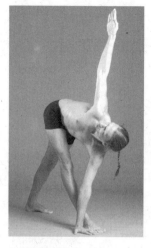

Parivrtta Trikonasana

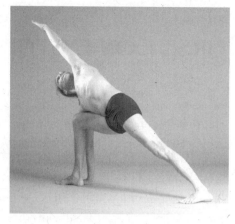

Utthita Parshvakonasana

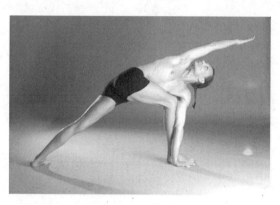

Parivrtta Parshvakonasana

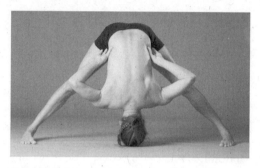

Prasarita Padottanasana A

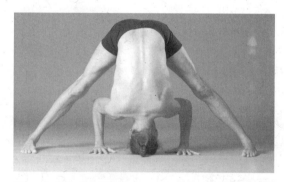

Prasarita Padottanasana B

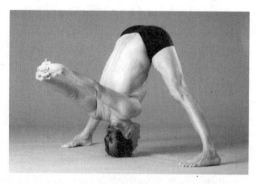

Prasarita Padottanasana C

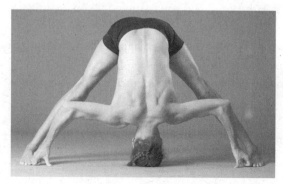

Prasarita Padottanasana D

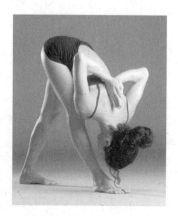

Parshvottanasana

FIRST CONNECTIVE SECTION

This first section opens up the Intermediate Series by repeating some themes of the Primary Series, such as twisting and forward bending. In addition to strongly engaging the *bandhas*, the section stimulates *apana* (downward vital air), thus counteracting and balancing the overly *pranic* (upward flowing vital air) nature of the backbend sequence that follows.

Pashasana

NOOSE POSTURE

Drishti Over your shoulder

OVERVIEW: *Pashasana* exercises the oblique abdominis muscles by combining trunk flexion and twisting. It increases the *vayu apana* and thus improves elimination.[4] The left sides of the posture is performed first, and no *vinyasa* is performed between the left and the right sides of the posture, since the *vinyasa* movement has a lifting and thus *pranic* effect that counteracts the *apanic* effect of this posture.

Pashasana is one of the first postures to be dropped from the Intermediate Series when the practitioner is pregnant or when a beginner's version of the posture must be used.[5] (The majority of students performing this posture for the first time do not get anywhere and are not sure how to begin the process of improving.)

Pashasana is an energetic continuation of *Utkatasana* in the Primary Series.

4 *Vayus* are the ten vital airs, of which the second is the vital downward current *apana*, related to elimination.
5 There are rumors of an *asana* group that was practiced when termination of a pregnancy was desired. In ancient society, a pregnancy was sometimes aborted when it was prophesied by a reliable authority that the child to be born would bring great evil to society. *Pashasana* is said to be able to bring about an aborting effect when performed in a particular sequence together with other postures.

CONTRAINDICATION: It is advisable to not perform intense twists during pregnancy.

Vinyasa Count

Vinyasa One
We begin standing in *Samasthiti* after completing *Parshvottanasana*, the last standing warm-up posture.
Inhaling, raise your arms and look up.

Vinyasa Two
Exhaling, fold forward, placing your hands on either side of your feet.

Vinyasa Three
Inhaling, straighten your arms, flatten out your back, and look up.

Vinyasa Four
Exhaling, jump back into *Chaturanga Dandasana* and lower slowly.

Vinyasa Five
Inhaling, transit into Upward Dog.

Vinyasa Six
Exhaling, transit into Downward Dog.

These first six *vinyasas* are identical with those of *Surya Namaskara* A.

Vinyasa Seven
Jump the feet up to land between the hands, as you do in *Utkatasana*, and squat down.[6] If you are unable to squat and balance while keeping the knees together, it may be due to tight and shortened calf muscles, shortened Achilles tendons, and/or hypomobility of the ankle joint. The most common

6 Notice the similarity of *Pashasana* with *Utkatasana*, the first posture of the Primary Series. *Pashasana* is a continuation of *Utkatasana*.

predisposing factor in females is the frequent wearing of high heels; high muscle tension is often involved in males.[7] To rectify this problem, place a folded towel underneath your heels. The use of a folded towel or blanket is preferred to tilting forward and balancing on your toes, since with padding under your heels you can still ground down through your heels and lengthen the calf muscles and Achilles tendons. This lengthening is essential to perform drop-backs (dynamic movement from *Samasthiti* to *Urdhva Dhanurasana* and return) while keeping the heels down and your feet parallel.

Turn now to the left (the opposite direction to all other twists so far), and place your right arm outside your left knee. Ideally you would go into the posture on one breath. If you find that difficult, access the posture as was taught in *Marichyasana* D (see *Ashtanga Yoga: Practice and Philosophy*, p. 85). Exhaling, contract your external and internal obliques to let your arm slide outward on your knee. Inhaling, press your arm firmly into your knee to prevent it from sliding back out as your chest expands. On the next exhalation, contract your obliques further to again reach deeper. Repeat this until your right shoulder is on the outside of your left knee.

Once your shoulder is outside of your knee, internally rotate your right arm and, flexing the elbow, reach around both knees and interlock your hands (called "binding"). If you tend to fall over backward once bound, you can lift your sit bones higher away from the floor to shift your weight toward your toes. With a gradual increase in flexibility, you will be able to sit back down.

With increasing flexibility and the shedding of any extra pounds, you may eventually take the left wrist with your right hand. Straighten your left arm and lift your left shoulder back over your legs, using your rhomboids and latissimus dorsi muscles on the left.

7   The average male has higher muscle tension than the average female, which leads to greater speed and more strength. Note the gender performance gap in many athletic disciplines at the Olympic games. The reason lies in our evolutionary past — that is, the male body was designed to club the sabertooth tiger and the mammoth. *Disclaimer*: The author does not wish to express the opinion that males are more suited than females for any activities other than the two aforementioned.

Breathe deeply into the chest, drawing the inhalations all the way up to the manubrium (top part of the sternum).

Use your arms as a lever to work deeper into the posture and your breath to progress deeper into the twist. Let your sit bones descend as the sternum and the back of the head reach away from the sit bones and the spine lengthens.

Please note that twisting trunk flexion is also involved in bringing your shoulder toward the opposite knee. This action is performed by the external and internal oblique abdominis muscles and in combination with the rectus abdominis muscle. *Pashasana* requires as much strength as it requires flexibility; in fact, it is one of the prime generators of abdominal strength in the Intermediate Series. Do not attempt any further intermediate postures before you can bind *Pashasana* on both sides without the help of a teacher.

Look over your left shoulder and take five deep breaths. On the last exhalation, come out of the posture.

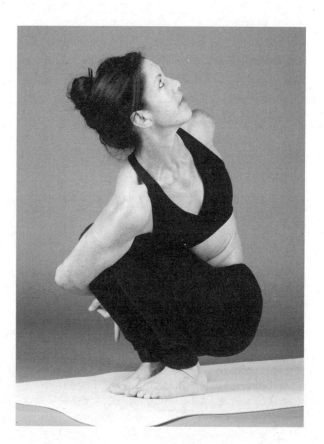

Pashasana

Vinyasa **Eight**

Inhaling, repeat *Pashasana* on the right side. Take five breaths, and exhaling, place your hands down on either side of your knees.

Vinyasa **Nine**

Inhaling, lift up into an arm balance. Ideally this is done without pushing off with your feet but rather using your arms, abs (rectus abdominis), and the power of the inhalation. This is the same movement that is used for exiting *Utkatasana* in the Primary Series, but lifting is more challenging here since we are squatting much lower.

Vinyasa **Ten**

Exhaling, float back into *Chaturanga Dandasana*, making sure that your forearms stay perpendicular to the floor, your hands are beside your waist, and your feet are dorsiflexed. In *Ashtanga Yoga: Practice and Philosophy*, this vertical-forearm approach was presented as the advanced version of *Chaturanga Dandasana*. The beginner's version, when the hands of the practitioner are placed under the shoulders, should no longer be necessary for a practitioner of the Intermediate Series. We might use the beginner's version in the initial months of practice, but if done year after year without being corrected, it will lead to a front/back imbalance of the shoulder muscles.

THE PARADOX OF ACTIVE RELEASE

When performing any posture, the actions that have brought us into the posture must be halted, and the opposite actions must be employed to capture the posture and hold us in it. We work isometrically (that is, the muscles stay the same length: *iso* = same, *metric* = length). To maintain the posture, one must cultivate a harmonious relationship between the agonist and antagonist muscles. This enables the practitioner to maintain the posture while continually exploring its depths, playing the opposing actions of the muscles toward increased flexibility and strength. (For a more detailed description of the "active release principle," see *Ashtanga Yoga: Practice and Philosophy*, p. 73).

The beginner's version places too much emphasis on both pectoralis muscles and fails to bring the latissimus dorsi and the lower trapezius sufficiently into play. An imbalance of the shoulder musculature predisposes the practitioner to shoulder injuries.

Vinyasa **Eleven**

Inhale into Upward Dog.

Vinyasa **Twelve**

Exhale into Downward Dog.

ACTIVE RELEASE TECHNIQUE: Use your oblique abdominis muscles and your pectoralis major and minor gently, as if you are trying to pull yourself out of the twist, but resist this action using your arms, your latissimus dorsi, and your rhomboid on the right side. You will find that your abs and pectoralis muscles will stretch and your chest will open more, which will be most beneficial in backbending.

Practice Exercise

If you do not seem to progress in this posture, try this simple practice exercise.[8]

Lie on your back and, inhaling, bend your left knee and lift your right shoulder off the floor; bring them as close together as possible. Exhaling, lie back down. On the next inhalation, repeat the exercise using your right knee and your left shoulder. Continue alternating sides until you feel your abdominal muscles fatigue. Perform this exercise daily and feel how range of motion and endurance significantly increase. The muscles performing this movement are the same muscles used in *Pashasana* (the external and internal oblique abdominis), which form the second and third layer of the abdominal muscle group. Become aware of their function when performing this exercise and then carry this awareness into your *asana* practice.

---

8 We suggest performing all additional exercises, such as warm-up and research postures, outside of the *vinyasa* practice. There is a subtle magic to following the sequence composed by the ancient seer Vamana. Its meditative flow would be interrupted by the insertion of additional exercises.

If you are unable to clasp your wrist with the opposite hand ("binding") in this posture, consider the following possible reasons and remedies:

- **Weak abdominal muscles:**
  Perform the practice exercise and put more effort into your *vinyasas*.
- **Excess deposits of adipose tissue on thighs and abdomen:**
  Exercise more and eat less. The so-called bad fat around the waist has been a long-standing joke in Ashtanga circles. Biomedical science today considers fat around the waist to be a better indicator of the likelihood of cardiovascular disease than body mass index (BMI). In other words, it matters more where you deposit fat rather than whether or not you have excess adipose tissue. There is "bad fat around the waist," after all.
- **Short femur (thighbone) compared to length of spine:**
  If you have to bend down in this posture much more than other students, a relatively short femur is likely the cause. You will have to train your abs more and gain more flexibility than students who don't have this condition. If it is any consolation, you will find jumping through without touching down, jumping through with straight legs, lifting into *Upavishta Konasana* B without letting go of your feet, and doing drop-backs without lifting your heels all easier to learn than those students who have longer femurs. In *Pashasana*, you may wish to increase the height of the padding under your feet to accommodate your short femur.

Krounchasana

HERON POSTURE

Drishti Up to the foot

OVERVIEW: *Krounchasana* is an energetic continuation of *Triang Mukha Ekapada Pashimottanasana* in the Primary Series. It is a surprisingly intense forward bend.

Vinyasa Count

Vinyasa Seven

From Downward Dog, jump through. If floating through without touching the floor has become easy for you, jump through with the right leg folded back, as you do when jumping into *Triang Mukha Ekapada Pashimottanasana*. This is done by bending the right heel to the right sit bone while jumping through and keeping the knee pointing straight ahead rather than letting it point out to the side. The left leg remains straight during the jump-through.

Upon landing, lift the straight left leg in front of you until you can reach the foot with your outstretched arms. Keeping the left leg straight in this transition will provide more training for your abs and hip flexors, which you will need once you get to the more difficult postures in this series.

Now, reach around your foot, and take your right wrist with your left hand. You will intensify the stretch by doing so, but if you have to bend your back to do it, take the left wrist with the right hand instead. Make sure that your folded right leg points straight ahead and does not veer out to the right. There is no point in faking a good forward bend if you have drawn your right knee out to the side and subsequently medially (internally) rotate your thigh. As in *Triang Mukha Ekapada Pashimottanasana*, also in *Krounchasana* the folded leg needs to point straight ahead and rotate externally to ground the outside of the right sit bone.

Point your left foot now, as in all extreme forward bends (see *Ashtanga Yoga: Practice and Philosophy*, p. 71), to protect your knees (cruciate ligaments) and the origin of your hamstrings, and look up to your foot.

Vinyasa Eight

Exhaling, bend your arms, draw your leg into your chest, and place your chin on your shin. This is done by lifting the chin and arching the neck. Make sure that your chin does not jut forward, which not only looks ugly but also impinges on the nerve supply to the brain and in the long run on the functioning of your intellect. You can subtly alter your mental matrix by changing your breathing pattern; your body

JUMPING THROUGH WITH STRAIGHT LEGS

If your hamstrings have become very long and your legs are not long compared to the length of your torso, you may learn to start jumping through with a straight left leg. To gauge whether your flexibility is sufficient and your build is suitable, go into *Pashimottanasana* and extend your palms beyond your feet. If you can extend your palms at least two inches (five centimeters) beyond your feet, you fulfill the prerequisite for jumping through with straight legs.

Go now into *Padangushtasana* with your back only a few inches away from a wall. Lean your back lightly against the wall, place your hands flat on the floor, and exhale. Engage the *bandhas* fully, and as you inhale, push your hands into the floor and lift your feet off the floor (do this only when you are fully warmed up; we never do any strenuous exercise without being warmed up). If your flexed feet clear the floor by a few inches, you will be able to jump through with straight legs. You are exactly in the position that you need to be to transit through at the peak of the jump-through. Let's call this position "downward facing *Pashimottanasana*."

Now go into Downward Dog. Bend your legs and, inhaling, jump your sit bones in a wide arc up into downward facing *Pashimottanasana*. As your sit bones reach the highest point of their trajectory, close your forward bend like a folding knife, until your knees touch your chest. Keep your arms straight and your feet flexed, and if necessary, elevate your shoulder girdle (engaging upper trapezius and levator scapula) to move the last inch or two. Let your feet swing through slowly, and as your heels come through, lower your sit bones slowly behind you. As your sit bones descend, swing your legs out to the front to fade out the momentum. Complete the inhalation as you arrive in a *Dandasana* position, but hover above the floor. Beginning the exhalation, lower down like a helicopter and land gently, without any impact.

If you can't lift off in downward facing *Pashimottanasana* because of lack of strength, you may still be able to perform the movement using momentum only. The jump-through with one leg straight is slightly easier than with both legs, as you can compensate slightly by lifting the hip of the straight leg higher.

position influences your personality, emotional reality, and choices.[9] An individual lets the chin jut forward during times of conflict, when getting ready to attack, and crucially when he or she wants to communicate this readiness to attack to opponents. The protruding chin communicates willpower, the resolve to let one's chin plough through resistance like a Russian icebreaker. In yoga, we need to draw the chin back in line with our shoulders to make the head stay in line with our hearts and to prevent our divine vision from being reduced to ambition. Success in yoga happens not through achievement but through an insight of what is here already and always has been. We therefore need to keep the chin where it is and focus on drawing the knee toward the heart.

Lift the crown of the head up to the ceiling, and draw the shoulder blades down the back. Bend your elbows as required. Attempt to re-create the curve in your low back, and continue to stretch your left

hamstring. Prevent the right thigh from escaping to the right, and keep it pointing straight ahead. Continue the external rotation of the right thighbone to keep the outside of the right sit bone grounded. Look up to your foot, and take five breaths.

ACTIVE RELEASE TECHNIQUE: Engage your right hamstrings, lightly pressing your foot against your hands, and counteract this action with your arms. The stretch will be distributed more evenly over the entire belly of the hamstrings rather than pulling on their origin, the ischial tuberosity. You will stretch deeper and more effectively using this method.

Keep your hips square to the mat, and laterally (externally) rotate your right thigh to ground the outside of the right sit bone. If the hamstrings of the left leg are not fully stretched, you may need to internally rotate your thigh gently (this situation needs to be assessed by a qualified teacher).

Keep lifting your heart up to your foot, draw your shoulder blades down your back, and take five deep breaths.

9　This has been shown through the work of Wilhelm Reich, Alexander Lowen, Jack Painter, and others.

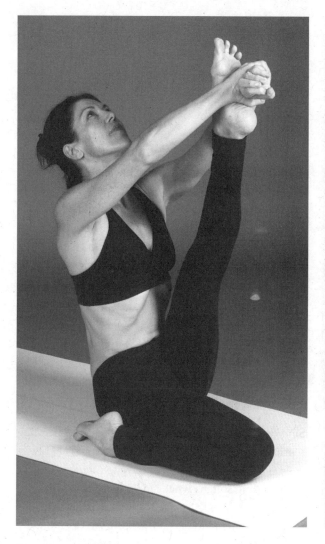

Krounchasana, vinyasa seven

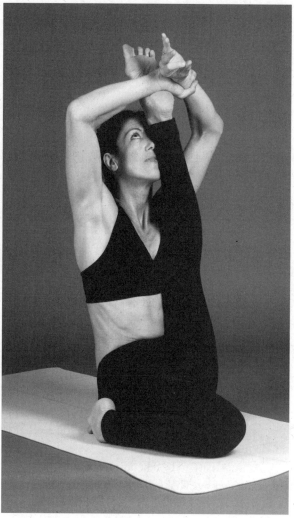

Krounchasana, vinyasa eight

Vinyasa Nine

Inhaling, straighten your arms, draw your leg away from your chest, and look up.

Exhaling, keep the leg in position, and place your hands on either side of your hips.

Vinyasa Ten

Inhaling, lift up into an arm balance, folding the left leg in the process. Don't just hop back into *Chaturanga Dandasana*. The jump-back has two counts: *vinyasa* ten, inhale up; *vinyasa* eleven, exhale back into *Chaturanga*. Don't be satisfied if you cannot yet lift. Challenge that notion. If you are good at the flexibility aspect of *Krounchasana*, great. Now it is time to explore its strength. You need to lift higher than *Bakasana*, obviously, with your knees

off your arms. The alchemy of *asana* is found between the extremes of strength and flexibility. Try every day to lift one centimeter or half inch higher. You will then be prepared when you encounter the strength postures in this series.

Vinyasa Eleven

Exhaling, float back into *Chaturanga Dandasana*.

Vinyasa Twelve

Inhale into Upward Dog.

Vinyasa Thirteen

Inhale into Downward Dog.

Vinyasas Fourteen to Twenty

Repeat *Krounchasana* on the left side.

BACKBEND SEQUENCE

Here begins the group of eight intermediate backbends that form the first essential sequence of the Intermediate Series. Backbending, when linked together with leg-behind-head postures, makes the spine supple and strong and purifies the *nadis* and chakras, which run along the central energy channel (*sushumna*). Illustrating this point, the Northern Indian school of yoga calls *Urdhva Dhanurasana* "Chakrasana," a name that points out the capacity of backbending to open and charge the chakras.[10]

Backbending is related to openness and vulnerability. *Openness* is here defined as the ability to receive what is offered. It relates to what Sigmund Freud called the "oral phase" in the maturing process of the individual, when saying yes, receiving, and being open are the predominant responses. When an infant is breastfed, the contact to the environment, solely represented by the mother, is made through the oral orifice.

A propensity to backbending is often accompanied by what Wilhelm Reich and later Alexander Lowen called an "oral character."[11] The oral character is related to relativism or, in yogic terms, excess *prana* flowing through *ida*, the lunar or left nostril. The relativist and the oral character tend to say yes to the position of another individual and accept it, even if that position could potentially be dangerous and should be rejected. The character tends to find it difficult to reject in others and themselves behavior that is wrong.

The oral character is not as apt at standing its ground, taking a position in life, or defending what is right and of questioning and opposing what is wrong. If the whole population consisted of individuals with oral tendencies, no despots or dictators would ever have been overthrown, and no revolutions would ever have been staged, in the social, scientific, spiritual, or any other arena.

Thus, backbending is most effective when it is matched and balanced with an improvement in opposing actions and posture groups, such as leg-behind-head and arm balances.

Backbending is *pranic* in that it supports the "up-breath," the upward flow of energy that is related to the inhalation. What is generally called "oral" in psychology is in yogic terminology produced by the vital air *prana*.[12]

It is thought that insufficient bonding with the mother leads to the inability to take a receiving stance later in one's life. In our experience, individuals with an open backbend find it easy to accept others without judgment, and there is at least anecdotal evidence that progress in backbending is related to acquiring a more open and sympathetic character. Since it improves our feminine qualities, backbending seems to help us to see value in the opinions of others even if these opinions are contrary to our own. As backbending softens what can be called the "armor" or "cage" of the heart — that is, the rib cage — it makes us compassionate and helps us to open our hearts to those disadvantaged or in need.

However, not everyone who has an open backbend is a genuine, loving human being, and not every stiff backbender is a selfish, hung-up miser. One's backbending seems to improve if one imagines the qualities and attributes associated with backbends while performing them.

Shalabhasana

LOCUST POSTURE

Drishti Nose

OVERVIEW: With *Shalabhasana*, the group of eight intermediate backbends begins. Apart from

---

10 Schools stemming from Shri T. Krishnamacharya are collectively referred to as the "Southern Indian school of yoga."
11 Alexander Lowen, *Körperausdruck und Persönlichkeit* [The Language of the Body] (Munich: Koesel Verlag, 1981), p. 197*ff.*

12 The term *prana* refers generally to life force and more specifically to the up-breath, one of the ten vital airs.

Mayurasana, which functions very similarly, *Shalabhasana* is the only backbend that is fully active; in other words, we use only the back extensors to get into the posture and do not counteract this with the opposite action. In all other backbends, we work against the strength of our arms and legs to deepen the backbend. Here we work only against gravity. For this reason, *Shalabhasana* is the first of the backbends. Its purpose is not to encourage flexibility but to awaken and strengthen the back extensor muscles for the backbends that follow. Strong back extensors are essential in the leg-behind-head postures and arm balances that follow the backbend sequence.

Vinyasa Count

We reached Downward Dog when exhaling in *vinyasa* twenty of *Krounchasana*. As the initial *vinyasa* of *Shalabhasana* is accompanied by an exhalation, we perform an additional inhalation in Downward Dog to link the two postures together.

Vinyasa Four

Exhaling, lower into *Chaturanga Dandasana*. Please note that we pick up the *vinyasa* count here at *vinyasa* four rather than *vinyasa* seven. We do so in the next four postures, all of which we enter by lying on the belly. This also means that if you do a full *vinyasa* practice (coming to standing between all postures and thus linking them with a *Surya Namaskara* A–like movement), you would simply lie down from *Chaturanga Dandasana* in *vinyasa* four and transit through Upward and Downward Dog only on exiting the posture. If you are following the half-*vinyasa* format (jumping back between the right and left sides of a posture but not coming to standing after completing a posture), which is the form of practice commonly done today, no difference will be apparent when entering a posture from *vinyasa* four.

At the end of the exhalation, lie down on your belly with your arms next to your trunk, palms facing up and fingers pointing toward the feet. Make sure that you keep your *bandhas* firmly engaged when lying on your belly; otherwise energy (*prana*) will flow out into the ground. This happens because the Earth is receptive, and energy flows from the higher to the lower potential. For the same reason, the yogi usually turns both hands and feet upward to the sky to receive *prana*.

Vinyasa Five

With the commencement of the inhalation, lift your legs and torso off the floor and point (plantar flex) your feet. Gaze toward the tip of your nose and avoid taking your head too far back. Let your neck harmoniously continue an arch with the rest of your

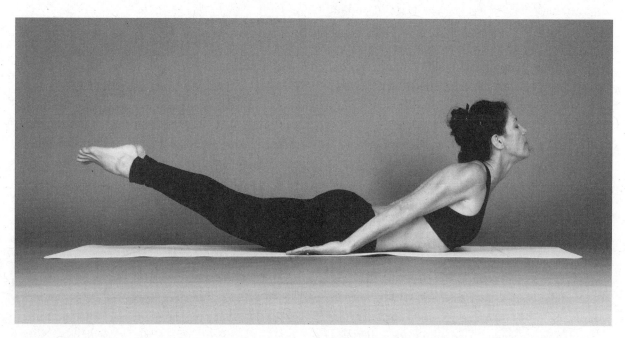

Shalabhasana A

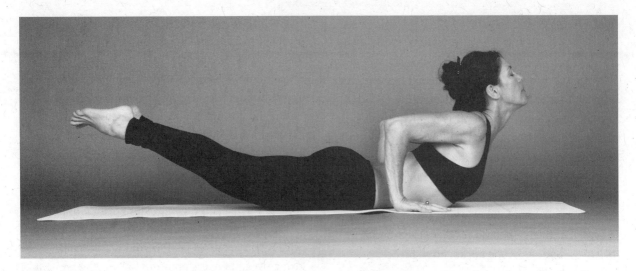

Shalabhasana B

spine. With few strong muscles in the front, the neck is the part of the spine most susceptible to hyperextension (overstretching backward). Hyperextension of the neck can result in headaches and wrist, shoulder, and other pains.

Keep your legs straight by engaging the quadriceps muscles, but use your glutei and your hamstrings to lift your feet as high as possible without bending your legs.

Lift your chest as high as you can by engaging erector spinae and quadratus lumborum. Roll the shoulders down the back, using latissimus dorsi (see *Ashtanga Yoga: Practice and Philosophy*, p. 26), and lift them away from the floor, using your rhomboids (see p. 73). Keep the lower abdomen firm and draw a significant portion of your breath up into your chest. This is essential in all backbending postures, as otherwise the chest will stay dormant and will not open.

Exhaling, lower down; place your hands next to your waist, palms facing down, fingers pointing forward. Place your hands far enough back so that your forearms are perpendicular to the floor, as in *Chaturanga Dandasana*.

Inhaling, lift your chest, head, and legs off the floor again and repeat all previous instructions. Put renewed emphasis on lifting the chest and drawing the shoulder blades down the back. Without moving your hands, draw them back toward your feet. This action helps to engage the latissimus dorsi and lower

trapezius muscles and keep the shoulder blades anchored down, preventing an overactivation of the upper trapezius muscle. *Shalabhasana* A and B are covered under one heading, as they do not have an individual *vinyasa* count.

Vinyasa Six
Inhale into Upward Dog.

Vinyasa Seven
Exhale into Downward Dog.

Bhekasana
FROG POSTURE
Drishti Nose

OVERVIEW: *Bhekasana*'s purpose is to lengthen the quadriceps. Note that the focus during the unfolding backbend series will slowly move from the thighs, which are targeted in *Bhekasana*, upward to the psoas, which is mainly stretched in *Dhanurasana* and *Ushtrasana*, to finally arrive at the upper chest area with *Kapotasana*.

Vinyasa Count
Vinyasa Four
Exhaling, lower into *Chaturanga Dandasana*. At the end of the exhale, lie down on your belly and bend your legs so that your feet come close to your

buttocks. Place your hands on the tops of your feet, palms facing down and fingers pointing forward, in the same position as in the second phase of *Shalabhasana*. Your soles and palms will now face downward and your toes and fingers forward toward your head. If you cannot get into this position, your limitation is likely to be stiffness either of the quadriceps, preventing you from flexing your knees enough, or of the pectoralis minor, preventing you from rolling your shoulders back enough to place your hands up on your feet with your palms facing down; more likely it is a combination of both. You may warm up and stretch both muscles outside of and prior to your *vinyasa* practice by means of the research postures suggested on pages 110–11.

Vinyasa Five

Press your feet down toward the floor and, inhaling, lift your chest off the floor, repeating with your torso the action performed in *Shalabhasana* B.

Draw your shoulder blades down your back, breathe deeply into your chest, and look toward your nose. The main purpose of the posture is to lengthen the quadriceps in anticipation of more difficult backbends. Focus first on getting your heels and feet down to the floor, and once that is achieved, work on lifting your chest high. You will get ample opportunity to work on opening the chest in the later postures.

Keep your femurs (thighbones) in a neutral position while you work your feet down to the floor to stretch centrally through the quadriceps. While you work your feet down to touch the floor on the outsides of your thighs, there is the tendency to internally rotate the femurs. You can recognize that situation when your soles and heels face inward (toward your thighs) and the tops of your feet face outward. If this is the case, externally rotate the femurs so that the heels face straight down. Remember that this posture is like a double *Triang Mukha Ekapada Pashimottanasana* done face down. As in that posture, we need to externally rotate the femurs here as well.

Attempt to keep your thighbones parallel, so that the knees are not wider apart than the width of the hip joints. If you widen the legs more, you will

emphasize the stretch of the vastus lateralis, the outermost head of the quadriceps. There is no need to touch the knees together. This may place undue strain on the knees.

If you feel knee pain when performing *Bhekasana*, a slight misarticulation of the femur or the tibia is most likely the cause. Come up to sitting, flex your knee joint, and then perform a kicking movement (in a sensible fashion). When you come close to 180 degrees of leg extension, relax the thigh muscles so that the momentum "gapes" the knee joint slightly. This means that for a short period the interjoint space will be increased. The ligaments will now pull the bones back together, which usually results in a more precise articulation. If you still experience pain, there is likely to be an underlying knee problem or a misalignment of the pelvis, and it is advisable not to go deep into *Bhekasana*. Address the problem by performing *Virasana* (see *Ashtanga Yoga: Practice and Philosophy*, p. 57) on a pile of blankets and decrease the height gradually over days. If necessary, have the alignment of the pelvis checked and corrected by a qualified musculoskeletal professional.

When done correctly and sensibly, *Bhekasana*, *Virasana*, and *Supta Virasana* all tend to improve the tracking of the patella. A maltracking patella is often caused by a mis-tone among the three vasti, a condition that is often alleviated by performing the three postures just described.[13]

During the posture, focus on stabilizing the lower abdomen and lifting the heart out to the front, thus lengthening out through the low back. Look toward the nose, and take five breaths in *Bhekasana*.

ACTIVE RELEASE TECHNIQUE: Engaging the quadriceps, press the back of your feet up against the resistance of your arms as if you were trying to straighten your legs. This will distribute the stretch evenly over the entire belly of the quadriceps.

---

13 The quadriceps has four heads — the two-joint muscle rectus femoris (which also flexes the thigh at the hip), the vastus lateralis, the vastus medialis, and the vastus intermedius — all of which insert into the patellar tendon. If one of the three vasti muscles is more toned than the others — most often the vastus lateralis — the patella will be pulled laterally.

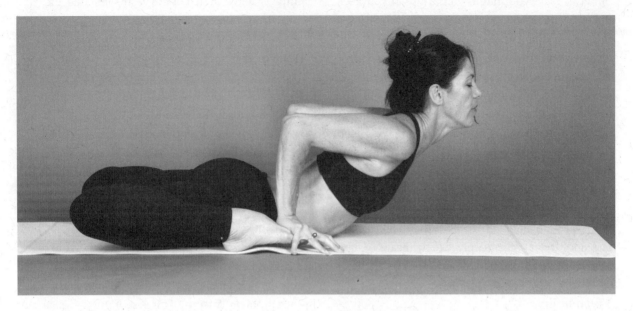

Bhekasana

BEGINNER'S VERSION: If you find it challenging to go straight into the full version of *Bhekasana*, warm up your legs one at a time. Rest on your left elbow and lift your chest. Bend your right leg and, using your right hand, press your foot down toward the floor. You can use your arm more effectively now, since your chest is lifted while propped up on your left arm. As you press your foot down, gently rotate your femur in both directions to stretch various portions of the quadriceps. Use the active release

method by pressing your foot up against the resistance of your hand. Once you have reached your maximum stretch, repeat on the left.

Once you have become proficient in *Bhekasana*, omit the beginner's version and go straight into the full posture.

WARM-UP AND RESEARCH POSTURE:

1. First lie in *Supta Virasana* to stretch the quadriceps. Then, with elbows pressing into

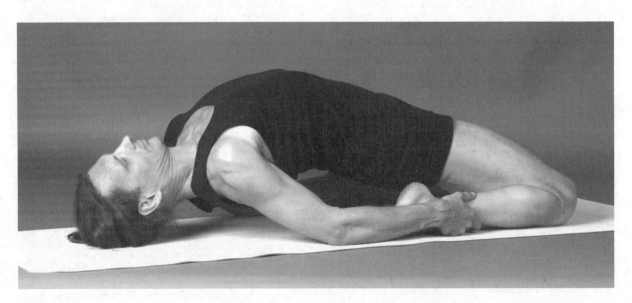

Releasing the quadriceps

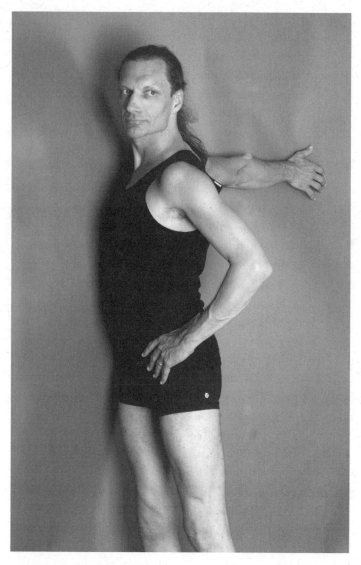

Stretching the pectoralis minor

the floor, lift your hips as high off the floor as you can. Breathe into the quadriceps and perform the preceding active release, using the resistance of the floor against your feet instead of your hands.

2. Your ability to perform *Bhekasana* might be impeded by a tight pectoralis minor. Try out the following passive stretch: Stand upright facing a wall and place your palm against the wall. Then turn your chest away from the wall while the entire length of the arm stays in direct contact with the wall. Check that you feel the stretch in your pectoralis minor rather than hyperextending your elbow. This passive horizontal abduction will improve your shoulder flexibility.

Exhaling, let go of your feet and straighten your legs, placing the feet down flexed and hip-width apart. Place your palms down next to your waist.

PASSIVE STRETCHING

The efficacy of passive stretching is due to muscle creep. *Muscle creep* is a phenomenon that happens when a constant load is applied to a muscle over time, causing the muscle to lengthen, or "creep." A stretch must be held for at least twelve minutes for muscle creep to take place; otherwise, the natural elastic recoil properties of the muscle tissue will cause the muscle to return to its original length. This return to normal is called *hysteresis* and involves the adaptive remodeling of muscles and their connective tissues. To get the most results from a stretch in the shortest amount of time, apply some resisted contraction to the stretch; this requires contracting the muscle group that you're stretching. For example, in exercise 2 above, you would press your hand into the wall for six seconds, then relax your arm, leaving your hand where it was. Then you would move more deeply into the stretch, pressing your hand into the wall for twenty seconds or five slow breaths. You would repeat this until you couldn't move any further into the stretch, an indication that the muscles had lengthened as much as they were going to for that day. This type of stretching is called "proprioceptive neuromuscular facilitation" (PNF) and has various forms. PNF relies on the proprioceptive properties (those that do not rely on visual clues) within the muscles to relax or inhibit the muscle. This achieves a more effective stretch.

Vinyasa Six
Inhaling, lift into Upward Dog.

Vinyasa Seven
Exhaling, move into Downward Dog.

Dhanurasana

BOW-SHAPED POSTURE

Drishti Nose

OVERVIEW: The first active backbend. It stretches the quadriceps and psoas and opens the chest.

Vinyasa Count

Vinyasa Four
Exhaling, lie down on your belly.

Vinyasa Five
Bend your legs and take hold of your ankles. Inhaling, lift your chest off the floor by attempting to straighten your legs.

Keep the lower abdominal wall engaged by using *Uddiyana Bandha*. If done correctly, you will rock back and forth on the upper abdomen with your breath. Holding *Uddiyana Bandha* should prevent the diaphragm from distending the lower abdomen and causing the whole of the torso to rock.

Keep drawing the shoulder blades down the back to open the chest. Breathe deeply into your chest to soften and open your rib cage. *Dhanurasana* focuses its stretch on the hip flexors, chiefly the psoas but also the rectus femoris. The rectus femoris is the fourth head of the quadriceps (*quadriceps* means "four heads"). It is the only two-joint muscle of the four, traversing the hip joints and knee joints (the other three heads, the three vasti, traverse only the knee joint and are mere leg extensors). Isolate the three vasti from the rectus femoris as we did in *Pashimottanasana* in the Primary Series. The rectus femoris eccentrically releases here to deepen the backbend, while the three vasti are powerfully used to straighten the leg at the knee; that is, the vasti concentrically contract to deepen the backbend, which in turn opens the chest more.

Try to keep your feet and knees hip-width apart and not any wider. The rule of thumb in all backbends is that the legs should be kept parallel, as if you were standing. If you leave too much space between the knees and bring the big toes together, the femurs (thighbones) will externally rotate. This position shortens the piriformis and other external hip rotator muscles. The piriformis inserts onto the anterior (front) aspect of the sacrum. When the piriformis becomes hypertonic (overactive), it has the potential to "jam" the sacrum. Since the sacrum acts as one of the pumping mechanisms for cerebrospinal fluid (CSF), and CSF in many ways ensures proper protection and function of the brain and spinal cord, we need to avoid external rotation of the femurs during backbending, since it can lead to a disruption of the flow of cerebrospinal fluid to the brain and thus diminishes intellectual, physical, and spiritual potential. One of the first symptoms of a jammed sacrum is low back, sacroiliac, or buttock pain. The safest way to avoid this in *Dhanurasana* is to keep the same amount of space between your feet and your knees that you have between your hip joints (8–10 inches or 20–25 centimeters).

For students who have good proprioceptive awareness, this way of doing *Dhanurasana* may be accessible. Many students, however, do not have well-developed proprioception, which means that if they cannot see what they are doing or cannot view themselves in a mirror, they arrive at only a very vague replication of the given instruction. Since we should never turn the head in a backbend — in fact, we should never combine backbending and twisting — and we generally do not espouse the use of mirrors for yoga (since they draw *prana* and awareness to the surface and increase identification with the body), I suggest that such students place the big toes together and the knees slightly apart (mediating between the feet and the hip joints).

Although the feet and knees are placed together in some advanced backbends, such as *Vrshchikasana*, *Viparita Shalabhasana*, and *Viparita Dandasana*, this should not be done in intermediate practice. It presupposes that the student is proficient in nutating the sacrum, a movement that is covered under *Kapotasana*. Once students are proficient in the

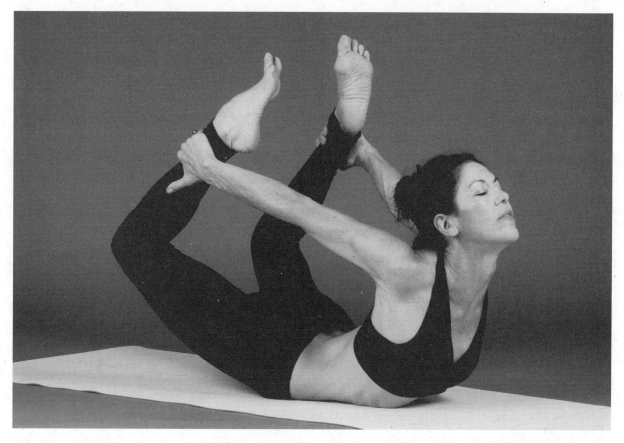

Dhanurasana

advanced backbends, they may place their feet and knees together in intermediate backbends without causing any harm.

Gaze toward the tip of the nose to avoid taking the head too far back, and take five breaths.

Exhaling, lower down to the floor, flex your feet, and place your palms down next to your waist.

ACTIVE RELEASE TECHNIQUE: Rather than focusing on your arms, focus on your abdominals and the straightening of the legs. This will further lengthen the psoas and the quadriceps.

Experiment also with slightly engaging the pectoralis minor when deeply in the posture. Once it is engaged, use the strength of your legs against the (gentle) resistance of your pectoralis minor to roll your shoulder back and stretch the pectoralis minor further. This will prove helpful once you encounter postures such as *Supta Vajrasana* that require anterior shoulder flexibility.

WARM-UP AND RESEARCH POSTURE: Experiment with holding your shins close to your knees, rather than your ankles. The closer you manage to get to your knees, the more you can carry the stretch into your chest.

Vinyasa Six

Inhale into Upward Dog.

Vinyasa Seven

Exhale into Downward Dog.

Parshva Dhanurasana

SIDE BOW POSTURE

Drishti To the side and to the nose

OVERVIEW: A continuation of the theme explored in *Dhanurasana*. Here we take the stretch slightly more into the chest, as we don't have to work against gravity.

Vinyasa Count

Vinyasa Four

Exhaling, lower into *Chaturanga Dandasana*.

Vinyasa Five

Take hold of your ankles and lift again into *Dhanurasana*, expanding fully into the posture with your inhalation.

Vinyasa Six

Exhaling, roll onto your right side, maintaining the backbend. Keep the same distance between the knees and feet as you had in *Dhanurasana*. There is no point in touching the knees together here if your knees do not touch in *Samasthiti*. Rishi Vamana explains the *drishti* here as *parshva*, which means to the side and not up to the ceiling looking over your shoulder. If the focal point were meant to be up to the ceiling, the *rishi* would have called it *urdhva* (upward). It is anatomically unsound to turn your head in backbending, as you can easily put your neck muscles into spasm doing so, especially if you have scoliosis or a lateral muscle imbalance in which your neck muscles are shorter and tighter on one side. If you overuse these muscles by twisting your neck in a backbend, especially by holding the neck's weight against gravity as in *Parshva Dhanurasana*, you might upset your existing compensatory pattern and manifest whiplash symptoms. Simply maintain the position of your head in relation to the spine that you had in the previous posture without attempting any contortions.

Lying on your side, work on straightening your legs, and breathe deeply into your chest. Draw your shoulder blades down your back and roll your shoulders far back to stretch your pectoralis muscles. Continue all actions performed in *Dhanurasana*.

The focus in *Dhanurasana* and *Parshva Dhanurasana* is on stretching the hip flexor group, with special emphasis on the psoas. Additionally, in *Parshva Dhanurasana* the body weight borne on each shoulder helps to stretch the pectoralis muscles and open the shoulders laterally across the chest.

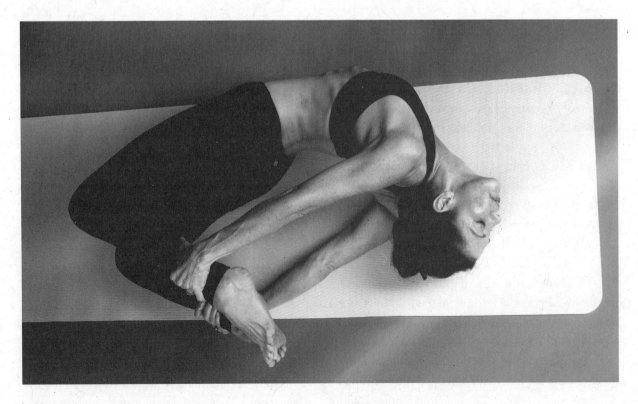

Parshva Dhanurasana

WARM-UP AND RESEARCH POSTURE: Again, experiment with holding the shins rather than the ankles, as close to the knees as possible, to gain more flexibility.

ACTIVE RELEASE TECHNIQUE: Use the strength of your quadriceps to straighten your legs. Slightly engage your psoas to work against the quadriceps. You can now carry the stretch deeper into the psoas by alternately engaging quadriceps and psoas.

Engage pectoralis minor and major as if you were trying to come out of the posture. Use the strength of your legs to open your chest further and stretch both pectoralis muscles.

Vinyasa Seven
Inhaling, roll back up into *Dhanurasana*.

Vinyasa Eight
Exhaling, roll over on your left side and repeat *Parshva Dhanurasana* on the left.

Vinyasa Nine
Inhaling, roll back up to the middle and hold *Dhanurasana* for five more breaths. It will be tiring, but nevertheless work intensely. The gaze here is again to the nose.

Exhaling, lower into *Chaturanga Dandasana*.

Vinyasa Ten
Inhale into Upward Dog.

Vinyasa Eleven
Exhale into Downward Dog.

Ushtrasana

CAMEL POSTURE

Drishti Nose

OVERVIEW: With *Ushtrasana* commences a sequence of kneeling backbends. Backbending on the knees may initially feel like your legs have been cut off. It does pose an extra challenge for the student to work the legs sufficiently to support the *bandhas* and an elongation of the spine. Actively press the front of the feet and shins into the floor, and without tensing the inner thighs or changing the distance between the knees, sufficiently squeeze the knees together to create an upward vector. The energy created from the legs must inspire a lift of the pelvic floor (*Mula Bandha*) and *Uddiyana Bandha* in the low abdomen, initiating the lengthening of the spine in the back-bend. A failure to do this will result in the knees widening and the lumbosacral junction being unsupported.

In *Ushtrasana* the main focus is on lengthening the quadriceps and psoas by pushing the pelvis forward.

CONTRAINDICATION: If you suffer from an acute whiplash, you should avoid all backbends on your knees for now. A chronic whiplash condition can be alleviated in this position by depressing the shoulder girdle using the lower trapezius and latissimus dorsi muscles. A whiplash often involves a spasm of the upper trapezius and levator scapula. Those muscles are shortened here and are thus susceptible to aggravation.

Vinyasa Count

Vinyasa Seven
Inhaling, jump forward to a kneeling position with your knees and feet hip-width apart and your feet pointed. Kneel with your torso upright and place your hands on your hips.

Vinyasa Eight
Exhaling, arch back and place your hands on your feet with your fingers pointing toward your toes. Try to place the heels of your hands onto the soles of your feet with your fingertips close to your toes rather than placing your hands up on your heels. You will intensify the opening of your chest that way. Engage your hamstrings and gluteus maximus to drive your pelvis forward. Bringing your hips over your knees, or even in front of your knees, is essential for fully utilizing this posture. Draw your shoulder blades down your back to deepen the arch of the chest and also to release the trapezius.

Ushtrasana primarily targets the psoas and the low back. Make sure to keep your abdominals engaged to avoid "hanging" on your L5 (fifth lumbar) disc. "Hanging" is used to describe the tendency to direct the stretch into the softest and weakest part of the lumbar spine. The junction of the fifth lumbar vertebra with the sacrum has the greatest mobility in extension of any spinal vertebra and is therefore the most vulnerable. Additionally, extra stress is incurred at all vertebral segments where the spinal curves change direction; here the spine shifts from the lordotic curve of the lumbar spine to the kyphotic curve of the sacrum.

Experiment with gently internally rotating your thighbones and/or gently engaging your adductors to deepen your backbend. Neither action should be overdone, as each can lead to a tight tensor fascia lata or tight adductors. It is, however, important to create an upward vector from the knees that supports the upward lifting of the *bandhas* in the lower abdomen and ascends the entire length of the spine.

Breathe deeply into the upper part of the chest, the manubrium, to make sure that you open there as well. Relax your neck and let the head hang downward. Use the additional weight of the head to carry the opening further up into your chest. Take five breaths in *Ushtrasana* and gaze toward the nose.

ACTIVE RELEASE TECHNIQUE: Contract your quadriceps and your abs, as if you were trying to come up and out of the posture. Press your feet firmly into the floor as if to straighten your legs. Counteract this by firmly gripping your feet with your hands. This will allow the quadriceps and the psoas to stretch more deeply.

Press your hands into your feet as if to flex the humeri and as if to sweep your hands over the floor and out to the front. Counteract this action by continuing to drive your pelvis forward.

Vinyasa Nine

Inhaling, come upright, driving your pelvis forward, and place your hands on your hips.

Exhaling, place your hands on the floor on either side of your knees. Avoid sitting down on your heels, as your energy will then drop.

Vinyasa Ten

Inhaling, lift up into an arm balance with your feet way off the ground and your arms straight. Hold this *vinyasa* for the duration of the inhalation. Do not go straight from *vinyasa* nine to *vinyasa* eleven. This is an intricate part of *Ushtrasana* and is often missed by students. Backbending always needs to be complemented with back stabilization. Never develop flexibility that is not counteracted and supported by strength. You might look good in the first few years of doing yoga, but after that, physical problems due to an increasing imbalance will arise. Some students practice for many years and wonder why their overall condition deteriorates rather than improves. Apart from faulty technique, the culprit here is often an increase in flexibility without a corresponding increase in strength. Lay good foundations for the future by developing your strength in the same way as your flexibility. (Ways of improving *Lollasana*, an arm balance similar to this one, appear in *Ashtanga Yoga: Practice and Philosophy*, pp. 70 and 90.)

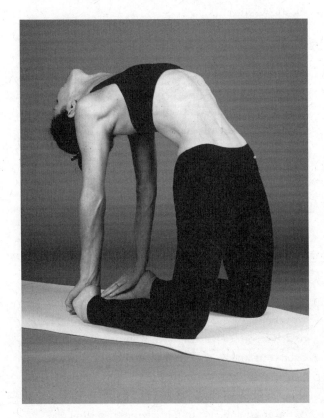

Ushtrasana

116

Vinyasa Eleven

Exhaling, float back into *Chaturanga Dandasana*.

Vinyasa Twelve

Inhale into Upward Dog.

Vinyasa Thirteen

Exhale into Downward Dog.

Laghu Vajrasana

LITTLE THUNDERBOLT POSTURE

Drishti Nose

OVERVIEW: The main focus of this posture is to strengthen the quadriceps in preparation of *Kapotasana*.

Vinyasa Count

Vinyasa Seven

Inhaling, jump forward to a kneeling position with your torso upright and your hands on your hips. Again, develop a strong base with your legs as described in *Ushtrasana*.

Vinyasa Eight (full version)

Exhaling, lean backward and place your hands on your ankles, thumbs inside and fingers outside.

Keeping your arms straight, lean back further until your head touches the floor, all the while maintaining as much back arch as possible. Don't drop all of your weight onto your head; touch the floor only lightly. Keep your hips as high as possible and your quadriceps engaged by pressing the front of the shins into the floor (as if you were to straighten your knees). By carrying most of your weight with your quadriceps rather than leaning your head onto the floor, you will be able to reverse this movement and come back up after five breaths. This may initially be very challenging. If you find you are unable to come back up, try the beginner's versions on the next page.

In the process of leaning back, carry the weight in the quads, thereby working them eccentrically, so that they work against gravity and are being lengthened as they contract. This is the most effective way to strengthen any muscle. Keep the *bandhas* firmly engaged and keep some adduction and internal rotation of the thighs so that your knees do not flare out to the sides.

Draw your shoulder blades down your back and breathe into your chest.

Take five breaths and look toward your nose to prevent overstretching your neck.

If you are unable to perform the complete posture as described above, try the following.

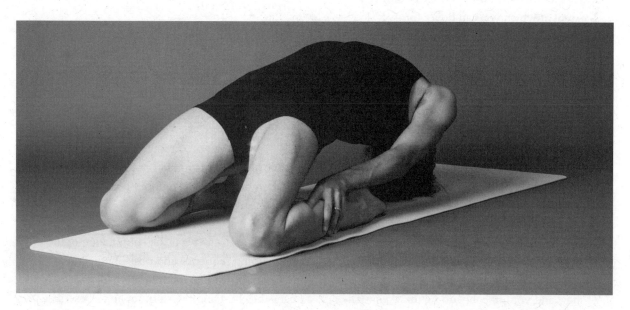

Laghu Vajrasana

Beginner's Versions

Performing the full version of *vinyasa* eight requires not only strong quadriceps but also a strong ligamental structure of the knee, especially strong cruciate ligaments (which prevent forward travel of the femur on the tibia or vice versa). If you previously had an injury or strain of the cruciate ligaments, do not perform the full version yet but let your knees slowly get stronger over months of practice.

- To make your quadriceps stronger, use the following method: First, hold your calves closer to your knees and see whether you can perform the whole sequence, including coming back up, keeping your arms straight.
- If you still can't come up, bend your arms in *vinyasa* nine and press your elbows powerfully against your heels and bounce up, using momentum. This way you can use your arms to make up for missing leg strength. Once you can do that, gradually, over months, fade out your arm involvement and let the quadriceps take over.
- If even with the use of your arms, you still can't come back up, try the following method: In *vinyasa* eight, don't place your head all the way down but lower only to an extent at which you can hover for five breaths and then reverse the movement and lift back up. Memorize this point and return to it the next day. Once you get confident, lower just a few centimeters or inches more. This way — again gradually, over months — you will improve your ability to eccentrically lengthen and concentrically contract your quadriceps until you can reach the floor. There is no therapeutic effect to lowering and then collapsing on the floor. You won't get stronger or any closer to performing *Kapotasana* that way.
- If you do not progress with the preceding exercises, your quadriceps is probably too short and you probably do not have enough range of movement. You will then need to do extra stretching exercises for the quadriceps, such as assuming *Supta Virasana* daily for an extended period.

ACTIVE RELEASE TECHNIQUE: Engage the quadriceps as if to straighten the legs to stand up. Stay in the posture, working your arms to counteract the action of your legs. This action will eccentrically lengthen the quadriceps.

Vinyasa Nine

Hook the inhalation firmly into the *bandhas*, contract your quadriceps, and come up, placing your hands on your hips.

Exhaling, place your hands on the floor on either side of your knees.

Vinyasa Ten

Inhaling, lift up into an arm balance (*Lollasana*) with your feet way off the ground and your arms straight. Hold this *vinyasa* for the duration of the inhalation. Again, this is important to counteract the backbend.

Vinyasa Eleven

Exhaling, float back into *Chaturanga Dandasana*.

Vinyasa Twelve

Inhale into Upward Dog.

Vinyasa Thirteen

Exhale into Downward Dog.

Kapotasana

PIGEON POSTURE

Drishti Nose

PREREQUISITE: Full version of *Laghu Vajrasana*. Do not attempt *Kapotasana* without properly performing *Laghu Vajrasana* beforehand.

OVERVIEW: *Kapotasana* is the culmination of the backbending sequence and possibly the most important posture in the Intermediate Series. It fully opens the chest and the sternum area. Described below are two versions: an intermediate version for those new to intense backbends, and then a version for advanced students, which involves nutation (forward bowing) of the sacroiliac joints.

Vinyasa Count — Intermediate Version

Vinyasa Seven

Inhaling, jump forward to a kneeling position with your torso upright and your hands on your hips. Keep your feet and knees roughly hip-width apart. You can place your feet slightly closer together than your knees to make it easier to "walk" around the outside of your feet with your hands in *vinyasa* eight. To place the feet together and the knees apart in *Kapotasana*, however, is not recommended for intermediate students, as it will externally rotate the femurs (thighbones). Externally rotated femurs in turn will tend to "jam" the sacrum into a counter-nutated position (see the section on sacroiliac joints in chapter 6, pp. 65–68).

The following backbend movement is very complex and ideally starts at the top of the torso, the manubrium or upper heart area, and then runs in a wavelike motion through the spine and terminates at the sacrum. The wavelike motion can also be initiated from the sacrum flowing upward, but in that case the upper chest area may not be sufficiently open.

If your chest is not yet completely open (for most of us it won't be at this point in our practice), lift your chest by pressing your hands onto your hips. Lift your heart as high as possible and grow as tall as you can. Imagine the entire front of your torso being sucked up to the sky, while the posterior aspect of your trunk flows down to the Earth. If necessary, you may take several extra breaths to achieve this effect. We first need to aim for quality in this complex posture, and once this is achieved we will reduce the time required. If we do not invest the necessary time in the posture now, after years we may still have nothing to show but the ability to do the entire posture in the required five breaths but without any inherent quality.

As your backbend deepens, steer away from just folding your pelvis backward and jutting the pubic bone forward. This method is an easy way out; it will carry the stretch only into the softest part of your spine but not into those areas where you are stiff and inflexible. One axiom of physical yoga is to support the areas where we are weak and open those where we are tight and closed. If you merely jut the pubic bone forward, you will not only stop the heart from opening but also put undue pressure onto your low back and sacroiliac joints.

Drop the pubic bone downward and toward the coccyx by engaging *Mula Bandha*. Rather than folding the pelvis backward, lift the front of the whole pelvis and the front of the torso up to the ceiling. Check that you are not clenching your buttocks to avoid externally rotating your femurs (thighbones). Clenching the buttocks means the gluteus maximus and piriformis muscles are fully engaged. The gluteus maximus along with the hamstrings performs hip extension (the action necessary for backbends). When the knees are bent, the hamstrings are shortened and thereby less powerful. The gluteus maximus is needed to initiate the action of hip extension as we raise our pelvis upward with our knees bent. The lower fibers of the gluteus maximus muscle also perform external (lateral) rotation of the femur, as does the piriformis muscle. This rotation puts more pressure on your sacroiliac joints because it squeezes the ischia (sit bones) together and prevents nutation of the sacrum, another necessary motion for harmonious back-bending. (This is covered in detail on p. 67.) It is therefore necessary to not excessively clench the buttocks while in a backbend position. Of course, as with all actions in yoga, this action can be taken too far; the glutei need to maintain a certain core tension, so do not relax them completely.

To prevent the clenching of the lower fibers of the gluteus maximus and of the piriformis, beginning and intermediate students and all those who experience discomfort during backbending should try internally rotating the femurs gently during all backbending postures. This action will prevent overactivation of the lower fibers of the gluteus maximus, piriformis, and other deep external rotator muscles in the buttocks, enabling the low back to lengthen and the sacroiliac joints to move freely.

You can achieve a similar effect in backbends by

engaging the adductors to squeeze your thighs together. Place a block between your knees — or at least imagine one there — to try to bring about this effect. However, this action is recommended only for those whose low backs or sacra are very unstable and who have tried internal (medial) rotation of the femurs with no success. The disadvantage of squeezing the knees together in backbending is that the action may be performed to such an extent that it will tighten your adductors. For this reason, inward rotation of the femurs is preferred, and it should be replaced with squeezing the knees together only if it has failed to achieve its objective.

Vinyasa Eight

Exhaling, extend your arms over your head, and arch backward, keeping your arms straight and hands shoulder-width apart. Let the backbend start from the uppermost thoracic vertebrae. Imagine that you are arching back over a bar that extends across your upper back, behind your shoulder blades, rather than behind your low back. This will help you to distribute as much of the backbend as possible through your thorax, where you are armored and need to open, instead of your low back, where you are soft and unprotected. Observe the weight distribution in your legs. Notice that with the weight distributed forward toward the knees, the stretch is taken further up the spine. As you take the weight back toward the feet, the stretch moves down to the low back. In this way, shift your weight to accentuate the stretch in areas of tightness. Draw your shoulder blades down your back, and as you arch backward, lift your heart up toward the ceiling to increase your back arch. Strongly use your abdominal muscles to keep space between the spinous processes of the lumbar vertebrae to create more length in the spine, allowing you to arch back further. Use both the abdominal muscles and the lifting of the heart up toward the ceiling to lengthen through your low back.

As your head and arms travel backward, let the pelvis draw forward. Let this movement come from the front of the pelvic bone rather than from the pubic bone. Use the drawing forward of the anterior superior iliac spines of the ileum, rather than the pubic bone, to stretch the quads.

As your pelvis draws forward and your hands come closer to the floor, continue to lift your heart to the ceiling, creating more space beneath you. Continue to draw the anterior aspects of all vertebrae apart from one another, drawing the spine as long as possible. Ideally, of course, you would perform all of this on one exhalation. If this is not possible, take as much time as necessary to study the movement closely and to experience and feel all aspects of the movement. There is an entire universe in this movement. If you hurry through it, you will not awaken your spine properly. Depending on your muscle tone, it might be necessary to hang in the posture with straight arms parallel to the floor, pointing to the back end of the mat for several breaths, until you have isolated all individual functions and awakened your chest. Take that time. Once you have understood the posture, perform it in one breath, returning to the original vinyasa count of the Rishi Vamana.

Once your hands touch the floor, walk them in a little toward your feet. Now attempt to extend the arms to further open the chest and armpits. Reach your elbows toward the floor and walk your hands in to reach your feet. If you find that challenging, try walking one hand in a little and then the other, repeating until you reach your limit. Rather than lifting your entire hand off the floor, creep along the mat with your fingers, as a caterpillar would move: place your fingertips firmly on the floor, lift the heels of your hands off, flex your hand, and place the heel of your hand down close to your fingers; then lift the fingertips off, extend the fingers, and place the fingertips down closer to your toes. This way you will never lose traction on the floor. If you are slipping and don't get in closer, the fabric of your mat may not be suitable. If necessary, use a mat that provides more traction.

Once you reach your feet, don't make the mistake of walking up your soles. Instead, walk with your hands around the outsides of your feet. If this is too difficult, place your feet slightly closer together. Once you reach the limit of your flexibility, walk your hands inward to get hold of your feet, heels, or even ankles. Ground your elbows and forearms firmly into the floor.

While you breathe deeply, think of the inhale as gently extending (arching) your thoracic spine, while the exhale lightly extends your lumbar spine. Even when you stand upright, breathing will always result in a gentle resonance frequency going up and down your spine, which is a sign of spinal health. In Kapotasana, use this tendency to exaggerate the arch in your upper back during inhalation and your low back during exhalation. Over time, using this method creatively will get you much deeper into your backbend.

Gaze toward the nose and take five deep breaths in *Kapotasana* A.

If you are very flexible in backbending, try to go to your heels or ankles directly without touching your hands to the floor. To do that, hang in the backbend until you gain maximum arch. Let your hands hover next to your ears. Then reach for your heels in a rapid movement. Do this first one arm at a time, in which case you need to be careful to not twist your spine in the course of the movement. As mentioned earlier, you should never combine backbending and twisting, especially during dynamic movements. Once you have learned the movement one hand at a time, practice it with both hands at once.

Still in *vinyasa* eight, inhale and let go of your

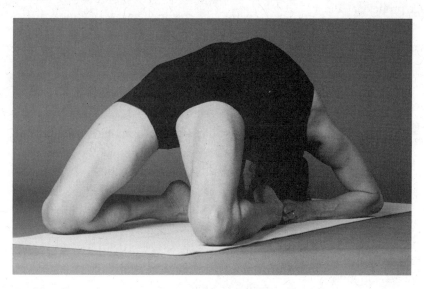

Kapotasana A

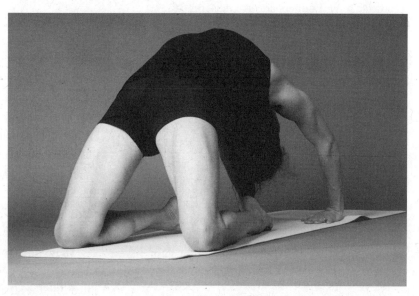

Kapotasana B

feet. If you need to, walk your hands out slightly, but the further you get away from your feet, the less deep the ensuing *Kapotasana B* will be. *Kapotasana B* is a more advanced and more intense version than A. However, if you walk your hands out too much, it will be less intense.[14] Place your hands firmly on the floor, shoulder-width apart, fingers pointing toward your knees, and straighten your arms. Look toward your nose and hold *Kapotasana B* for five breaths. Place even more emphasis on opening the chest than in the A version.

The method described thus far is suitable for most students who are new to the Intermediate Series and those who are of average proficiency in backbending. Typically this method will allow you, after due practice, to clasp your toes or even the balls of your feet with both hands, which is a sufficient proficiency for this series.

If you are comfortable with deep backbends and want to prepare for the much deeper backbends of the advanced sequences, you will need to add an additional element to the posture, which is the nutation of the sacroiliac (SI) joints. It is recommended that you stay away from consciously altering the position of your sacrum in the first two years of yoga practice (there are enough other valuable things to work on), or if you have any form of discomfort in the sacral or SI joint area. In those cases it is wise to let the sacrum take the position it would take without conscious interference.

If you want to add the additional approximately five degrees that sacrum nutation offers and are proficient in all postures of the Intermediate Series, including the leg-behind-head and strength postures, then study the information on pages 65–68 pertaining to the sacroiliac joints closely before you proceed. The information described therein is an analysis of what a "natural backbender" will automatically do when performing postures like *Kapotasana* or other difficult backbends.

Next we describe the advanced method of

backbending in *Kapotasana*. The added five to ten degrees of nutation at the sacrum may make the difference between reaching the feet and reaching the heels or ankles in *Kapotasana*.

Vinyasa Count — Advanced Version

Vinyasa Seven

Inhaling, jump forward to a kneeling position with your torso upright and your hands on your hips.

Stabilize your pelvic bowl by slightly engaging your hamstrings. This will counteract the hip-flexing tendency of the psoas.

Reduce the tension in your rectus abdominis (abs) to permit the ensuing increase of lumbar arch. It is now evident why this is an advanced method; we recommend that primary and intermediate students use the full force of their rectus abdominis to take the extension out of the lumbar spine and carry it into the chest and the quads.

Engage your psoas and draw the upper, frontal rim of the sacrum, called the promontory, into nutation. Richard Freeman refers to this action as creating a slight suction in the cave of the sacrum. He locates the cave of the sacrum anterior to the sacrum in the space formed by its kyphotic shape. We can identify the cave of the sacrum as the gross equivalent of the storage location of *kundalini* energy in the subtle body; this is why the sacrum is known as the sacred bone.

Increase your nutation by strongly engaging *Uddiyana Bandha*, thus drawing your anterior superior iliac spines toward each other. At the same time, spread your sit bones, meaning draw the ischia apart from each other. If you previously squeezed your knees together or squeezed an imagined or real block between your thighs, you will need to leave this technique behind now, as it draws the ischia together and the anterior superior iliac spines (ASISs) apart and thus prevents nutation of the sacrum. Replace squeezing the thighs together with internally rotating the thighbones.

These three movements — nutation of the sacrum, drawing the ASISs toward each other, and spreading the sit bones — are really only one movement that we approach in three different ways.

---

14 One can entirely take out the intensity by walking the hands out further (which is not suggested). In other words, some students will think, "More intense? What are you talking about?" They are the ones who walk out their hands too far.

It is helpful, however, to consciously do them consecutively.

Do not mistake the engaging of the psoas with tilting the pelvis forward. The pelvis is fixed in space by the remaining tension in the rectus abdominis, the hamstrings, and of course the quadriceps, quadratus lumborum, and others. If you were to tilt your pelvis forward, letting it follow the movement of the sacrum, you would then counter-nutate your sacrum.

Vinyasa Eight

Once your sacrum is fully nutated, arch the entire rest of the spine as described in the version for intermediate students. Exhaling, take your arms overhead and begin to arch backward toward the floor. Do this ever so slowly, and use the character of the exhalation to increase the extension in your low back.

Keep monitoring the tension in your rectus abdominis, and slowly eccentrically lengthen both the rectus and psoas muscles. As the backbend deepens, it will feel as if your spine is wholly suspended by the psoas.

As you proceed to arch further into *Kapotasana*, keep releasing your gluteus maximus (buttocks). Clenching it has the tendency to draw the ischia together and the ilia apart by externally rotating your thighbones, thus encouraging counter-nutation.

Keep also releasing the adductors (insides of the thighs). The largest adductor (adductor magnus) inserts on the femur and originates on (apart from the pubic bone) the ischium. Engaging it will draw the ischia together and produce counter-nutation. Most of the adductors also laterally rotate the femurs (thighbones); their engagement, too, tends to draw the ischia together.

The only adductor of use for us here is the gracilis, which originates at the pubic bone and medially (inwardly) rotates the femur. Maintain medial rotation of the femur by lightly engaging the tensor fascia latae (a hip flexor) and semitendinosus and semimembranosus (two hamstrings).

Depending on your level of flexibility, place your hands on the floor, walk around the outsides of your feet to your limit and then reach in to take your heels, or take your heels one at a time while you hang in midair. If this is your method, take care to laterally twist the spine as little as possible. Even an

ever-so-slight scoliosis will come with vertebrae that are extended, rotated, and flexed laterally at the same time. If you perform a vigorous movement in the direction of an already existing pattern, you might entrench your pattern further, setting the foundation for trouble to come.

Use your inhalations to further open your low back and your exhalations to open your chest more. A student who has naturally less open shoulders or chest can walk the hands toward the feet as close as possible, then straighten out the arms (*Kapotasana* B position) for a moment, maintain the height gained, and again walk the hands in toward the feet.

Stay in *Kapotasana* A for five breaths and gaze toward your nose.

Inhaling, let go of your feet, walk your hands out slightly, place your hands firmly on the floor shoulder-width apart, fingers pointing toward your knees, and straighten your arms. The less you walk your hands out, the more opening you will demand of the trunk and shoulders. Look toward your nose and hold *Kapotasana* B for five breaths.

Vinyasa Nine (for both intermediate and advanced methods)

Inhaling, engage your quads and come up on your knees again. Coming out of the backbend, reverse the movement that got you into it. Start from the pelvis and let the movement travel in a wavelike motion up the spine, and lift the head last.

If you find it difficult to come up that way, bend your arms slightly and, inhaling, push off the floor to come up with momentum. Keep your arms straight and over your head as you push your pelvic bone (again, not the pubic bone) forward during the upward movement to maintain your backbend as you come up.

At the end of the inhalation, place your hands on your hips.

Exhaling, place the hands down on the floor on either side of your knees. Don't place your hands too far forward, as you will use your legs too much in the subsequent jump-up.

Vinyasa Ten

Inhaling, lift up into an arm balance with your feet way off the ground and your arms straight. Hold

123

this *vinyasa* for the duration of the inhalation. This is important to counteract the backbend.

Vinyasa Eleven
Exhaling, float back into *Chaturanga Dandasana*.

Vinyasa Twelve
Inhale into Upward Dog.

Vinyasa Thirteen
Exhale into Downward Dog.

Supta Vajrasana
RECLINING THUNDERBOLT POSTURE

Drishti Nose

PREREQUISITE: Reaching your toes in *Kapotasana* without the help of the teacher. Do not start performing *Supta Vajrasana* before you have properly learned *Kapotasana*. Use all your energy first to learn *Kapotasana* properly.

OVERVIEW: *Supta Vajrasana* combines the back-bend movement of *Kapotasana* with a full lotus position. At this point all the lessons learned in the Primary Series will pay off, or lack thereof will show up. Unless one is constitutionally very flexible or lean, one will not get past this point without the internal rotation pattern of the femur learned in the Primary Series. *Supta Vajrasana* directs the intensity of the backbend into the lotus position and opens it further. It functions as a warm-up for the more challenging lotus and half-lotus postures later in the sequence, and chiefly for *Karandavasana*.

Vinyasa Count
Vinyasa Seven
Inhaling, jump through to *Dandasana*.

Vinyasa Eight
Exhaling, fold into *Padmasana*, placing the right leg first and then the left leg on top.

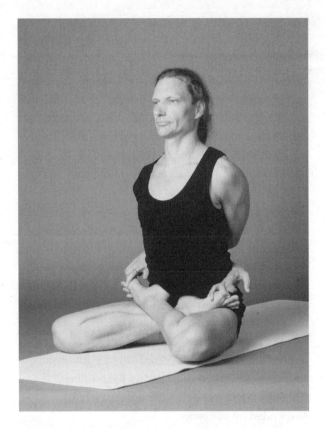

Baddha Padmasana

OBSTACLES TO BINDING IN *SUPTA VAJRASANA*

If binding is difficult, try the following:

- Stretch your pectoralis minor and major muscles regularly or get the teacher to stretch them while you are in the posture by drawing your arm backward. This will bring your hands closer to your feet.
- Draw your feet higher up into the groin by internally rotating your femurs more and by bringing the knees closer together. This will bring your toes closer to your hands.
- Place the right elbow over the left one. If that doesn't work, spray your elbows and forearms with water so that the elbows can slide over each other.
- Dispose of excess adipose tissue on your waist.

Reach around and bind the foot on top first. In our case, usually the left foot is on top, so we reach around and bind with the left arm first. Then reach

PLACING THE RIGHT LEG FIRST INTO LOTUS

As stated already in *Ashtanga Yoga: Practice and Philosophy*, the reason to place the right leg into lotus first is to accommodate the asymmetry of the abdominal cavity. According to Yoga Shastra, placing the right leg first into *Padmasana* and the left leg on top purifies liver and spleen, while placing the left leg first does not produce any desirable result. *Padmasana* right-side-first is also thought to stimulate insulin production.

Pranayama techniques involving *kumbhaka* (breath retention) and alternate nostril breathing generally start with the first *kumbhaka* after an inhalation through *surya*, the right nostril. The reason this is done is that the *surya nadi*, which powers the solar mind, promotes structured learning, refining, controlling, achieving, and perfecting. This also means, for example, that you will memorize more details when reading a textbook when breathing through your right nostril. A more intuitive form of learning (which won't get you far when going to university) or visionary insight is possible when breathing through *ida*, the left nostril, which powers the lunar mind.

A similar relationship exists not only for the breath but also for the body. As *pranayama* is generally started with the right nostril, so is *asana* generally done on the right side first,[15] which is also reflected in placing the right leg into *Padmasana* first.

One might think that doing all lotus postures with the right side first could have an adverse effect on the balance of the hips, leading to a permanently torqued pelvis. It appears, though, that this effect is counteracted by the leg-behind-head postures such as *Supta Kurmasana* in the Primary Series and *Dvipada Shirshasana* in the Intermediate Series, in which the left leg is placed in position first. Evidence supports the conclusion that students who practice a complete Primary or Intermediate Series seem to not be harrowed by pelvic imbalance.[16] The situation appears to be different with those students who stay at *Supta Vajrasana* for a very long time without mastering this posture. They thereby do not receive the next postures from their teachers and do not progress to the safety of the hip-balancing *Dvipada Shirshasana* and *Yoganidrasana*.

If you belong to this group, there might be ground to do the lotus postures on one day with your right leg first and on the next day with your left leg first. Another option would be to get your teacher to select some lotus postures in your practice that you could do with the left side first. Once you have progressed to intermediate leg-behind-head postures, I suggest going back to doing *Padmasana* exclusively with the right leg first. The only time my pelvis was torqued was when I sat for long periods of *pranayama* in *Padmasana* with my right leg first, while at the same time my intermediate leg-behind-head postures were disabled through a shoulder problem. I solved the problem by sitting not in *Padmasana* but rather in *Siddhasana* during my *pranayama*.

around with your right arm, placing the right arm on top of the left one, and bind the right big toe.

Holding on to both big toes, you are now in *Baddha Padmasana*. *Supta Vajrasana* is a backbend in *Baddha Padmasana*.

Inhaling, lift your chest and arch your back. The

same principles apply here as in *Kapotasana*. Let the arch commence from your T1 vertebra, and from there let it travel down the spine in a wavelike motion.[17] Let your clavicles curl back over your shoulders as if wanting to meet your shoulder blades. Draw your shoulder blades down your back and wrap your chest back over them. As you arch back, attempt to cross your elbows past each other. Imagine that you are arching back over a bar that extends right behind your shoulder blades. Expand

15 There are exceptions, such as *Pashasana* and two-sided leg-behind-head postures, in which you place your left leg first.
16 Apart from those who continue to drink coffee. Coffee is a stimulant that mobilizes and expels *prana* that otherwise is used to stabilize the pelvis. This is not a moralistic statement but is based on observation. Over the years, most of my students who had a tendency to have a twisted or imbalanced pelvis were those who insisted on continuing their coffee habit. Decaffeinated coffee or tea does not appear to have the same destabilizing effect.

17 We don't start from the cervical spine as it is too soft and lends itself too easily to extension. It will automatically emulate the backward arch attempted in the thoracic spine and usually too much so.

the front of your chest by stretching your intercostals. Rather than just folding your pelvis back, drop your pubic bone down together with the coccyx and lift the ASISs upward rather than letting them drop backward. Keep extending out of the top of the back of the head to transfer the stretch from the cervical spine into the thoracic spine, maximizing back arch.

Vinyasa Nine

The ideal scenario is described first and then a more beginner-friendly version is introduced.

Exhaling, arch back and place the crown of your head on the floor behind you. Attempt to touch the crown of your head as close to your buttocks as possible. To prevent landing with a thud, fade the movement out by lifting your knees off the floor. Once your head is down, place your knees back down. Stay for five breaths and look toward the nose.

Inhaling, lift your knees off the floor with a rapid movement, then flex your hip joints to lift your head off the floor. Once your chest is up, place your knees back down on the floor.

This version takes a lot of flexibility. If you are not yet flexible enough, ask the teacher to place his or her legs over your knees, or if you practice alone, stick your knees under a sofa.

If your teacher keeps your knees in position, check first whether both knees are on the floor while sitting in *Padmasana*. If one knee is airborne, place a

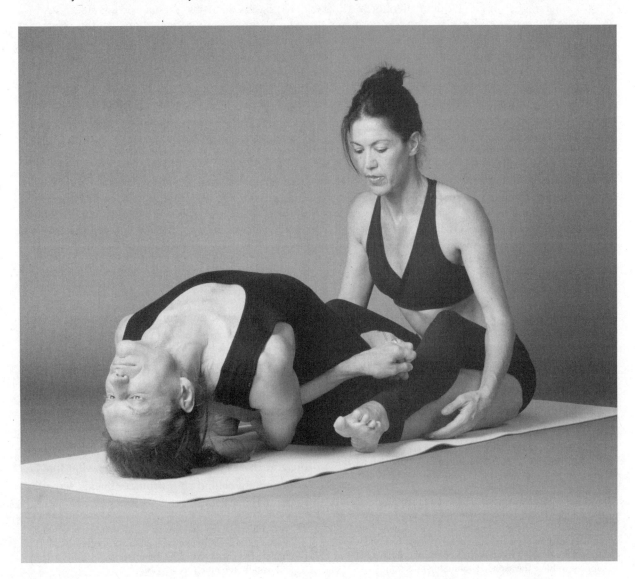

Supta Vajrasana

126

folded towel under it, so that when the teacher places his or her legs on top of yours, your knee is not pressed down to the floor. If you can't get your knee down by yourself while in lotus or half-lotus using your leg muscles only, do not allow someone else to press it down. The pressing down of the knee will result in unwanted friction in the knee or your opposite buttock will lift off, in which case the pelvis can become torqued.

Once your knees are securely in place, start arching back. If your hands start to slip, use some rough cotton cloth to keep your toes bound. In no case are you to let go of your hands. If you let go, you are not doing *Supta Vajrasana* but only *Matsyasana* (counter-posture for shoulder stand in the finishing sequence). Part of the journey of *Supta Vajrasana* is to strengthen your hands enough for the advanced arm balances. If you let go, the energy cycle will be interrupted and the posture rendered useless. Instead, arch back only to an extent where you still can hold on, and then come back up even if your head does not reach the floor. Reaching the floor is not the defining element; bending back in *Baddha Padmasana* is the defining element. If you let go of your feet, you are no longer bound (*baddha*) and you are doing *Matsyasana*, which is part of the finishing series and not the Intermediate Series. Go to your limit of flexibility, and if possible rest your head on the floor for five breaths. As you arch back, hold on to your toes and draw your feet further up into the groin while bringing your knees closer together and internally rotating the thighbones. A great part of *Supta Vajrasana*'s effectiveness lies in its ability to open your lotus further by rapidly switching between internal and external rotation of your thighbones.

Inhaling, come up, and exhaling, place your head back down. If you cannot perform the final version of *Supta Vajrasana*, for training purposes you can repeat this movement four more times synchronized dynamically with the breath, using a significant amount of momentum.

The purpose of this sequence within *vinyasa* nine is to emphasize femur rotation. Apart from arching the back and strengthening the hands, the other theme of *Supta Vajrasana* is to improve the lotus by leading us deeper into femur rotation. It is an expansion of the material covered in the Primary Series, and once we reach *Karandavasana*, we need to be proficient in femur rotation. In other words, it needs to either happen here and now or it never will. As you lower your head down and arch back, you need to internally rotate your femurs (thighbones), which will let your feet slide higher up into the groin and thereby move closer to your hands. As you lift your torso and come up, you need to externally rotate your femurs. The more you can rotate, the more open the lotus becomes. Eventually, with sufficient external rotation, one could potentially slide into lotus position in midair. The flexibility you gain here will be instrumental in properly performing postures such as *Mulabandhasana* (the most extreme internal hip rotation) and *Kandasana* (the most extreme external hip rotation) later on. Both these postures are used to trigger the rising of *kundalini*, to which extreme movements of the femur seem to be linked.

On the fifth exhalation, keep your head on the floor for another five breaths.

Inhaling, come up and place your hands on the floor on either side of your thighs.

Advanced practitioners may use the nutation of the sacrum described here also in *Supta Vajrasana* to increase back arch.

Vinyasa Ten
Inhaling, lift off the floor.

Vinyasa Eleven
Slide out of *Padmasana* in midair and float back into *Chaturanga Dandasana*. This movement was described in *Ashtanga Yoga: Practice and Philosophy* (pp. 98–99) and is not covered here in detail. Perform this movement only if you do not suffer from a knee condition such as a cruciate or collateral ligament sprain or menisci tears. If any knee pain is present, simply sit on the floor, gently fold out of lotus, and jump back.

Vinyasa Twelve
Inhale into Upward Dog.

Vinyasa Thirteen
Exhale into Downward Dog.

SECOND CONNECTIVE SECTION

This second connective section consists of three postures: *Bakasana*, which is an *apanic* (energetic downward flow) strength posture, and two twists, *Bharadvajasana* and *Ardha Matsyendrasana*. This section separates the backbend sequence from the leg-behind-head sequence. Remember that the only leg-behind-head posture in the Primary Series was introduced by a nearly identical section (two twists and two strength postures), whereas in the Advanced A Series, arm balances and backbends are separated by a section of advanced twists and *apanic* strength postures.

Bakasana counteracts the backbend sequence and has a similar *apanic* effect to *Pashasana*, which came before the backbend sequence. Through its kyphotic strength, it takes any excess backbend out of the low back and ignites the *bandhas* for the upcoming leg-behind-head sequence. Twists are the ideal link between backbends and leg-behind-head postures as they contain *pranic*-lordotic elements (as with backbends) and *apanic*-kyphotic elements (as with leg-behind-head postures).

Bakasana

CRANE POSTURE

Drishti Nose

OVERVIEW: *Bakasana* is an important counter-posture to the just completed backbending sequence. It activates your trunk flexors and counteracts excessive back extension. It also sets the tone and prepares for the upcoming leg-behind-head sequence.

Vinyasa Count — A Version

Vinyasa Seven
Inhaling, jump forward into a semi-squat with your feet landing just in front of your hands. Bend your arms and, going up onto your toes, place your knees up into your armpits. Make sure that you use the fronts of your knees rather than your shins and that you place them all the way up into the armpits rather than halfway down on the arms. The feeling is more of wrapping the arms around the knees as opposed to climbing the knees up onto the arms. This action will activate the shoulder-stabilizing muscles and provide strong support for this arm-balancing posture. Because you lift your entire body weight with your shoulder and arm muscles, the stabilization of the shoulder joint is essential. Draw the shoulder blades toward each other, draw them down the back, and suck them onto the back of the chest. These actions engage the shoulder-stabilizing muscles, the rhomboids and middle trapezius, the lower trapezius and latissimus dorsi, and the serratus anterior and subscapularis, respectively. Make sure that you consciously engage those muscles a split second before your shoulders bear weight. Do not expect that they will work miraculously or through divine intervention. Take responsibility for your shoulders. If you do not use these stabilizing muscles enough, you are likely to develop a front/back imbalance — that is, you will use the pectoralis muscles too much. Doing so may lead to shoulder injuries, as covered in detail on pages 74–77.

Still inhaling, shift your weight forward toward the roots of your fingers, and lift your feet off. Touch your big toes together and tuck up your heels tight under your sit bones. Now straighten your arms and, using breath and *bandhas*, lift your sit bones as high as you can. This movement strongly relies on the anterior deltoid, latissimus dorsi, and lower trapezius muscles. It improves your ability to anchor and stabilize the shoulder blades on the back.

To lift your sit bones that high while keeping the knees in the armpits takes a considerable amount of trunk flexion. You will need to develop your abdominal muscles here, which will also benefit your jump-backs and jump-throughs. You will be

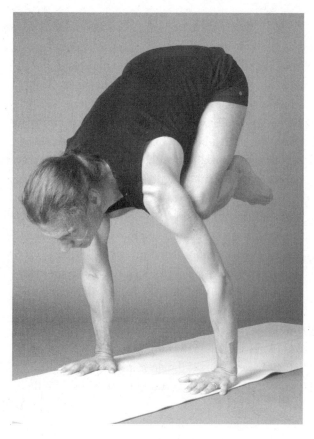

Bakasana

surprised how beneficial the effect of this posture is if you lift high and straighten your arms.

Hold *Bakasana* A for five breaths and look toward your nose.

Vinyasa **Eight**

While inhaling, lift your knees even higher up your arms, if possible.

Exhaling, float back into *Chaturanga Dandasana*.

Vinyasa **Nine**

Inhale into Upward Dog.

Vinyasa **Ten**

Exhale into Downward Dog.

Vinyasa **Count — B Version**

Vinyasa **Seven**

Inhaling, jump forward and, without touching the floor, land straight with your knees in your armpits. The synchronization of breath and movement is important here. In Downward Dog, bend your legs

with the exhalation and jump with the beginning of the inhalation. Aim the fronts of your knees right at your armpits, and do not just land with your shins on your arms. Land in the middle of your inhalation, with your arms bent slightly as you land. Imagine that the inhalation creates a vacuum in your armpits into which the knees get sucked. With the remainder of the inhalation, intensify that suction, straighten your arms, and lift as high as possible. The most common reason one does not achieve this important transition is that the inhalation is completed before one lands on the arms. Land with your lungs still half-empty; otherwise, your puffed-up chest will be in the way, and you will not be able to utilize the elevating quality of the inhalation upon landing.

This is a very important posture and should not be treated lightly. If your feet keep touching down, you have not developed adequate shoulder, abdominal, and/or *bandha* control. You also need to make sure that you jump not forward but rather up, as if you were jumping into a handstand. Focus on the trajectory that your sit bones make and not that of your feet. First go way up, and only after your sit bones are almost over your hands, consider landing. At this point you bring trunk flexion into play, which sucks your knees, thighs, and feet toward your abdomen. In other words, the landing is not a function of gravity or dropping down but of shoulder and abdominal strength. As soon as you hand the landing over to gravity, you will do nothing but drop down.

Another cause of failing to keep the feet off the floor is carrying the weight too far back in your hands upon landing in your armpits. In the moment of landing, you need to carry the weight somewhere between your fingertips and the roots of your fingers. You fade out the movement by pressing your fingertips firmly into the ground. You will be able to do that if you exercise your hands strongly in postures like *Bhekasana* and *Supta Vajrasana*. If you hold your weight between the heels of your hands and the roots of your fingers, you will fall backward and touch your feet down. Bringing your weight forward can produce the fear of falling forward. If you feel that you are about to fall, rapidly bend your elbows backward to drop your sit bones and place the crown of your head or forehead down as in *Bhujapidasana* rather than landing disgracefully on your face.

You will also make this transition more easily if you initially choose a short stance in Downward Dog. This will make the jumping and catching of your weight less risky. After you have learned the transition with a short Downward Dog, slowly extend your stance.

You may also temporarily abandon the official focal point of the nose with a temporary practice *drishti*. Look toward a point on the mat that is about twelve inches (thirty centimeters) in front of your hands. If you tend to fall back to your feet after landing on your arms, then shift your gaze forward a couple of inches (about five centimeters) more and try again. The more you lift your gaze, the more your weight will distribute from the heels of your hands toward your fingertips, thus making it more likely that you will catch and balance your weight upon landing.

If after all attempts you can't shift the weight forward in your hands, you might need some extra training for your hands and deltoid muscles.

Do not go on to the next posture before you have learned this important transition.

Vinyasa Eight
Inhaling, lift up and off your arms.
Exhaling, float back into *Chaturanga Dandasana*.

Vinyasa Nine
Inhale into Upward Dog.

Vinyasa Ten
Exhale into Downward Dog.

Bharadvajasana
POSTURE DEDICATED TO RISHI BHARADVAJA
Drishti To the side

OVERVIEW: *Bharadvajasana* is a twist that at face value is no more difficult than the twists in the Primary Series. It separates the backbends from the leg-behind-head postures and arm balances that follow.

Vinyasa Count
Vinyasa Seven
Inhaling, jump through to *Dandasana* and fold the left leg back, the front edge of the tibia (shinbone) facing straight down, as if you were doing *Krounchasana* or *Triang Mukha Ekapada Pashimottanasana*. You may also fold your left leg back in midair as described under *Krounchasana*. Sit down with your folded left leg parallel to the straight right leg.

Vinyasa Eight
Exhaling, place your right leg into half-lotus, using the safety precautions listed in *Ashtanga Yoga: Practice and Philosophy* (p. 55). Draw your right knee out to the right, forming a 90-degree angle between both thighs. Place your left hand, palm facing down and fingers pointing to your left knee, under your right knee and start twisting to the right. Let your left sit bone come off the floor if necessary. With your right arm, reach around your back and bind your right big toe.

Firmly ground your left hand, which will draw your left shoulder out to the right. Use your right arm, bound to your big toe, to draw your right shoulder around your back and out to the left. Continue to twist as you breathe, and work on grounding your left sit bone.

Rotate your left thigh externally to ground the left sit bone. Rotate your right thigh (the one in half-lotus) internally and let the thighbone reach out of the hip socket to release your adductor muscles. Novices to lotus postures often suck the thigh into the hip as a reflex action. This, however, tightens the adductors and decreases your lotus flexibility. The failure to overcome this reflex often forms the beginning of a history of knee problems. To overcome this reflex, let your thighbones reach out of the hip sockets in all lotus and half-lotus postures.

Look over your right shoulder and breathe deeply, allowing the diaphragm to descend down from the chest, broadening the ribs. Use the exhalation to grow tall and allow your spine to spiral around to the right. Draw your shoulder blades down your back, extend out of the crown of your head, with your chin dropped, and ground your sit bones.

ACTIVE RELEASE TECHNIQUE: Your primary effort in this posture is to work your arms to get deeper into the twist. Do this until you have reached your maximum twist, maintaining a level of sensibility and without resorting to crude strength. Alongside that strong primary effort of twisting, a slightly weaker secondary effort consists of using your trunk muscles to counteract the effort of the arms. While your arms twist your trunk to the right, let the trunk muscles attempt to twist back to the left as if you were trying to exit the posture. The trunk muscles will now be eccentrically lengthened, and your twist will deepen.

Take five breaths and look over your right shoulder. Exhaling, swing around and place your hands down on either side of your legs, ready to lift off. You may jump straight out of the posture.

CONTRAINDICATIONS: First, if you feel discomfort in your knee, straighten your right leg and jump back as done in *Krounchasana*. Second, if there is the smallest amount of doubt that you have built up a level of strength equivalent to your current flexibility, straighten both your legs into *Dandasana*, ready for a normal jump-back as done in the Primary Series, without touching the feet to the

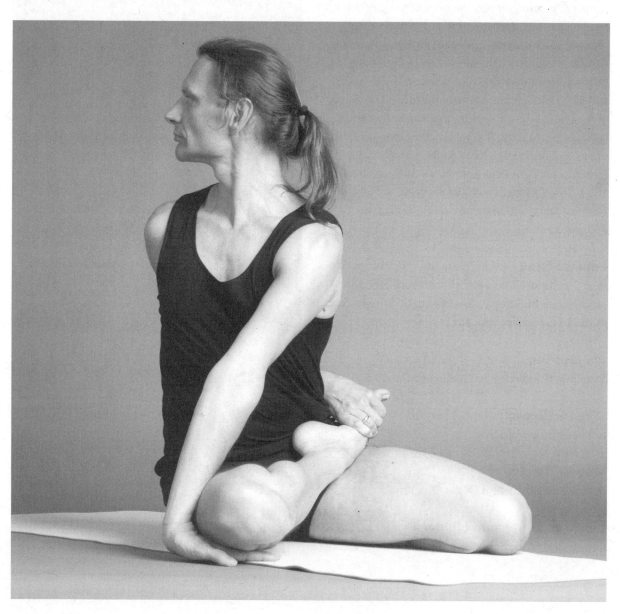

Bharadvajasana

floor. I particularly recommend this movement to females. Put effort into establishing a balance between strength and flexibility. Do not chase excessive flexibility, especially for the purpose of looking good in the postures. Excessive flexibility leads to instability and may be much harder to rectify than excessive stiffness. Without the necessary stability, recurring back pain can become an obstacle to consistent practice.

If you jump straight out of the posture, you can cheat by pushing off with your left foot, which will result in insufficient exercise for your abdominal muscles. You can use this shortcut if you are already sufficiently strong. If not, this way of jumping back results in a slow decrease of strength during the years of practicing the Intermediate Series, since you will have to practice the more strength-building Primary Series only once per week once you have added on enough intermediate postures. This is one of the major traps of the Intermediate Series, and it needs to be avoided. If you lose core strength, practice of the Intermediate Series will lead you, from a yogic perspective, down a dead-end street. If you balance strength with flexibility, your body will show its appreciation by providing decades of dedicated service.

Vinyasa Nine
Inhaling, lift up into *Lollasana* with your feet clearly off the floor. Build up extra strength by lifting a few millimeters higher every day.

Vinyasa Ten
Exhaling, float back into *Chaturanga Dandasana*.

Vinyasa Eleven
Inhale into Upward Dog.

Vinyasa Twelve
Exhale into Downward Dog.

Vinyasas Thirteen to Eighteen
Repeat *Bharadvajasana* on the left side.

Ardha Matsyendrasana
POSTURE DEDICATED TO MATSYENDRANATH, HALF-VERSION
Drishti Side

OVERVIEW: *Ardha Matsyendrasana* is an easy version of a difficult posture that occurs in the Advanced A Series. Its purpose here is not to challenge the yogi but to connect and separate[18] the backbends from the

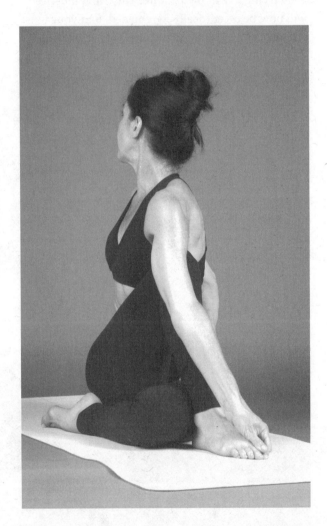

Ardha Matsyendrasana

18 Only what is separate can be connected. The embracing and thus resolving of paradoxes such as this is an integral part of yoga.

leg-behind-head postures and to create some nonintensive downtime before the next difficult posture is undertaken.

CONTRAINDICATION: If you have scoliosis you will notice that twisting in one direction is easier than the other. The angles of the facet joints mean that rotation will accompany the lateral curve of a scoliosis, the whole spine forming a spiral that adds immense strength to an otherwise stressed structure. Rather than twist to the end range of your predominately flexible side, work only on increasing flexibility on the side with less rotation to inspire a better balance. In other words, take care to not drive yourself deeper into your tendency, but rather aim at counteracting it.

Vinyasa Count

Vinyasa Seven
Inhaling, jump through to *Dandasana*.

Vinyasa Eight
Exhaling, bend both legs, lifting the knees off the floor. Place the left foot outside of the right buttock and the left knee on the floor in front of you, so that your knee points straight ahead. Draw the right hip back, unsquaring the hips, as when attempting to bring both hip joints in line with the left knee. Point (plantar flex) your left foot and keep the toes close to your right buttock. Do not assist the balancing in the posture by flexing (dorsi flexing) this foot. Place the right foot outside of your left thigh with the knee pointing up to the ceiling.

Twist to the right, and place your left shoulder outside of your right knee. Take the inside of your right foot and the big toe with your left hand. Rotate your humerus (arm bone) internally so that the elbow faces outward, away from your leg. If you have the crease of your elbow facing outward, pressure will be added to your elbow, tending to hyperextend it.

Reach around your back with your right arm and take hold of your left thigh. Draw the right sit bone down toward the floor and continue to twist as you breathe. Draw your shoulder blades down your back as you lift your heart and the back of your head up to the ceiling.

Bring the back of your head in line with your spine; don't let your chin jut forward.

Let your spine grow long by reaching the top of your head and your sit bones in opposite directions. Use the strength of your arms to move deeper into the twist.

Gaze over your right shoulder and take five breaths.

ACTIVE RELEASE TECHNIQUE: We employ the same technique as in *Bharadvajasana*. Engage your trunk muscles gently in a secondary effort, as if you were trying to get out of the twist, but counteract this with an even stronger primary effort of your arms. Your trunk muscles will eccentrically lengthen and you will be able to work deeper into the twist.

Exhaling, swing around and place your hands down on either side, ready to lift off. Again, you may jump straight out of the posture or transit through *Dandasana*, attempting to clear the floor with your feet.

Vinyasa Nine
Inhaling, press up into an arm balance and hover there for the remainder of the inhalation.

Vinyasa Ten
Exhaling, float back into *Chaturanga Dandasana*.

Vinyasa Eleven
Inhale into Upward Dog.

Vinyasa Twelve
Exhale into Downward Dog.

Vinyasas Thirteen to Eighteen
Repeat *Ardha Matsyendrasana* on the left side.

LEG-BEHIND-HEAD SEQUENCE

Leg-behind-head postures, the second essential sequence of the active element, are some of the most important, effective, and beneficial yoga postures. Their importance is reflected in the fact that each progressive Ashtanga Vinyasa Series contains more leg-behind-head postures than does the previous one. Whereas the Primary Series contains only one leg-behind-head posture, the Intermediate Series increases the number to three, the Advanced A Series has six, and the Advanced B Series contains an unprecedented eight leg-behind-head postures — a third of the entire series.

The purpose of all leg-behind-head postures is first to open the hip joints and then to strengthen the spine and the chest. All this can be done without any adverse effects if we analyze the posture and proceed cautiously but steadily. If we proceed with undue haste and without understanding the underlying anatomy, we might fall back and progress much more slowly in the long term. Nearly all difficult postures can be mastered if they are precisely broken down into their constituent phases, as discussed later in this section.

Leg-behind-head postures open the hip joints, a process that continues in the Advanced Series through the extreme hip rotations. This process releases life force from its reservoir at the base of the spine, its ascent leading to divine involution.[19]

Leg-behind-head postures are also instrumental in developing the organs of the thoracic cavity (that is, the heart and the lungs); they make the rib cage strong and supple through the weight and pneumatic pressure that they apply.

Finally, together with backbending, leg-behind-head postures return the spine to a state of vibrancy and fluidity, so that it may be the pathway for the ascent of Shakti. During backbending, the spine is extended, but in a deep, advanced backbend the trunk extensors need to be released, and it is the trunk flexors that open the backbend more deeply. Leg-behind-head postures are the counter-postures to intermediate and advanced backbends. Unless a student is extremely flexible, his or her spine will be in flexion. However, the correct action in these postures is to use the back and neck extensors to return the spine to a neutral or upright position against the weight of the leg being carried behind the head. This makes leg-behind-head postures an important training for trunk extensor muscles.

In addition to trunk and neck extension against resistance, the other important action in leg-behind-head postures is the support from the abdominal cavity. Having supported from below with *Mula Bandha*, we now bear downward with the respiratory diaphragm and inward with the abdominal muscles. The result is a strong increase in intra-abdominal pressure that will protect the low back when all exercises up to this point are performed to a satisfactory level.

Do not attempt leg-behind-head postures if your teacher does not deem you ready. If you are ready and perform these and the later, advanced leg-behind-head postures daily, you will develop abdominal muscles as strong as steel. This will ensure that your low back will always be in excellent condition. The increase in intra-abdominal pressure just mentioned massages the organs of the abdominal cavity, producing a superb fluid exchange, with stale fluid being expelled under pressure. In this way your organs are flushed and vitalized.

19 The term *evolution* comes from the Latin *evolvere*, which is *volvere*, "to roll," with the prefix *ex*, meaning "out." Evolution, or the "rolling out" of the species and the entire world of manifestation, is seen by yoga as a down-and-out process from consciousness (*sahasrara* chakra) to the earth element (*muladhara* chakra), a process during which knowledge of the divine self is lost. To regain this knowledge, the yogi lets life force ascend back up through the chakras to recognize divinity at the *sahasrara* chakra. As this in-and-up movement reverts the direction of evolution, it is called *involution*.

The dynamics between deep backbending and leg-behind-head postures, which inform the core theme of many of the Ashtanga sequences, can be called the most important and effective aspect of this *asana* practice. Since leg-behind-head is the counter and complementary theme to backbending, there should be no practice of deep backbends without a competent practice of leg-behind-head postures.

If backbending can be likened to what Freud called the "oral phase," then leg-behind-head represents the anal dimension. Freud related saying no and defining yourself by setting boundaries with contracting the anus and relating to the father. Typically, a child learns not only to willfully postpone defecation and thus become independent of diapers during the anal phase but also to define him- or herself by saying no.

While backbending stretches the front of the body (the oral orifice is located at the front) and increases our ability to say yes, leg-behind-head strengthens the back of the body (the anal orifice located at the back) and improves our ability to say no. Depending on our level of flexibility, an enormous weight might be placed on our back and shoulders. It will make our back very strong but also increase our ability to shoulder the weight of responsibility. Since we learn to erect our spine tall against resistance, leg-behind-head teaches us to stay unperturbed in the face of corrupting influences. It also teaches us to defend our rightfully held positions in life if they are under attack. Leg-behind-head generally has a "male," "manly," or heroic influence on our psyche and balances the softening, feminine influence of backbending.

As leg-behind-head forces energy downward, it improves the "down-breath," the vital air *apana*. The psychological dimension of *anal*, related to saying no, is in yogic terms powered by *apana*.

Leg-behind-head has a toning influence on the pelvic diaphragm, the muscles that form the pelvic floor. This influence is due to pneumatic pressure in the thorax and hydraulic pressure in the abdomen that occur when one places one's leg behind one's head, combined with the radical external rotation of the femur present in those postures. This theme is continued when practicing the Advanced Series with the extreme hip rotations, which are designed to access the energy reservoir at the base of the spine.

Make sure to study closely the section in chapter 6 on the hip joints and their limitations of movement (pp. 69–71) before attempting any leg-behind-head postures. Every individual is different, and the practice needs to be adapted to the needs of the individual. If your hip joints are stiff or you encounter too much resistance on the way into the posture, then practice the following set of warm-ups daily.

Warm-Ups

For some students, practicing leg-behind-head for five breaths per day on each side will not result in the opening desired. The following warm-ups are designed to speed up the opening process in leg-behind-head postures. For maximum effect, they may be included right before the leg-behind-head sequence. Do this for a limited time — that is, until you have achieved the desired effect. Although some yogis sneer at the idea of warm-ups, dismissing them as a modern flourish, performing warm-ups is preferable to desperately cranking your leg behind your head without the necessary opening and hurting yourself, particularly your intervertebral discs, in the process. If somebody suggests that maintaining a traditional practice is more important than the integrity of your spine, you would do well to question that person. Once you are able to perform the leg-behind-head postures without a warm-up, return to the traditional series as quickly as possible. If you cannot perform the warm-ups during your practice, you can do them outside of your practice. However, you need to take extra care if you do this, since you will not be warmed up from having done the first half of the series.

WARM-UP 1: Go into *Chaturanga Dandasana*, keeping your arms straight, and draw your right leg up so that your right knee is under your right shoulder and your right foot is approximately under your left shoulder. Please note that your right knee is only about 90 degrees flexed. If you flex it much more and place your foot further down under your chest or hip, it will not be a simulation of a leg-behind-head posture but instead that of a lotus posture and consequently will not contribute to your leg-behind-head flexibility. Lean forward, gently drawing both hips down toward the floor. Make sure that your hips stay square, by drawing the right hip down toward your left foot.

Continue to lean further forward, simultaneously drawing your right shoulder down on your right knee and your left shoulder down on your left foot, ideally until they touch. You don't need to use strength; instead allow gravity to draw your chest and torso down to the floor. If you feel discomfort or pain at the lateral aspect (outside) of your right knee, put more emphasis on laterally rotating your right thighbone. Your limitation in leg-behind-head might be due to an inability to effectively laterally (externally) rotate your femur. This is often the case on one side only. If you detect this, study the Primary Series postures more deeply, particularly *Triang Mukha Ekapada Pashimottanasana* and *Janushirshasana* B, that require you to laterally rotate your femur on the side where you feel knee pain.

If you are able to sufficiently laterally rotate your femur, you should be able to feel a significant sensation in your right hip joint. Hold the posture for five breaths if done during your *vinyasa* practice or several minutes if done isolated, and then repeat on the left side. Make sure that you keep your hips square at all times, being careful not to hold the pelvis in a torqued position.

WARM-UP 2: Lie on your back and draw both feet toward your head, keeping them bent up at approximately 100 degrees. Lift your head and your hips off the floor, engaging your trunk flexors. Point your right foot and draw it behind your head. Make sure that you keep your left foot close to your head. At this point of your practice, extending the leg and bringing it into a position resembling the advanced posture *Kashyappasana* will most likely twist your pelvis. Therefore avoid doing so.

Exhale, flex your neck and upper thorax more, and draw your foot as far down your back as possible. To do this in this posture is less perilous and strenuous, as you don't have to keep your spine upright against gravity. In fact, gravity will assist you in getting your leg behind your head. The only thing you need to maintain is tension in your abdominal muscles.

Once your leg is sufficiently behind your neck, extend your neck gently and draw your head down toward the floor. You will feel that this tends to lift your hips further off the floor. Pointing your foot toward your head, straighten your left leg completely and draw your left foot toward your chin. Use your back extensors to straighten your spine, which will draw your hips back down to the floor. You will again feel a significant opening sensation in your right hip joint. This posture is similar to the first warm-up but is much more strength-oriented and therefore should be done after the first one. Its great advantage over the

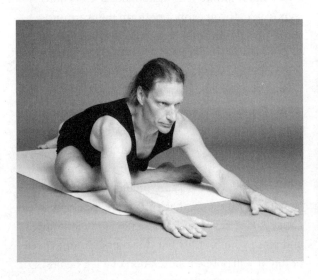

Leg-behind-head warm-up 1

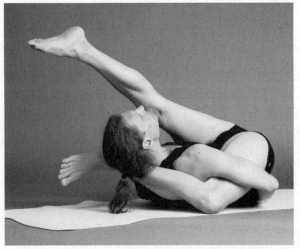

Leg-behind-head warm-up 2

first warm-up is that it increases your core strength. Unless you are extremely flexible, you need to look at leg-behind-head as core-strength training.

WARM-UP 3: This warm-up is suitable to be done only outside of the *vinyasa* practice. Lie on your back, bend up your left leg, and place the left foot next to your left hip. Make sure to keep your hips level and square. Draw your right foot up toward your forehead. Place a heavy sandbag (ideally 20 pounds or 10 kilograms) on your right foot.

Ekapada Shirshasana

ONE-LEG-BEHIND-THE-HEAD POSTURE

Drishti Nose in upright version; up to the foot in final version

OVERVIEW: *Ekapada Shirshasana* is the entrance to a whole universe of leg-behind-head postures. It is easier than *Dvipada Shirshasana* and *Yoganidrasana* because you place only one leg at a time. Practice it well before moving on.

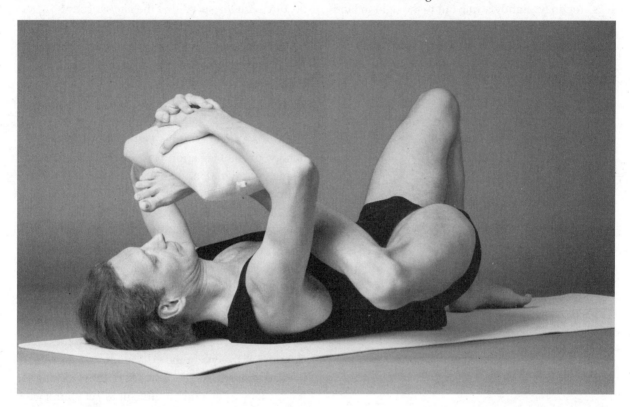

Leg-behind-head warm-up 3

Balance it there to capacity, stabilizing it with one or two hands if necessary. If you place a pillow under your head, this becomes a comfortable reading posture. Again, feel the opening of the hip joint and breathe into it.

You may also act as if you were trying gently to lift the sandbag away from your chest by internally rotating your femur (thighbone). Do this only to the extent that your effort is overcome by the weight of the sandbag. You will now feel a deeper opening of your hip joint.

CONTRAINDICATIONS: Forward head-posture, acute sacroiliac-joint injuries, twisted pelvis, weak low back, weak neck muscles, and weak abdominal muscles.

Vinyasa Count

Vinyasa Seven

Inhaling, jump your right leg around the outside of your right arm while bringing your left leg through as in any conventional jump-through. This jumping of the right leg is the same as in the transition into

Bhujapidasana in the Primary Series, except that in *Bhujapidasana* we perform the movement simultaneously with both legs. It is wise, therefore, to start exercising by jumping straight into *Bhujapidasana* without touching down at an early point, as suggested in *Ashtanga Yoga: Practice and Philosophy* (p. 90), because this will prepare us for many transitions to come. If *Bhujapidasana* has been done to satisfaction, *Ekapada Shirshasana* should hold no surprises for us.

Make sure that you clear the floor with both legs. You may slightly swing out to the right to land your right thigh on your right arm. This can be achieved, for example, by bending the left arm slightly just before landing while keeping the right arm straight.

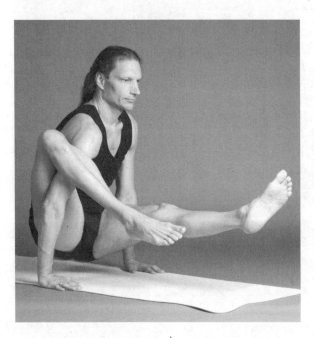

Jumping around the right arm without touching the floor

Sit down with your left leg straight in front of you, your right knee on your right arm, and your hips square. As you place your leg behind your head, keep your left leg straight to anchor your pelvis. If you bend up your left leg, you will more readily be able to compensate for lack of hip joint flexibility by tilting the pelvis backward. We will try to avoid this tilt as much as possible while learning leg-behind-head. Tilting the pelvis places considerable stresses on the lumbar facet discs as well as the sacroiliac joints. This constellation also diverts movement away from the hip joint and will thus not force you to open it. Remember that Ashtanga Yoga of Patanjali starts with *ahimsa*, meaning "non-harming." To not harm with speech, thought, and action includes your own body. Teachers knew this in the great days of yore, and the practice therefore adapted to the needs of the students. Today much of this knowledge is lost, and many believe it is the student who must adapt to the practice.

Since not all students will be able to get into this posture with the speed that the *vinyasa* count requires, we give, in the interest of non-harm, a step-by-step breakdown into five phases for beginners. As you get more proficient, delete or amalgamate unnecessary steps until you arrive at the original *vinyasa* count.

PHASE 1 — PLACING KNEE BEHIND SHOULDER

Bend your right leg approximately 90 degrees,[20] and taking your right foot with your left hand, lift your right knee over your right shoulder by laterally rotating your femur (thighbone).

Flex your spine forward slightly and at the same time draw your right knee behind your shoulder, using the strength of your left arm. You can bring your right shoulder forward if that makes it easier (we will draw it backward once the leg is in position). Use your breath to do so, bending forward on the exhalation, placing the knee behind the shoulder at the end of the exhalation, and growing tall and sitting up on the inhalation, thus opening the hip joint. If you find it difficult to get your knee behind your shoulder, repeat the same movement several times, each time lifting your leg a little higher onto your shoulder.

At the end of phase 1, you will need to have your right knee firmly behind your shoulder. Your shoulder will carry a significant part of the weight of the leg and in this way will take pressure off the neck. You need to understand that leg-behind-head

---

20 The exact amount is determined, as with so many things, by the ratio between the length of your legs and your spine. If you have short legs, your hip joints will need to become more flexible. On the other hand, if your legs are long, it will become difficult to hook the shin below the C7 vertebra. An average leg length is ideal for leg-behind-head postures.

postures are partially strength postures. They will make your spine strong. Trying to do them with only flexibility will lead you nowhere.

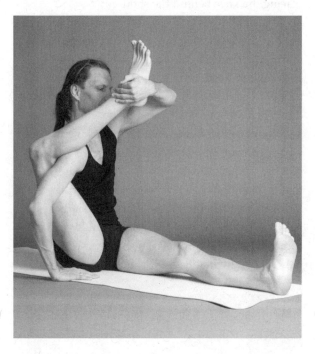

Placing the knee behind the shoulder

If you can't get your knee on your shoulder, the cause could be one of the following four scenarios:

1. In all leg-behind-head postures, the femur (thighbone) is first flexed, abducted, and laterally rotated and then adducted (drawn toward) to place the leg behind the head. In this final movement, the femur is drawn toward the ilium (hip bone), which is part of the pelvic bone. The closer the femur can get to the ilium, the further you will get the leg behind your head. Anything that gets in between your femur and your pelvis will obstruct your progress. This "anything" is all too often adipose tissue (fat). Eliminating excess adipose tissue can make the difference between your experiencing despair in this magnificent posture or being at ease.
    Solution: Eat less and exercise more.
2. Leg-behind-head postures are a peculiar mix of hamstring flexibility and hip rotation. A satisfactory amount of hamstring flexibility needs to be acquired by practicing

the Primary Series before commencing the Intermediate Series.

The longer your legs are, the less hamstring flexibility is required, as you will bend your legs more to get into the posture. As you know from forward bending, bending your legs at the knees takes the stretch off your hamstrings. Due to the lateral rotation of the femur, it is only the most lateral of the hamstrings, the biceps femoris, that experiences a significant stretch in this posture. The tendon of the biceps femoris can sometimes get caught close to its origin at the ischial tuberosity (protuberance of the sit bones). Shaking out the leg or making a gentle kicking movement often resolves this predicament.

Please note that the biceps femoris is in most individuals the hamstring that obstructs forward bending the least. Antagonistic to the other two hamstring muscles (semimembranosus and semitendinosus), it performs external rotation. Novice students may find it difficult in *Pashimottanasana* to keep the big toes together, to extend out through the inseam of the legs, and to keep the thighbones from rotating externally, all at the same time.
Solution: Improve forward bending by putting renewed emphasis on the Primary Series.

3. Unless your hip joints are already extremely flexible, all leg-behind-head postures involve a significant amount of trunk flexion. As in most *Marichyasanas*, curl your trunk forward to hook your shoulder around your upright knee, and then extend your spine, working against the resistance of the posture.[21]

    The more you are able to flex your spine, the more you can draw your leg down your back. This action can be performed only by strong trunk flexors —

---

21 *Marichyasanas* A, B, C, and D are part of the Primary Series.

that is, the abdominal muscles. Strengthening the abdominals demands that you relentlessly attempt to clear the floor with your feet in all *vinyasas*. Don't be surprised if this does not happen in the first year of practice. Most students will need to perform jumping through and jumping back roughly about fifty thousand times to become proficient.

The trunk flexors need to be accompanied by similarly strong trunk extensors. Apart from leg-behind-head postures, *Shalabhasana* and *Mayurasana* are the main strengthening postures of the trunk extensors in the Intermediate Series. *Solution*: Put more emphasis on *Navasana* and cleanly jumping back and through.

4. The most important factor in performing leg-behind-head postures is the flexibility of the hip joints. Please note that it is a different form of flexibility than that required in lotus postures and the deep hip rotations like *Mulabandhasana, Kandasana, Ekapada Yogadandasana*, and so on.[22] There are students who are flexible in lotus postures and stiff in leg-behind-head postures, and vice versa. If you find your hip joints to be stiff, it is worth spending some time warming them up, preferably outside of your *vinyasa* practice. These warm-ups typically take some time and would interfere with the sequencing and rhythm of your *vinyasa* practice. *Solution*: Practice leg-behind-head warm-ups outside of your *vinyasa* practice.

In many cases a combination of several or all four of these solutions needs to be applied. Be persistent. The outcome is worth the effort.

After duly practicing these warm-ups to satisfaction, disposing of excess adipose tissue, and improving forward-bending flexibility and abdominal strength, you will likely be able to keep your leg behind your head in an upright position.

22 These three postures are extreme hip rotations, which form part of the Advanced Series.

PHASE 2 — PLACING LEG BEHIND HEAD

To place the leg behind the head, we use the same steps and breathing technique we used when placing the knee behind the shoulder.

Exhaling, draw your head forward and place your leg behind your head. Still holding your foot with your hand, feel the weight of the leg on the back of your head. With your next exhalation, bend forward again, and with your hand, draw your foot down behind your head. Inhaling, extend your neck and your back, drawing your head backward. This will open your hip joints further and give you a bit more space for the next exhale. Exhaling, draw the foot an inch or two (a few centimeters) further down the back, and inhaling, draw your head and chest backward again. Repeat these steps until you have come to your limit for that day. Always work patiently and without aggression.

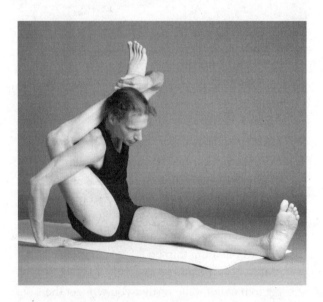

Placing the leg behind the head

PHASE 3 — TAKING SHIN BELOW C7

If you are ready to go further, we will now take the shin below the C7 vertebra (its spinous process is the large protrusion at the base of your neck). Passively, meaning by using your left hand, laterally rotate your right femur further, and flex your knee joint. Then draw your foot behind your head and down behind your neck. Ideally you will hook your shin below your C7 vertebra. If you manage to get your leg that low, it will likely feel as comfortable as

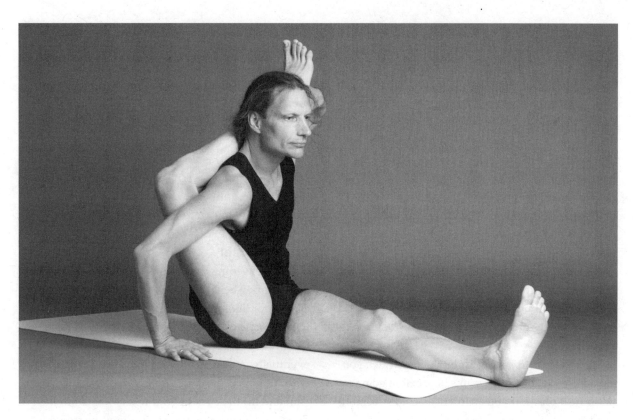

Placing the shin below C7

carrying a large backpack. The weight of your leg is carried by your shoulders and your rib cage, which are designed to carry significant loads.

If you can't get your leg that low, the sensation in the posture will be similar to someone pushing your head under water from behind. Indeed, it will make you feel as if you're drowning in a leg-behind-head posture. This is due to the weight of your leg being carried by your neck only, which is not designed to withstand such a heavy load. If you imagine your C7 vertebra as the axis of a lever, you can appreciate the vast difference it makes if you carry the weight of your leg right at or below C7 versus much higher up. If your leg is pressing against the back of your skull, for example, you will have to carry several times the weight that you would if you carried it below C7. It is possible to carry your leg on the back of your skull, but you need to be quite athletic in order not to experience any adverse effects from it. In many students, over time this results in cervical spine dysfunction, combined with a strain of the trapezius and levator scapulae muscles.

PHASE 4 — ASSUMING THE PRAYER POSITION

To keep the leg in position, we now take the head back, which will let the foot slide further down the back. With your leg safely behind your shoulder and lower cervical or ideally thoracic spine, you can let go of the foot, which until now was held up by the guiding left hand. Before you let go fully, brace your abdomen. This action includes not only all four abdominal muscles but also the psoas, quadratus lumborum, and all layers of the erector spinae — that is, all the muscles that maintain the integrity of the low back under load. Place your hands in prayer position and gaze toward your nose.

Keep the right foot pointed and keep the hamstrings of the right leg engaged, which aids in keeping the leg behind the head and takes pressure off the neck muscles. Do not attempt to straighten the leg that is behind your head, as this would increase the load on your neck. (This may be done by advanced and very flexible students and then constitutes "active release.")

141

Lift your heart and draw your shoulder blades down your back. Gently draw your chin backward to support your neck. Draw your right shoulder back against your right knee to take weight off your neck. Lift the back of your head up toward the ceiling to grow as tall as possible. Ground down through your sit bones to elongate and lengthen in the posture. Remember that because yoga works mainly with subtle spinal energy (*kundalini*), we are not concerned as much with the position of the limbs as with the integrity and proper function of the spine and associated *nadi* (energy channel) system.

Keep your left leg straight by pulling up on the kneecap without letting the thigh rotate laterally. Extend out through the heel and the bases of the toes and gently press the heel of the left foot into the floor.

If you need to open your hip joints further, you are advised to take five breaths here before going on to the next phase. If you are proficient at leg-behind-head, look at this phase as a transition only and directly proceed to phase 5. If you choose to stay here for five breaths, you may experiment with looking toward your third eye instead of your nose. This encourages you to take your head back further, which encourages the leg to slide further down the back.

PHASE 5 — BENDING FORWARD

PRECAUTION: Move into phase 5 only if you can sit in the upright version of *Ekapada Shirshasana* with apparent ease and prayer-position hands for five breaths. Needing the help of the teacher or your own hand to keep your leg behind your head indicates that the support strength of your spine and abdomen as well as your flexibility are not yet sufficient to go further. In this case, continue with the program until your teacher deems you ready rather than going on to the next phase.

Vinyasa Eight

Exhaling, keeping your spine as straight as possible and your leg behind your head, fold forward and clasp your left foot with both hands as in *Janushirshasana* (a posture of the Primary Series). Continuing to exhale, place your forehead and eventually your chin on your left shin. Do this without jutting the chin forward. Instead, drop your chin and lift the back of your neck away from the floor as you suck your chest through toward your left knee. This movement is designed to further open your right hip joint. It is the equivalent of sitting up tall in the upright version.

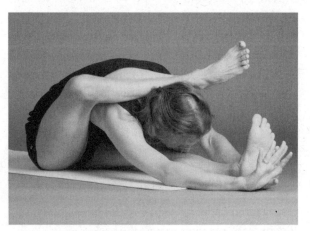

Ekapada Shirshasana, vinyasa eight

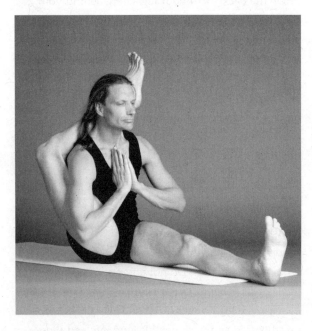

Ekapada Shirshasana, vinyasa seven

If flexibility permits, let your chin slide forward on your shin, elongating your spine. Draw your shoulder blades down your back and your elbows out to the sides. Make sure to ground your right sit bone and extend backward through both sit bones.

Draw your left sit bone into the floor, and extend out through the bases of all toes of your left foot. Extend the crown of your head and your heart toward your left big toe.

Gaze toward your nose and, once you have progressed enough, up toward your left foot. Take five breaths in this full version of *Ekapada Shirshasana*.

Vinyasa **Nine**

Inhaling, let go of your left foot and come upright, again placing your hands in *Anjali Mudra* (prayer position).

Exhaling, place your hands down on either side of your hips, ready for lift up.

Vinyasa **Ten**

Inhaling, lift your sit bones off the floor and, keeping your right leg behind your head, draw your straight left leg into your torso until your shin comes close to your chin. Point your left foot and look up to your toes. Note that this transition posture is similar to leg-behind-head warm-up 2 (p. 136). There you performed it lying on your back, whereas here you balance on your arms and have to work against gravity. However, here this posture is only a transition and is held merely for the duration of the inhalation. It is nevertheless the most taxing part of *Ekapada Shirshasana* and must be performed cleanly before going on to the next posture.

ACTIVE RELEASE TECHNIQUE: Please note that this method is only for practitioners already proficient in leg-behind-head postures.

Medially rotate your femur and attempt to straighten your leg. Counteract this with your core muscles by sitting upright and drawing your head, neck, and right shoulder backward. Superficially, this will take you out of the posture, but if your support structure is sound, it will open your hip joint more and increase the lateral rotation of your femur.

Vinyasa **Eleven**

As you initiate the exhalation, flex your neck slightly and sweep your right leg off your back. At

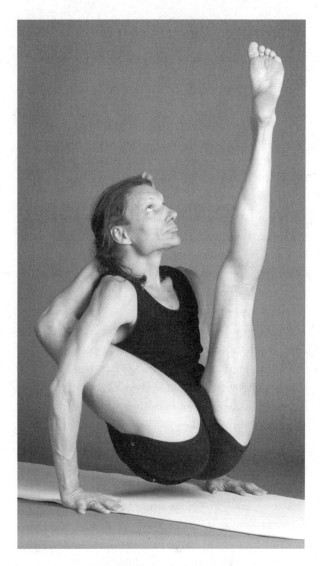

Ekapada Shirshasana, vinyasa ten

the same time, flex your left leg, drawing your knee into your chest, and jump back into *Chaturanga Dandasana*. Perform this movement without touching your feet down before landing in *Chaturanga Dandasana*.

Vinyasa **Twelve**

Inhaling, lift into Upward Dog.

Vinyasa **Thirteen**

Exhaling, transit into Downward Dog.

Vinyasas **Fourteen to Twenty**

Repeat *Ekapada Shirshasana* on the left side.

Dvipada Shirshasana

TWO-LEGS-BEHIND-THE-HEAD POSTURE

Drishti Nose

OVERVIEW: *Dvipada Shirshasana* is the most difficult leg-behind-head posture in the series. With the left leg placed into position first, the *asana* balances *Supta Vajrasana*, where the right leg is placed first.

PREREQUISITE: Performance of all *vinyasas* of *Ekapada Shirshasana*, particularly *vinyasa* ten. *Dvipada Shirshasana* is much more difficult than *Ekapada Shirshasana*. If you do not find yourself relatively at ease in *Ekapada Shirshasana*, don't attempt *Dvipada Shirshasana*.

CONTRAINDICATIONS: Forward head-posture, acute sacroiliac-joint injuries, twisted pelvis, weak low back, weak neck muscles, and weak abdominal muscles. Also see the sidebar below, "Taking Responsibility."

Vinyasa Count

Vinyasa Seven

Inhaling, jump both legs around your arms in the same fashion that you enter *Bhujapidasana* in the Primary Series. As stated in *Ekapada Shirshasana*, by the time we are practicing the Intermediate Series, we need to be capable of jumping straight into this transitory posture without touching our feet down.

Keep the left leg on your left arm, and extend the right leg straight in front of you. Put first the left leg behind the head and then the right leg on top of the left one.

Vinyasa Eight

Place the left leg behind your head by laterally rotating your thigh, using all the steps and precautions described in *Ekapada Shirshasana*. The further you manage to get the leg down behind your neck, the easier it will be to carry the additional weight of the second leg. It will be impossible to carry both legs on the back of your head, whereas to carry them on or below C7 will be quite comfortable.

Hold the first leg in position by taking your head back, and place your left hand on the floor in front of you to keep your balance. Bend up your right leg, laterally rotating your thigh and, using your right hand, take your ankle or, flexibility permitting, your calf closer to the knee.

Exhaling, bend forward somewhat and lift your right leg behind your shoulder and then your right ankle behind the left ankle. Keep sufficient tension in your neck so that your left leg does not slip from behind your head. You may allow that in the initial stages of practicing the posture, but *Dvipada Shirshasana* is not properly executed until both legs

---

TAKING RESPONSIBILITY

If your low back tends to be unstable, on days when you are not sure whether you will be able to maintain the integrity of your spine due to weakness, practice only *Yoganidrasana* (yogic sleep posture, the next posture in the series) and leave out the more taxing *Dvipada Shirshasana*. Yes, true, the sequence is not to be changed, but Patanjali's dictum in *sutra* II.16, *"heyam duhkham anagatam,"* means that we need to avoid creating future suffering. If you intuitively feel that the performance of a particular posture on a particular day will be detrimental, then take the responsibility of your body into your own hands and do not perform it (particularly if you are an experienced practitioner). You may have heard that yoga looks at the body as a temple. How will you worship the Divine in this temple if you have defiled it through an injury because you wanted to live up to some ideal? It is your body — take responsibility for it! The human spine is the gross equivalent of the central energy channel of the subtle body, which is nothing but the royal pathway of the ascent of Shakti, which again is the manifestation of the Mother Goddess. Do not practice yoga to an extent that you damage your spine. Practice mindfully!

When you feel stronger, do *Yoganidrasana* first and then *Dvipada Shirshasana*. Once you are completely recovered, perform *Dvipada Shirshasana* before *Yoganidrasana*.

LEFT LEG FIRST

In *Supta Kurmasana* in the Primary Series, the left leg is placed first, and that order is also followed in the next posture in this series, *Yoganidrasana*. In general, whenever both legs are placed behind the head, the left leg is brought into position first, followed by the right.[23]

This is at odds with the arrangement in lotus postures such as *Padmasana* and *Supta Vajrasana*, wherein the right leg is brought into half-lotus before the left leg. As described in the sidebar on page 125, the reason we place the legs in this order and not the other way around is to accommodate the asymmetry of the abdominal cavity. Placing the right leg into lotus first leads to a purification of the liver and spleen, whereas the reversal of this order does not have this effect, according to Yoga Shastra.

Similarly, the placing of the left leg first into *Dvipada Shirshasana* accommodates the asymmetry of the thoracic cavity, which would not be affected if the order of the legs were reversed. Placing the left leg first into *Dvipada Shirshasana* particularly purifies and strengthens the heart, but the lungs also benefit from it.

There has been speculation that the reversed order of placement of the legs in leg-behind-head postures like *Dvipada Shirshasana* and *Yoganidrasana* would balance the lotus postures like *Supta Vajrasana* and *Karandavasana*. Although at first glance there doesn't seem to be much evidence of a balancing relationship between leg-behind-head postures and lotus postures, I have noticed over many years of teaching that those students who practice the entire Intermediate Series or the entire Primary Series do not seem susceptible to twisted pelvises. However, this problem repeatedly occurs among students who add on the Intermediate Series up to *Supta Vajrasana* and stay stuck for a long time either at *Supta Vajrasana* or at *Ekapada Shirshasana*.[24] In other words, they could not yet get the balancing effect of *Dvipada Shirshasana*.

Of course, doing *Dvipada Shirshasana* before you are ready is not the solution, as this could lead to all sorts of other problems. If you develop the problem of a twisted pelvis at this point, then and only then may you start to practice some of the lotus postures with your left leg first. A way of doing that would be to practice *Supta Vajrasana*, *Urdhva Padmasana*, *Pindasana*, *Matsyasana*, *Padmasana*, *Yoga Mudra*, and *Utpluthi* with the left leg first every other day, or to let your teacher pick which ones to do left side first.

You may be able to resume placing the right leg first once you start performing *Dvipada Shirshasana* and *Yoganidrasana* and experience their balancing effect.

are secured behind the head and stay there for the full breath count.

Drawing both legs as far down the back as possible ensures that your shoulders carry part of their weight rather than all of it pressing onto your cervical spine. Once proficient in the posture, point (plantar flex) both feet. In the initial stages, you might prefer to use flexion (dorsiflexion) of the feet; this makes it easier to hook the second foot onto the first. In the final version of the posture, however, the feet are to be plantar flexed.

Once both legs are securely in place behind the neck, engage your back extensors and straighten up as much as you can. Lift your chest and drop your pubic bone. Find your point of balance on your sit bones and place both hands into *Anjali Mudra* (prayer position). Take your head back as far as possible, which will let your legs slide further down, and look toward your nose. If you find it difficult to take your head back, place the tips of your index and middle fingers against your chin to support the action with your hands.

Take five deep breaths into your chest.

---

23 This does not apply in postures such as *Ekapada Shirshasana*, in which only one leg at a time is placed behind the head. These postures follow a completely different energetic structure.

24 It must be mentioned again that the overwhelming majority of students with pelvic obliquity, colloquially referred to as "twisted pelvis," are coffee-drinking females. Females generally have lower muscle tension than males, which means that their bodies are softer and more readily thrown out of balance. Coffee is a stimulant that expels and mobilizes *chi/prana*. This *prana* is used, among other things, to retain a subtle balance in the body. Coffee reduces the *pranic* stability of your pelvis. It appears from observation that decaffeinated coffee does not have this effect.

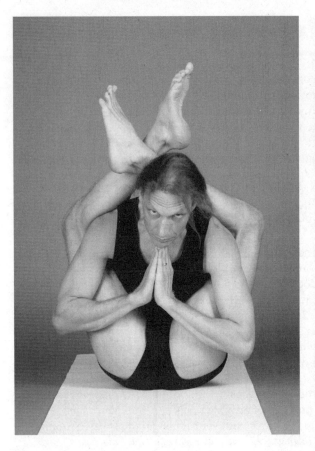

Dvipada Shirshasana A

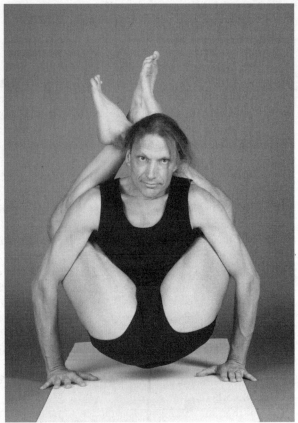

Dvipada Shirshasana B

Vinyasa **Nine**

Place both hands on the floor in front of you, and, inhaling, straighten your arms and lift your sit bones off the floor. Try to keep your feet pointed and breathe deeply into your chest. Take five breaths and gaze upward. This posture is considerably easier than *vinyasa* eight. The spine here is suspended from the shoulders, whereas in *vinyasa* eight you have to support your spine in an upright position against the force of gravity.

Use the combined effort of your back extensors and trunk flexors to draw your sit bones down to the floor as the crown of the head extends upward, thus putting your spine into traction. Although putting the spine into traction initially seems impossible, it is the key to effective leg-behind-head postures because it increases the space between the vertebrae and thus improves the flow of spinal energy (*kundalini*).

ACTIVE RELEASE TECHNIQUE: Please note that this method is only for established practitioners. Medially rotate your femurs and attempt to straighten your legs. Superficially this will take you out of the posture, but if your support structure is sound enough to keep your legs in position, it will take you deeper into the posture by increasing the lateral rotation of your femurs and increasing the hamstring stretch aspect of the posture.

At the end of the last exhalation, bend your head forward slightly and sweep both legs off your neck. Inhaling, straighten your legs, keeping them on your arms.

Vinyasa **Ten**

Exhaling, jump back into *Chaturanga Dandasana*.

Vinyasa **Eleven**

Inhaling, lift into Upward Dog.

Vinyasa **Twelve**

Exhaling, move into Downward Dog.

Yoganidrasana

YOGIC SLEEP POSTURE

Drishti Third eye

OVERVIEW: If you mastered *Dvipada Shirshasana*, *Yoganidrasana* should not pose many problems, as gravity works in your favor.

CONTRAINDICATIONS: Same as with the previous leg-behind-head postures but to a lesser extent here, since gravity works with us.

Vinyasa Count

Vinyasa Seven

Inhaling, jump through, and exhaling, lie down.

Vinyasa Eight

Inhaling, draw both feet up to your head, bending your legs. Exhaling, take the left leg and, pointing the foot, draw the knee behind your left shoulder and the foot behind your head down your back as far as possible. While doing so, engage your abdominal muscles to lift your chest somewhat and lift your head upward by flexing your neck. You now will have more space to draw the left leg down your back. Once your left leg is in position, secure it by drawing your head again down toward the floor and engaging your erector spinae muscles to extend your back.

Take your right leg and, while again pointing the foot, draw your right knee beneath your right shoulder. Hook your right ankle underneath your left ankle,

making sure that your left leg stays behind the head in the process. Do so by engaging your neck extensors. The further down your back you draw this second leg, the more comfortable the posture will be for you. If you can barely keep your feet behind your head, you will need to keep them flexed (dorsal flexion) to lock them in position. As soon as you have made enough progress, point your feet (plantar flexion).

Once both legs are in position, reach around your back with both arms and interlace your fingers or clasp your wrist with one hand.

Engage your trunk extensors to draw your hips and shoulders down to the floor. Let your abdominal muscles lengthen eccentrically as your sternum moves away from your pubic bone. Use your shoulders to draw your legs down to the floor. Engage your rhomboid muscles to broaden your chest and to suck it through the gateway of your legs up to the ceiling.

Lengthen the front of your torso and engage and shorten the back. Make your sit bones heavy and let them sink down toward the floor. Keep laterally rotating your thighs. Continue to take your head back; take five deep breaths and look toward your third eye.

Exhaling, let the feet come off from behind your head and straighten your legs, keeping your trunk and your hip joints flexed.

ACTIVE RELEASE TECHNIQUE: Please note that this method is only for established practitioners. Medially rotate your femur and attempt to straighten your leg. Superficially this will take you out of the posture, but if your support structure is sound enough, it will take you deeper into the posture by increasing the lateral rotation of your femur and increasing the hamstring stretch aspect of the posture.

Vinyasa Nine

Inhaling, perform *Chakrasana*; exhaling, roll over into *Chaturanga Dandasana*. This movement is described in *Ashtanga Yoga: Practice and Philosophy* (p. 107).

Vinyasa Ten

Inhaling, lift into Upward Dog.

Vinyasa Eleven

Exhaling, transit into Downward Dog.

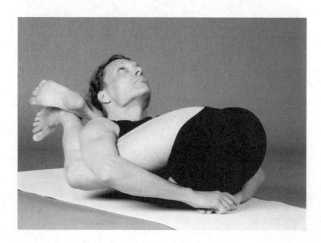

Yoganidrasana

THIRD CONNECTIVE SECTION

This section separates and connects the leg-behind-head and arm-balance essential sequences. It consists of only one posture, *Tittibhasana*, although this *asana* has three very strenuous versions. *Tittibhasana* links the leg-behind-head and arm-balance sequences by combining their characteristics. Its A version is an arm balance, its B version has a dynamic strength aspect, and its C version is very similar to a leg-behind-head posture. Please note the similarity of this posture with *Kurmasana* (*vinyasa* seven of *Supta Kurmasana*) and its Primary Series–like character.

Tittibhasana

INSECT POSTURE

Drishti Nose

OVERVIEW: With this posture the focus shifts from flexibility to strength and endurance. *Tittibhasana*, with its strong focus on engagement of the *bandhas*, creates a link between the upper and lower extremities. It is essential to establish this link before commencing the arm balances.

CONTRAINDICATIONS: Hamstring and/or low back injuries.

Vinyasa Count

Vinyasa Seven

Inhaling, jump around your arms as you did in *Bhujapidasana* and *Dvipada Shirshasana*. By now you will be proficient at doing so without touching your feet down. Jump off early in the inhalation and keep inhaling while the feet transit around the arms. Upon landing, you will still have some inhalation left to do; otherwise, your feet will drop down.

After you land, check that your knees are high up near your shoulders and not somewhere lower down on your arms. Your inner thighs need to be

touching the sides of your rib cage, without any gap. If this is not the case, do not hesitate to place your feet on the floor, straighten your legs as much as possible, and lever your shoulders under your knees one at a time. This is not an elegant choice, but the posture is inefficient if your knees are down around your elbows.

Once your thighs fit snugly against the sides of your torso, place your hands down, straighten your arms, and lift your feet off. Straighten your legs and plantar flex (point) your feet until your toes arrive at eye height. While in the posture, work your lumbar extensor muscles as if you were trying to re-create the natural lordotic curve in your low back. This action is immensely strengthening for the low back and counteracts the lack of lumbar extensor strength that results from prolonged sitting, especially with poor posture. Keep the legs strong and straight; engage the quadriceps by pulling up on the kneecaps and press your legs down onto your arms. This action deepens the forward flexion at your hip joint, while at the same time strengthening and protecting the hamstring muscles.

Gaze toward your nose and hold *Tittibhasana* A for five breaths.

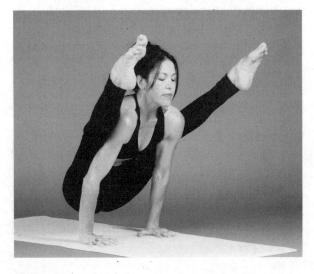

Tittibhasana A

Vinyasa **Eight**

Exhaling, keeping your legs as straight as possible, place your feet on the floor and lift your sit bones up, so that you come into a standing forward bend with your chest between your legs. Continue to exhale and draw your shoulders further under your knees, flexing your spine. Reach around your back and interlock your fingers or, better, take one wrist. Straighten your legs, and against their resistance extend your trunk as much as possible. Hold the posture for five slow breaths, gazing toward the tip of the nose. Make sure you contract your quadriceps strongly and breathe into your hamstrings to encourage their release.

Inhaling, lift your right foot, step forward and, exhaling, place it down. Repeat this movement four times, alternating between the left and right feet. Then take five steps backward, synchronized with your breath, alternating between the left and right feet. Keep your hands bound throughout the process.

Both parts together constitute *Tittibhasana* B.

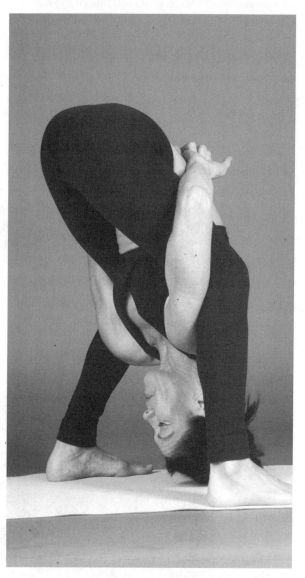

Tittibhasana B, walking

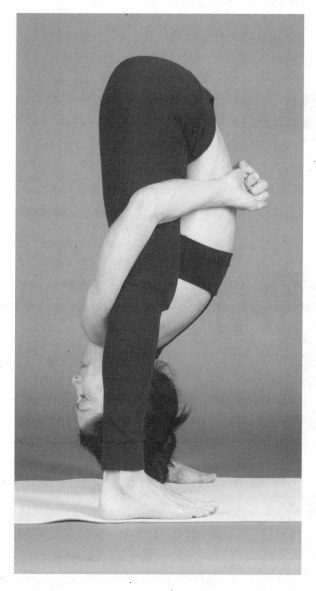

Tittibhasana B, standing

Vinyasa **Nine**

Exhaling, bring your heels together, ideally until they touch. Turn your feet out as much as possible. Pull your head and chest through, so that your calves touch your shoulders from behind. Now reach around your ankles and interlock your fingers. Attempt to straighten your legs again as much as possible until your quadriceps fatigue. This will help to improve the access to these important muscles in other postures.

Breathe into your chest, keep your abdomen firm, and release your hamstrings. *Tittibhasana* C is the most challenging part of the posture; it provides a mixture of forward bend and external rotation of the femurs. Gaze toward the nose and take five deep breaths.

ACTIVE RELEASE TECHNIQUE: This happens automatically in versions B and C.

Vinyasa **Ten**
Inhaling, place your hands down, lift your legs off the floor, and return to *Tittibhasana* A for the length of the inhalation.

Exhaling, fold your legs and transit toward *Bakasana*.

Vinyasa **Eleven**
Inhaling, lift as high as you can, straighten your arms, bring your big toes together, and tuck your heels up under your sit bones. If you want to make it more challenging, you can try to lift your knees off your arms into an arm balance.

Vinyasa **Twelve**
Exhaling, jump back into *Chaturanga Dandasana*.

Vinyasa **Thirteen**
Inhale into Upward Dog.

Vinyasa **Fourteen**
Exhale into Downward Dog.

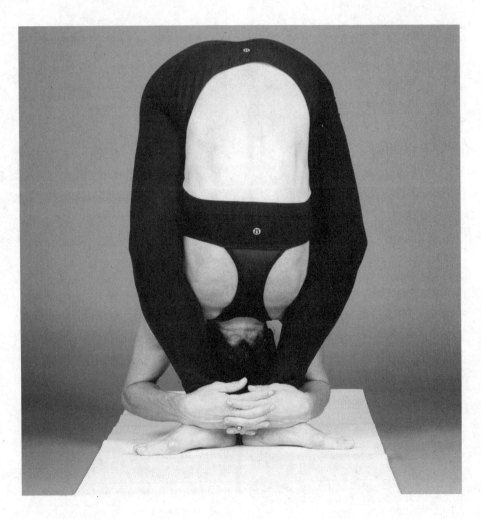

Tittibhasana C

ARM-BALANCE SEQUENCE

The third essential sequence of the active element is the arm-balance sequence of the Intermediate Series, a strengthening section that consists of four postures: *Pincha Mayurasana*, *Karandavasana*, *Mayurasana*, and *Nakrasana*. In the Advanced A Series, too, a strengthening section immediately follows the leg-behind-head section. Leg-behind-head postures are indeed an apt preparation for arm balances; their spine-stabilizing function emphasizes engaging the abdominal muscles.

With the intermediate arm balance sequence, the focus shifts for the first time to the shoulder girdle. During arm balances, the shoulders take center stage, as the hip joint has during the standing postures. If there is aberrant function or an imbalance of the shoulder muscles during the arm balances, it will become aggravated rather than improve with years of practice. Serious shoulder injuries can result, which can prove to be a formidable obstacle to one's practice. Analysis of the underlying problem and the application of specific therapeutic exercises can resolve most of these issues.

The ability to support one's weight on one's arms is related to one's ability to support oneself in all situations of life as well as the ability to be independent and autonomous of the opinions and judgments of others whenever required. The shoulder region is also instrumental in one's capacity to shoulder the burdens of life and responsibility. Arm balances can help those who suffer from lack of confidence. However, in today's world, everybody is seeking more confidence, but few people devote themselves to gaining more competence. Often we see people, even in public office, making decisions with great confidence. But when that confidence is not paired with sufficient, or even greater, competence, those confident decisions may result in great detriment to their makers and to the community as a whole. We should seek confidence only in areas wherein we know exactly what we are doing.

Standing postures and many sitting postures focus on the pelvic girdle; standing postures improve one's ability to "stand one's ground," and sitting postures, with their influence on the pelvic and abdominal region, can be used to sort out issues of the reproductive and metabolic systems. Leg-behind-head and backbending postures focus on the spine, abdomen, and thorax. Backbending greatly benefits the throat region, which is related to expressing oneself through voice. The heart-opening effect of backbends enables one to express oneself in a compassionate way.

Arm balances, however, place the spotlight on the shoulder girdle and the upper extremities — that is, the arms. The arms are related to giving to and modeling the environment to reflect one's ideas and needs. Arm balances can help to fortify one's actions with the necessary conviction, firmness, and steadiness so that one will be taken seriously by others.

On an energetic level, arm balances serve to complement the emphasis that the other postures place on other regions of the body; they lift energy up to the heart and above. Leg-behind-head postures, because of their kyphotic and *apanic* tendency, are important counterweights to back-bending postures, which are predominantly lordotic and *pranic*. In the same way, arm balances counteract and complement standing postures and, to a certain extent, sitting postures. Sitting postures are also counteracted and complemented by inversions, such as shoulder stand and headstand.

Grouped together, standing postures, sitting postures, and inversions make up most of the Primary Series and prepare the body for the alchemy of the more advanced postures. Standing postures and sitting postures, with their focus on the lower extremities, pelvic girdle, and abdomen, are in due time counteracted by arm balances, which emphasize the shoulder girdle and supporting rib cage. If standing postures are not counteracted with arm balances, advanced yogis can develop top/down imbalances — that is, a weak upper body in relation to the lower body — akin to those of dancers.

When one studies the composition of the various series of the Ashtanga Vinyasa method, another feature of arm balances becomes apparent. After the pelvic area is opened in the Primary Series, arm balances are used in combination with leg-behind-head postures and backbends to prepare the royal pathway of the spine for the ascent of Shakti. Leg-behind-head postures focus on the lower part of the spine, backbends mainly on the middle section, and arm balances on the upper part. The combinations and order in which the postures are practiced is important. Only in those prescribed sequences can the postures bring the desired effect. This preparation of the spine, the second objective of the *vinyasa* practice, takes up most of the Intermediate and Advanced A Series.

Once this effect is achieved, one enters the final phase: extreme hip rotations, which occur mainly in the later advanced sequences. These postures ignite *kundalini shakti* and send it up along its prepared pathway. The Ashtanga Vinyasa practice is therefore similar to *Kechari Mudra*, which is another physical method used to awaken *kundalini*. *Asana* practice, then, not only restores health to the body and tranquillity to the mind but also has a distinct alchemical quality, preparing the subtle body for *pranayama* and the awakening of *kundalini*.

Make sure to study closely the material in chapter 6 pertaining to the shoulder joint (pp. 71–77) before attempting any arm balances.

Pincha Mayurasana

FEATHERS OF THE PEACOCK POSTURE

Drishti Nose

OVERVIEW: With *Pincha Mayurasana* starts the strength section. This first posture focuses on stabilizing the shoulder blades (scapulae).

PREREQUISITE: *Kapotasana* and *Dvipada Shirshasana*. Students need to be proficient in *Kapotasana* before starting arm balances. If the humeri cannot be flexed enough to grab one's feet while arching back on the knees, arm balances will only further stiffen the shoulders.

When balancing on one's arms, the spine and abdomen need to be firm and steady enough to hold the weight of the legs and pelvis without dropping over into a backbend; this could injure the shoulder joints. Proficiency in *Dvipada Shirshasana* indicates that this firmness has been achieved.

CONTRAINDICATION: In case of an existing shoulder injury, jumping out of the posture (*vinyasa* nine) may need to be modified.

Vinyasa Count

Vinyasa Seven

Inhaling, hop forward, landing your knees next to your hands. Exhaling, place your forearms on the floor. Check that your hands are close to the front of the mat to ensure that upon exiting the posture your feet will still land on the mat.

Make sure that your elbows are shoulder-width apart and keep your forearms parallel throughout the performance of *Pincha Mayurasana*. Because beginners to the posture tend to place the elbows too far apart, we suggest that you initially check the stance in the same fashion as done in *Shirshasana* (headstand). Place your hands around the opposite elbows and make sure that your knuckles and fingers are outside of your elbows. Maintaining this precise distance between your elbows, now place your forearms parallel to each other and ground your hands down firmly, spreading your fingers. During the ensuing movement, make sure not to move your wrists toward each other or your elbows further apart.

Straighten your legs now and, walking your feet in toward your elbows as close as possible, lift your hips high over your elbows in the process. The further you can walk in, the less momentum you will need to get up into the posture, making it easier to fade out that momentum and come to a point of balance on your forearms.

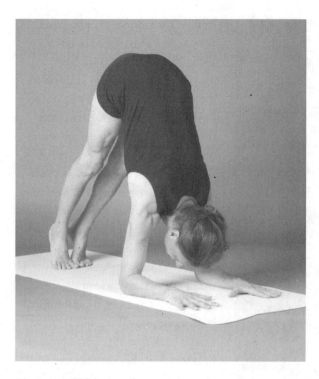

Pincha Mayurasana, set-up

Vinyasa Eight

Inhaling, lift your head and gaze toward a point between your fingertips. If you find it difficult to focus on a spot on your mat, consider placing a small object in your chosen location or mark a spot on your mat. Those whose balance is unstable will find this a welcome aid. Fixing your gaze to a spot makes it much easier to establish your balance.

Proceed now to kick up into the full posture one leg at a time. Students with extremely long hamstring muscles may be able to perform the movement without momentum — keeping the left foot on the floor, extending the right leg up and eventually over the head, and then using a pivoting action, lifting the second leg up to bring both legs together. For most students, this cannot be recommended. Usually one needs to twist the pelvis too much to achieve this transition, and when done always on the same side a muscular imbalance may result in pelvic obliquity.

It is therefore better to learn to kick up with straight legs, one leg after the other (scissor kick). Extend your straight right leg up into the air as high as possible without twisting your pelvis. Bend your left leg and, inhaling, push off the floor with your

leg, and raise the now-straight left leg up until both legs meet.

If you don't make it all the way up, lift your gaze slightly. The more you lift your gaze, the more you will extend your back and neck and subsequently the higher you will lift up. If you raise your gaze too much, you may drop over into a backbend. In the beginning, when the student is learning the posture, the teacher should spot the student and prevent him or her from overshooting the mark. Within a short time the student will have stored the memory of how much force is needed to reach the exact position and will be able to perform the movement without the help of the teacher.

It is not advisable to use a wall for this purpose. With the safety of the wall to catch him or her, the student may not attempt and thereby learn to use only the amount of force necessary to reach the balance position. The wall is an inert, *tamasic* object and cannot give you feedback as to whether you are using too much force when kicking up. Fine-tuning never occurs, and one becomes dependent on the wall as on a crutch. Students usually will become independent from the teacher from within a week to a month when learning *vinyasa* eight and similar postures. When employing a wall, this independence often never occurs.

Even if you kick up with momentum rather than flexibility, the continual use of the same leg may lay the foundation for a muscular imbalance in the pelvis. Finding one side much harder than the other points toward an already existing imbalance that needs to be rectified by giving preference to your weaker side. Once you have learned to kick up on one side, change sides and practice kicking the other leg up first.

Once you can kick up on both sides, you may practice swinging both legs up at the same time. To make this more accessible, start by bending both legs during transit. Once that has become easy, practice it keeping both legs straight and together in transit. Note, however, that this difficult movement requires much hamstring flexibility.

Once you are up in *Pincha Mayurasana* and have established your balance, engage your abdominal muscles to flatten out your low back. Straighten up,

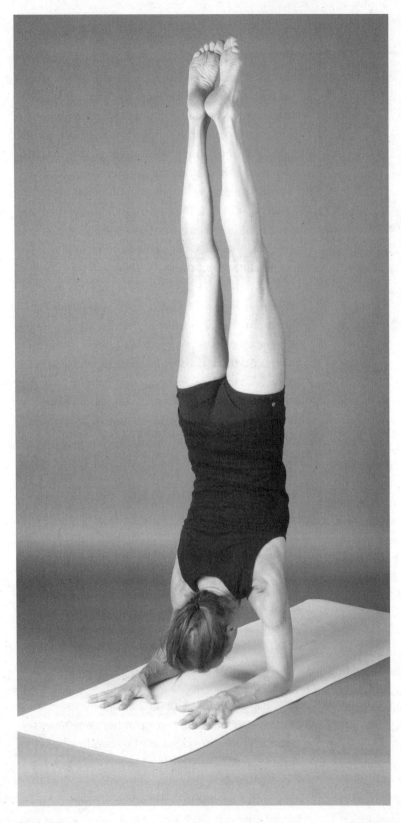

Pincha Mayurasana

humeri (arm bones) can be flexed fully (arms above head position) using the deltoid and triceps muscles.[25] Any residual stiffness in the shoulders needs to be removed first in Downward Dog and later through backbending before one is ready to attempt postures such as the present one. This is the reason that arm balances are practiced only after proficiency in backbending is gained. Starting the practice of arm balances with shoulder joints that are not yet fully opened usually means that deep backbends cannot be reached anymore, as any future back opening will be counteracted by the back-firming effect of the arm balances. For this very reason, the performance of postures like handstands needs to be postponed until one's backbend is open enough to perform postures like *Kapotasana*.

Once you have gained confidence, drop your gaze between your wrists and lower your head. The action of sucking your shoulder blades into your back brings the serratus anterior and subscapularis muscles into play. Make sure that your elbows do not turn out and that your wrists do not move closer together. If this occurs, you will need to more effectively engage your infraspinatus and teres minor muscles (often fused to one muscle). Infraspinatus externally rotates the humerus (arm bone) and is of course the antagonist to the internally rotating subscapularis. You will need to use infraspinatus concentrically (shortens during use) and subscapularis eccentrically

grow as tall as you can, and fully open your chest and shoulders. This is, of course, possible only if the

25 Remember that raising your arms above your head is called "flexing" the humerus and that extending the humerus is defined as "returning" from flexion.

(lengthens during use). In this way the subscapularis does not internally rotate; its origin sucks the medium borders of the scapulae (shoulder blades) into the back. This is an important detail for the stabilization of the shoulder joint. Do not allow a winged appearance of the shoulder blades.

Take five slow breaths while looking down on the nose. On the last exhalation, bend your hip joints by about 30 degrees. As you inhale strongly, hook the breath into the *bandhas* and extend upward, becoming as light as possible. At the peak of the inhalation, when you are most buoyant, flex both legs at the knee and then perform a kicking movement with both legs. This will reduce weight on your arms; since your hip joints are slightly flexed, the vector will go not only up but also slightly toward your elbows. Simultaneously execute a strong push with both hands, as if pushing the floor away from you. Once your hands lift off, pull them out and place them further toward the foot end of your mat. The further down you can place them, the softer your landing will be.

Vinyasa Nine

Exhaling, catch the weight of your body with your hands and lower down slowly, keeping the legs straight and flexing the feet before landing in *Chaturanga Dandasana*. This whole transition is very challenging, of course, but important. The key is coordination and timing. The key actions of kicking into the right direction, explosively pushing with one's hands, and pulling the hands out need to be performed almost simultaneously at the peak of inhalation. There is a brief moment during the descent of the legs when you feel you no longer have control of the weight of your legs and gravity takes over. You must observe this moment and, before your feet reach the floor, take the opportunity to move your hands and place them in their new position.

Vinyasa Ten

Inhale into Upward Dog.

Vinyasa Eleven

Exhale into Downward Dog.

Karandavasana

WATERFOWL POSTURE

Drishti Nose

OVERVIEW: *Karandavasana* is the most difficult posture in the series; however, progress is possible if its phases are precisely isolated. It is essential that we isolate the movements of the hip joints from the movements of the spine and the movements of the shoulder joints to succeed in this difficult posture. We will also learn the importance of being able to revert each phase of this posture before going on to the next.

PREREQUISITES: Taking your feet in *Kapotasana* shows that your shoulders are open enough to sustain that openness against the shoulder and back-stiffening tendency of this strenuous posture. Keeping hold of your toes during the entire transition in *Supta Vajrasana* without the aid of the teacher shows that your hip joints are flexible enough. Jumping out of *Pincha Mayurasana* in the prescribed method is important because you exit *Karandavasana* in the same way, but the transition is more difficult after having performed the much more strenuous *Karandavasana*.

CONTRAINDICATIONS: Knee problems, shoulder problems.

WARM-UP AND RESEARCH POSTURE: The following suggestions will prepare you for this difficult posture.

1. Lie on the floor face down with legs folded in *Padmasana* and arms extended over your head. Draw your hips and shoulders into the floor to target residual stiffness here.
2. When performing your cool-down postures, fold into lotus during *Shirshasana* (headstand). Although this transition is much easier than *Karandavasana*, it will highlight any difficulties in performing *Padmasana* without the help of your hands and in an upside-down position.
3. Hold *Pincha Mayurasana* for fifteen breaths instead of only five breaths, as that's how

long you will be in the various phases of *Karandavasana* initially (unless you are already proficient).

4. Hold *Urdhva Dandasana* (headstand variation) for ten to fifteen breaths. On the way in and out of *Karandavasana*, you will transit through a forearm balance with your hips extended over or even beyond the back of your head. At this point, many students fall out of the posture due to lack of strength. Holding *Urdhva Dandasana* for ten to fifteen breaths will prepare you.

As usual, you should practice variations outside of the *vinyasa* practice or, if you need to introduce them into the practice, then include them for only as long as necessary.

Vinyasa Count

Vinyasa Seven
Inhaling, hop forward to land on your knees. Exhaling, as in *Pincha Mayurasana*, place your forearms on the floor, straighten your legs, and walk your feet in.

Vinyasa Eight
Inhaling, move up into *Pincha Mayurasana* as described.

Vinyasa Nine
As with all complex postures, the key is to completely break the posture down into its constituents and isolate the respective phases of the movement. We use six phases here.

PHASE 1 — PLACING THE RIGHT LEG CORRECTLY
Exhaling, while balancing on your forearms, place first your right leg into half-lotus. You will need sufficiently flexible hip joints, which we acquired through the practice of such postures as *Baddhakonasana* and *Garbha Pindasana*, and strong lateral (external) rotators of the hip, which we acquired in *Janushirshasana* B and *Triang Mukha Ekapada Pashimottanasana*, all part of the Primary Series. Also, performing the prescribed femur rotations in *Supta Vajrasana* while holding on to your toes will have prepared you for this moment.

You need to strongly externally rotate your femur to get into lotus without the aid of your hands. If you cannot get your right foot far enough toward your left groin, you may use momentum to sweep your right foot over your left thigh.

Once your right leg is in half-lotus, bend your left leg and draw the left knee toward your chest and abdomen. This will bring your legs into a similar position as they are when performing *Marichyasana* D, only here you are upside down. The bent left leg will help to draw the right leg deeper into half-lotus. When you cannot get any further, alternately abduct and adduct the right thigh (which means to move the knee away from the center line of your body and again back toward the midline), while continuing to flex the right knee. This will make the right foot slide over the left thigh, and since you continue to flex the left thigh, the right leg will now slip deeper toward the left groin. Continue to flex the left hip to draw the left knee further toward your chest, until your right foot is firmly placed into the left groin.

If your right foot does not slide up into half-lotus, consider the same situation as in *Garbha Pindasana* regarding traction. The solution that worked for you there is likely to work for you here. To repeat, if you have a papery skin type (*vata* skin) you may find it beneficial to wear long tights. If you have thick, watery skin (*kapha* skin type), you will be better off wearing shorts and sprinkling water on your thighs and feet before you perform the posture. If your skin is oily (*pitta* skin type), you might consider an oil-based lubricant or emulsion. However, if you use this option, make sure not to use too much lubricant or make your skin too slippery. You will need a certain amount of traction to safely perform the posture's subsequent phases.

PHASE 2 — PLACING THE LEFT LEG CORRECTLY
Proceed with the next phase only if your right leg is in a stable position, deeply in half-lotus. Remember that when you sit on the floor to perform *Padmasana*, you never place the second leg into position before the first one is properly secured, so we will not resort to this while balancing on our arms either. Doing otherwise might endanger the knee joint of the leg that is on top.

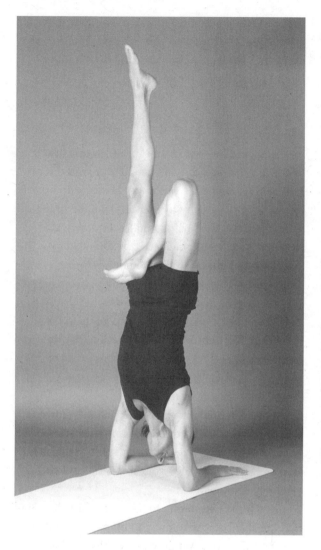

Forearm balance with right leg in half-lotus

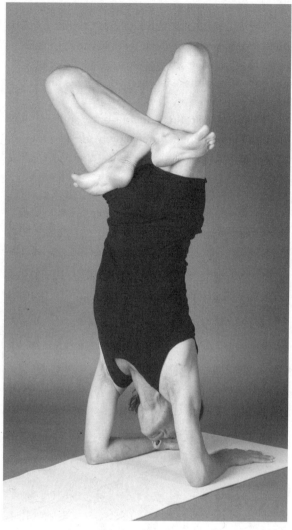

Forearm balance with both legs in lotus

Place the left leg into lotus by strongly externally rotating the left femur. For most students, it will be helpful to sweep the leg into position using momentum, especially if you have strong, bulging thighs. Once your left leg is in position, alternately adduct and abduct both thighs. Every time you move your knees together, strongly internally rotate your thighbones (this is similar to the femur movement performed in *Supta Vajrasana* in *vinyasa* nine). This will annul the previous external rotation and move your legs deeply into lotus. Both feet will need to be high up in the groin with the heels close together and the femurs almost parallel to move through the next phase of *Karandavasana*.

If you are new to this posture, I suggest that you stay here for five breaths, then extend your legs

slowly back up into *Pincha Mayurasana* and then exit as described under *vinyasa* nine of that posture. Do this for some time before you go on to the next phase.

These first two phases deal only with movements of the hip joints.

PHASE 3 — LOWERING THE LEGS TO THE HORIZONTAL PLANE

If you are a seasoned practitioner, then slowly flex your hip joints until your folded legs are parallel to the floor and your knees are at the same height as your sit bones. To do so, you need to extend your low back into the same position that you hold in *Urdhva Dandasana*, the variation of headstand wherein your legs are parallel to the floor. Holding

Urdhva Dandasana for a long time is good training for *Karandavasana*. As with *Urdhva Dandasana*, in this phase of *Karandavasana* you need to draw your sit bones over the back of your head. The defining moment of this phase is when you have a distinct backbend in your low back.

Balance here for five breaths or for longer if you want to build strength. Then slowly lift your knees up to the ceiling, sweep your legs out of *Padmasana*, and exit the posture in the same way as *Pincha Mayurasana*.

In this phase we added back extension to the movement of the hip joints.

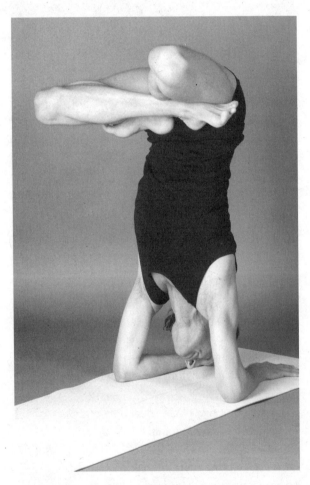

Forearm balance with horizontal lotus

PHASE 4 — STRAIGHTENING THE BACK

If phase 3 and the proper execution of its exit have become easy for you, then you are ready for the next step. Characteristic of phase 4 is that we completely annul the backbend that we created in phase 3, by dropping the knees further down. You may go as far as touching the thighs to your rib cage, but do not go further yet. Focus on stabilizing the shoulder blades using the latissimus dorsi, lower trapezius, and rhomboid muscles. Keep your humeri (arm bones) still completely flexed and resist the urge to lower down further.

Stay here for five breaths and then transit backward through the previous phases and out of *Pincha Mayurasana*. If you cannot lift back up out of phase 4, do not go any further but take the time to learn to do so. The further you lower down, the harder it will be to come back up. You need to imprint into your body the memory of lifting yourself up. Then you can try lifting up from a slightly lower point each day.

In this phase we flexed the hip joints to the maximum and returned the low back to neutral from extension.

PHASE 5 — FLEXING THE BACK

Once you can hold and lift out of phase 4, start to flex your trunk until your thighs are almost vertical. Your knees will now rest on your chest. If this is not the case, powerfully flex your hip joints and suck your knees into your chest.

Resist the temptation to drop down further. Stay here for five breaths before you lift back up out of the posture. If you can't hold this phase and just drop down to rest on your arms, chances are you won't be able to come back up.

In this phase we only flexed the spine. The hip joints were fully flexed in the previous phase and the shoulder joints will be extended in the subsequent phase.

PHASE 6 — EXTENDING THE HUMERI

In this final phase of the descent we add only the extension of the shoulder joint. Perform this action very slowly. Suck your knees up into your armpits rather than letting them drop down to your elbows. You will need very strong abdominal muscles to isometrically maintain the curl of your trunk. Fortunately, if you performed *Navasana* in the Primary Series with passion, your abdominals should be sufficiently strong. You also need to continue isometrically flexing your hip joints.

You will be able to draw your knees up into your armpits only when you have completed isotonic (contraction of muscles that involves their shortening) flexion of the hip joint and flexion of the trunk in the previous phases. We may call this the secret of successful execution of *Karandavasana*.

Make sure that you lower down in slow motion. To land heavily on your arms is not conducive to healthy knee joints. It would be the equivalent of receiving a kick against your knees from the front when sitting in *Padmasana*. If you collapse to the floor, landing on your derriere with a thud, your spine — and more important, what is attached to its other end, your brain — will bear the brunt of the impact.

After landing gently on your knees in a controlled fashion, stay in *Karandavasana* for five breaths, gazing toward your nose and keeping your knees sucked into your armpits.

Vinyasa Ten

Inhaling, strongly suck your thighs into your chest and at the same time flex your arm bones. To do so, imagine that you are lifting a heavy weight over your head. Focus on stabilizing your shoulder blades by drawing them down the back, engaging latissimus dorsi and lower trapezius. At the same time, draw the shoulder blades in toward the spine by engaging the rhomboids. Engage subscapularis and serratus anterior to suck the medial border of the shoulder blades into the posterior surface of the rib cage. Only when all of those actions are performed satisfactorily can the deltoid, triceps, and pectoralis major raise the heavy weight of the trunk effectively. Do not try to swing your legs up yet. This will move a large portion of your weight (that is, your legs) away from the axis around which you have to lift (that is, your shoulder joint) and thus increase the total weight you will need to lift.

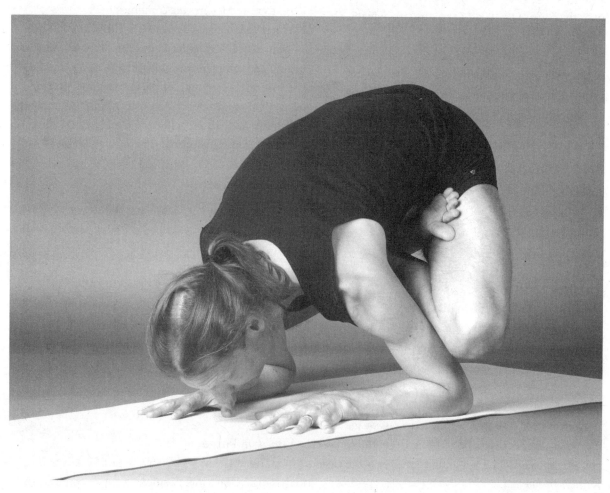

Karandavasana

If you tend to lose your balance — that is, fall toward the foot end of your mat — shift more weight into your hands. Continue to draw your knees into your chest by isometrically flexing your hip joints until your thighs are vertical to the floor. This is an exact reversion of phase 6.

Continue to suck the thighs into your chest and start to extend your back until it is in a neutral position. This is a reversion of phase 5.

Continue to extend your back by lifting your sit bones over the back of your head. Stop hip flexion and just slightly lift your legs off your rib cage. This movement reverses phase 4.

In the next phase we encounter a change of weight distribution, and many students lose their balance and fall out of the posture at that point. As we slowly extend the hip joints and lift the thighs toward a horizontal position, we need to create an arch in the low back and let the sit bones travel over the back of the head to balance the weight of the legs. This annuls phase 3.

Continuing the inhalation, extend the knees up to the ceiling and return the spine back to neutral. From here, straighten your legs out of lotus and transit out of the posture as described under *Pincha Mayurasana*, *vinyasa* eight.

Vinyasa Eleven

Exhaling, transit into *Chaturanga Dandasana*.

Vinyasa Twelve

Inhale into Upward Dog.

Vinyasa Thirteen

Exhale into Downward Dog.

We will continue the *vinyasa* count here to standing. The *vinyasa* count for the next three postures starts from the standing position, as you will either enter the state of the *asana* already in *vinyasa* five (which is normally the *vinyasa* for Upward Dog), as is the case for *Mayurasana* and *Nakrasana*, respectively; or you will begin the *vinyasa* count by placing your leg in half-lotus, as is the case with *Vatayanasana*.

Vinyasa Fourteen

Inhaling, jump forward to standing and look up. This *vinyasa* is identical with *vinyasa* three of *Surya Namaskara* A.

Vinyasa Fifteen

Exhaling, bend forward, placing your hands on either side of your feet, with your fingertips in line with your toes. This *vinyasa* is identical with *vinyasa* two of *Surya Namaskara* A.

Inhaling, come up to *Samasthiti*. This is the concluding posture of *Surya Namaskara* A.

Mayurasana

PEACOCK POSTURE

Drishti Nose

OVERVIEW: *Mayurasana* combines the features of an arm balance and an active backbend; it is essentially *Shalabhasana* balancing on your arms. Fully engaging your back extensors and shoulder stabilizers is essential for performing this posture effectively and safely. The posture is thought to cure abdominal diseases, reflecting the belief that the peacock can transform and neutralize poisons.

Vinyasa Count

We begin this and the next two postures with *vinyasa* one in *Samasthiti*. Exhaling, hop your feet hip-width apart and bend forward.

Vinyasa One

Place your hands between your feet, palms facing down and fingers pointing backward. Inhaling, straighten your back and look up.

Vinyasa Two

Exhaling, fold forward.

Vinyasa Three

Inhaling, raise your chest again and look up, arriving in the same position as *vinyasa* one.

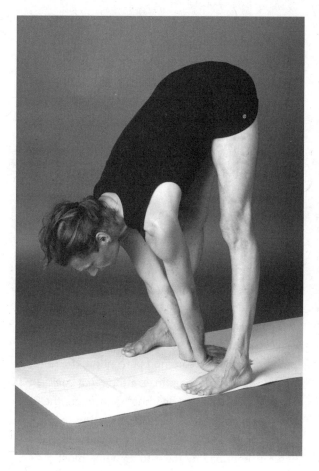

Mayurasana, vinyasa one

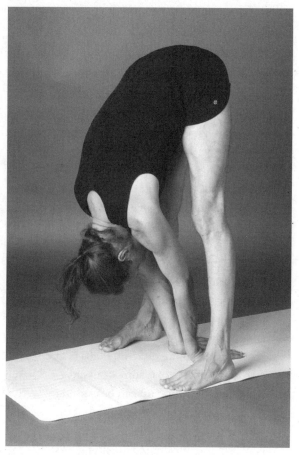

Mayurasana, vinyasa two

Vinyasa Four

Exhaling, hop back as if entering *Chaturanga Dandasana*. Bend your elbows in transit and bring them as close together as possible; ideally they will touch each other. Failure to do so means you will need to adduct the humeri (arm bones) the whole time, which means engaging the pectoralis major muscle. The weight of the chest will tend to drive the arms apart unless you can place your chest on top of your arms rather than in between them.

To enter *Mayurasana* the forearms must be firmly planted onto the chest and abdomen. This will give you the advantage of not having to flex the rib cage at the outset of the posture, which will make it easier later on to lift your chest and shoulders away from the floor. Those whose center of gravity is lower down, often females and people with long legs, need to make the thorax hyperkyphotic to place their elbows as low down as possible against the

contracted rectus abdominis muscle. This contraction acts as armor for the abdominal organs and provides a stable platform on which to mount the arms. Bend your elbows to form a right angle between your upper arms and forearms. Consciously engage and co-contract all stabilizers of the shoulder girdle and joints before you raise your weight into the air.

Vinyasa Five

Inhaling, shift your center of gravity forward, engage your back extensors, and lift up into what looks like a suspended *Shalabhasana*. Shifting your weight forward in this position means partially extending your elbows. The lower down the center of gravity in your body (when standing), the more you have to lift your chest forward in *Mayurasana* and extend your elbows to lift your feet off the floor. Bring your feet together and point them.

If you find it difficult to lift up, keep your head down and lift your feet only for five breaths. Once you have mastered this, lift your head by shifting your weight further forward.

If you still encounter problems, consider the following possible reasons and solutions.

- Make sure that your elbows don't come apart; this will make it much harder to lift. Strongly engaging pectoralis major will ensure that the elbows stay together.
- On hot days, your elbows may slip because you are sweating. In this case, place fabric between your elbows and abdomen to provide traction.
- Excess adipose tissue on thighs and buttocks will make you "bottom heavy" and thus you will have to lunge forward by extending your elbows more. This will make the posture much more difficult. If this is the case, dispose of excess adipose tissue.
- Difficulties in lifting up can be caused by weakness of the back extensors, but the latissimus dorsi, gluteus maximus, and hamstrings contribute to the lifting as well. Practice *Shalabhasana* to strengthen these muscles.
- Shifting your weight forward on slowly extending elbows requires considerable strength of arms and shoulders. If lacking here, practice jumping through from Downward Dog to *Dandasana*. Perform this movement with great passion, very slowly, gliding through *Lollasana* without touching down, into a suspended *Dandasana*, while still inhaling. Lower down only once, and commence exhalation.
- The abdominals need to provide a strong base to balance on. They are also important as antagonists of the back extensors. To strengthen your abdominals, hold *Navasana* longer and put more emphasis on clearing the floor when jumping through and jumping back.

Once you find *Mayurasana* easy, lift as high as you can and straighten your legs. Make sure that your shoulders don't round and collapse down toward the floor. To do so would court an imbalance of your shoulder muscles, as the more forward and down your shoulders are, the more emphasis will be shifted toward the pectoralis muscles that already bear the brunt of this posture. For a more holistic approach to using your shoulders, lift them away from the floor. This is achieved by drawing the shoulder blades down the back and in toward the spine, using latissimus dorsi, rhomboids, and lower trapezius. Also, make sure that your shoulder blades do not have a winged appearance in this posture. To prevent this, suck the medial borders of the scapulae into the chest by engaging serratus anterior and subscapularis.

To take the posture further, engage your erector spinae even more and arch up into a suspended *Shalabhasana*. This is the only posture apart from *Shalabhasana* in which we fully engage erector spinae. Contrary to common perception, the full engagement of erector spinae, although a back extensor, prevents backbending by drawing the spinous processes toward each other, thus shortening the back. As the erector spinae is therefore shunned by the astute yogi in most backbends, we should engage it in *Mayurasana* to its maximum capacity.

Look toward your nose and stay for five breaths. Exhaling, lower your feet.

WARM-UP AND RESEARCH POSTURE: *Shalabhasana* with arms extended overhead; if that's not enough, lie on your belly, place your feet under a sofa, and raise a barbell with your arms.

Vinyasa Six
Inhaling, place your feet on the floor and lift into what resembles an Upward Dog with your hands still in *Mayurasana* position.

Vinyasa Seven
Exhale into a Downward Dog–like position, apart from keeping your hands in place.

Vinyasa Eight
Inhaling, jump forward to standing, repeating *vinyasa* three of *Mayurasana*.

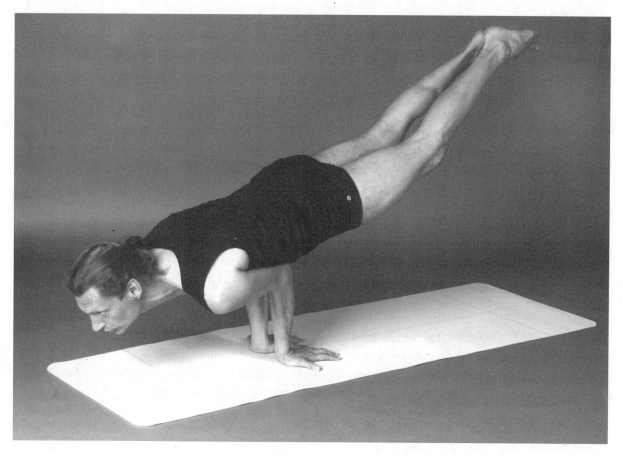

Mayurasana

Vinyasa Nine

Exhaling, bend forward, repeating *vinyasa* two of *Mayurasana*.

Inhaling, come up and hop your feet together, returning to *Samasthiti*.

Nakrasana

CROCODILE POSTURE

Drishti Nose

OVERVIEW: This movement, where the body is held close to the floor supported by all fours, resembles the movement of the crocodile. The same movement is performed in African dance, where it also is associated with the crocodile.

Vinyasa Count

Again we start from standing in *Samasthiti*.

Vinyasa One

Inhaling, raise your arms and look up.

Vinyasa Two

Exhaling, fold forward, placing your hands on either side of your feet.

Vinyasa Three

Inhaling, straighten your arms, flatten out your back, and look up.

These first three *vinyasas* are identical with those of *Surya Namaskara* A.

Vinyasa Four

Exhaling, jump back into *Chaturanga Dandasana* but keep your feet together.

Vinyasa Five

Inhaling, push off with all fours simultaneously and hop forward, landing on the exhalation. Repeat four

163

more times, each time moving further forward. Use the next five breaths to hop backward over the floor until you arrive in the same position that you started in.

The forward movement is easily achieved by plantar flexing your feet and pulling your hands across the floor toward your hips while becoming airborne. Both actions performed simultaneously will create forward propulsion. The lifting-off action, although done instinctually if the strength required is available, is more complex. You need to push your hands with high velocity into the floor, rapidly flexing your humeri (arm bones). This is a movement that is often employed in martial arts, such as boxing, karate, and so on. At the same time powerfully engage your hip flexors and push your feet into the floor. It is similar to the movement you would use to kick a ball, only it is performed with both legs simultaneously, while your body is horizontal. You need to synchronize your arm and leg movements to lift off effectively.

ADDRESSING DIFFICULTIES IN *NAKRASANA*: Strictly speaking, *Nakrasana* is the only posture in this series in which power is exercised, if we accept the definition that power equals strength multiplied by velocity. Other movements might exercise strength, but they are not rapid enough to exercise power.[26] For this reason, *Nakrasana* can pose a formidable challenge for some students.

If you cannot lift up at all after trying for a reasonable amount of time, isolate both movements and train them separately. You can train the arm movement by standing upright in front of a wall, facing it. Start with a distance of about two feet (sixty centimeters) and let your body fall toward the wall. Prior to impact, which at this distance would be quite mild, forcefully extend your arms and push your body away from the wall back to an upright position. Do this about ten to twenty times in quick succession. Once you find this exercise easy, extend your distance from the wall. At one yard's (one meter's) distance your arms will have to work much more.

A similar exercise benefit would derive from throwing a basketball against a wall from a short distance and catching it on the rebound. Do about forty fast repetitions. A more serious approach

26 The term *power* is used here strictly in a physical sense. The development of a "powerful personality" runs counter to the tenets of yoga.

THE TWO TYPES OF MUSCLE FIBERS AND YOGA

Muscles are made up of different types of fibers. Type 1 fibers are also called "slow-twitch" fibers because they do exactly that. Their contraction velocity is approximately one-tenth that of type 2, or "fast-twitch," muscle fibers; they produce less maximum force. Different muscles have a different proportion of type 1 versus type 2 fibers. For example, stabilizing muscles, which need to work a little all the time and provide tone, are made up of slow-twitch fibers. Conversely, a muscle like the biceps, which works only when we need to use it, is primarily composed of fast-twitch muscle fibers. Most muscles will have a combination of both fast- and slow-twitch fibers. Additionally, different people have different proportions of slow- and fast-twitch muscle fibers in their muscles. Muscle fibers, however, do adapt on the basis of the functional demands that are placed upon them. This means that power is a muscle characteristic that can be trained.

As almost all movements in yoga are slow, yogis don't exercise fast-twitch muscles enough. Similarly, they do not exercise power enough but focus excessively on strength and flexibility. As a result they often become very unbalanced toward the slow-twitch/strength and flexibility end of the spectrum. This is most common in extremely flexible females with low muscle tension. After decades of yoga, they often find they must move on to forms of exercise that are more based on power and fast-twitch. To prevent this imbalance from unfolding, yoginis must emphasize postures like *Nakrasana* that develop fast-twitch muscles and power. Without this understanding, those who find *Nakrasana* "too hard" are unlikely to invest the necessary passion to learn to perform it properly.

would be to take a weight, such as a medicine ball, in both hands and forcefully throw it away from you.[27] Don't choose a weight that is too heavy. It is the velocity of the movement that counts. And yes, be careful where you throw the weight.

You can simulate the leg movement by lying on your back and forcefully lifting one leg at a time off the floor. Make sure to fully brace your abdomen (strongly contract all layers of the abdominal muscles but principally the transverse abdominis) to protect your low back. Lift each leg only 20–25 degrees maximum, as this is the amount you move your leg in the posture to lift yourself off the floor, and do about twenty repetitions on each side.

Together with the previous three postures, *Nakrasana* can exacerbate an already existing shoulder injury. Our tendency is to overuse the muscles on the anterior surface of the thorax, particularly pectoralis minor and major, to the detriment of those on the posterior, the lower trapezius, rhomboid, and latissimus dorsi. Avoid that by strongly drawing your shoulder blades down the back and drawing them in toward the spine. This amounts to lifting the heart and puffing out the chest in the posture. If you have an existing shoulder problem, you may insulate your shoulder joint from impact in this posture and stabilize it by strongly squeezing your elbows in against the rib cage.

Synchronize your movements with the breath. Utilize the lifting quality of a deep inhalation to lift off the floor in *Nakrasana* and expel the air forcefully upon descent. Let the movement follow the rhythm of the breath and not vice versa. If necessary, experiment with taking a few rapid, forceful breaths first, and once their resonance frequency is established in the body add the vigorous, powerful movement of the extremities to arrive at the forward and backward lunging movement.

27 The throwing of weight is used as a training in martial arts, where not strength but strength times velocity counts. Do not try to catch the weight once it falls. The catching of a heavy falling object is the classic cause of a glenoid labrum tear, one of the slowest to heal injuries of the passive stabilization system.

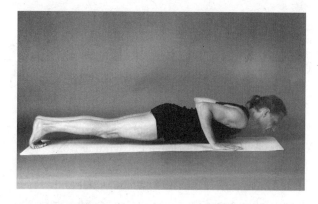

Nakrasana on floor

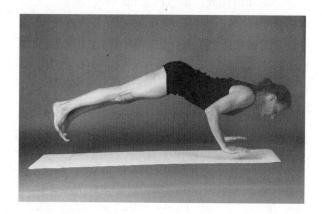

Nakrasana suspended

Vinyasa Six
Inhaling, move into Upward Dog.

Vinyasa Seven
Exhaling, move into Downward Dog.

Vinyasa Eight
Inhaling, jump forward to standing and look up. This *vinyasa* is identical with *vinyasa* three of *Surya Namaskara* A.

Vinyasa Nine
Exhaling, bend forward, placing your hands on either side of the feet with your fingertips in line with your toes. This *vinyasa* is identical with *vinyasa* two of *Surya Namaskara* A.

Inhaling, come up to *Samasthiti*. This is the concluding posture of *Surya Namaskara* A.

FOURTH CONNECTIVE SECTION

Here commences the fourth and last connective section of the passive element, extending from *Vatayanasana* to *Baddha Hasta Shirshasana*. The section fulfills two purposes. The first is to buffer and insulate the subsequent cool-down postures from the intensity of the arm-balance sequence. This is achieved through a mix of hip openers (*Vatayanasana, Gaumukhasana, Supta Urdhva Pada Vajrasana*), forward bends (*Parighasana*), and twists (again *Parighasana* and *Supta Urdhva Pada Vajrasana*), thus continuing the Primary Series–like characteristic of the connective sections.

The second purpose is to create a capstone for the series; when bricklayers construct an archway, they place the capstone last, and it gives the whole structure stability. Through the *amrita*-absorbing capacity of *Mukta Hasta Shirshasana* and *Baddha Hasta Shirshasana*, this connective section serves a similar function for the series.

Vatayanasana

WINDOW POSTURE

Drishti Upward

OVERVIEW: With *Vatayanasana* begins the energetic wind-down of the series. The next four postures utilize the heat created by the strength and endurance section to increase the flexibility in the hamstrings, hip joints, and shoulder joints.

PREREQUISITE: Proficient performance of *Supta Vajrasana* and *Karandavasana*.

CONTRAINDICATION: Knee pain and instability.

Vinyasa Count

Vinyasa One

Standing in *Samasthiti*, inhale and place your right leg into half-lotus as you would to perform the last

---

PROTECTING THE KNEE IN *VATAYANASANA*

Those new to this posture may wish to place some padding, such as a folded towel, under the knee. This protects the knee from the hard surface, but it also raises the right hip slightly, which can help the body get used to the odd geometry of the posture. Once you are experienced in *Vatayanasana*, discard this aid, but don't hesitate to go back to it during phases of knee sensitivity.

---

standing posture of the warm-up in the Primary Series, *Ardha Baddha Padmottanasana*. With your right hand, reach around your back and bind your right big toe.

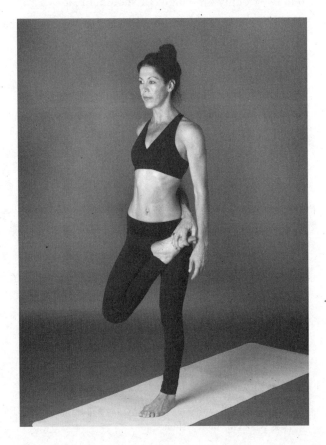

Vatayanasana, vinyasa one

166

Vinyasa **Two**

Exhaling, bend forward, placing your left hand next to your left foot, with your fingertips in line with your toes. Prevent your right hip from sagging by lifting the right knee out to the side until the hips are level, parallel to the floor. At the end of the exhalation, let go of your foot and place your right hand down on the floor in line with your foot and left hand.

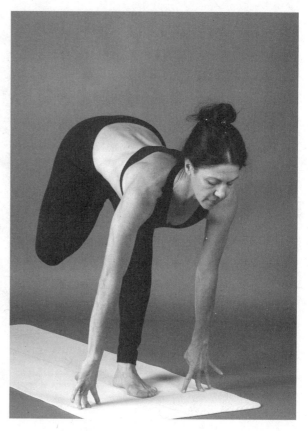

Vatayanasana, vinyasa three

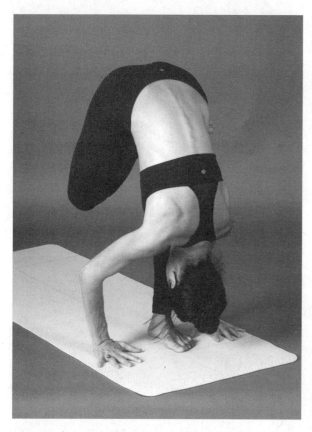

Vatayanasana, vinyasa two

Vinyasa **Three**

Inhaling, look up and straighten your back while leaving your hands on the floor.

Vinyasa **Four**

Exhaling, jump back into a *Chaturanga Dandasana*–like posture, but with your right leg remaining in half-lotus.

Vinyasa **Five**

Inhaling, move into an Upward Dog–like posture, keeping your right leg in half-lotus. Point your left

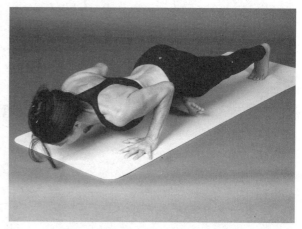

Vatayanasana, vinyasa four

foot and allow your right knee to touch the floor lightly. To avoid this you would need to lift your right hip upward (this would translate into drawing the pelvis backward in normal standing), a movement that should not be combined with the backbend in this posture as it could cause imbalance in your hips.

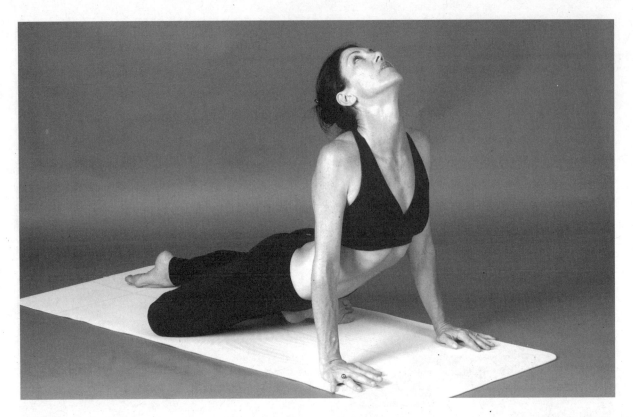

Vatayanasana, vinyasa five

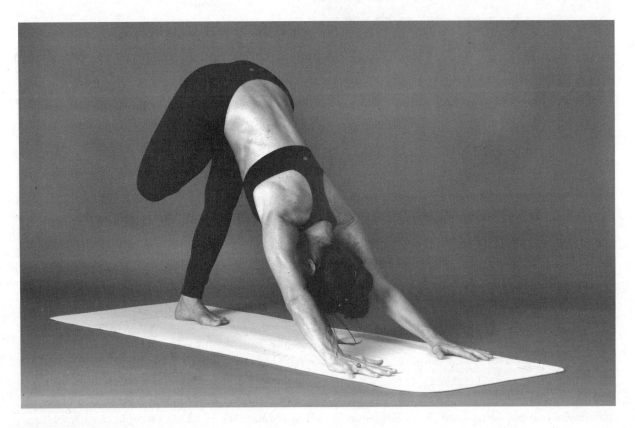

Vatayanasana, vinyasa six

Vinyasa Six

Exhaling, move into a Downward Dog–like posture, keeping your right leg in half-lotus.

Vinyasa Seven

Inhaling, hop forward, bending your left leg in the process, and turn your left foot out on the ball as far as possible, ideally 90 degrees, so that your toes point out to the left, and let your knee follow suit. Do not perform this movement with your ankle joint but rather through abduction of the femur. This may prove to be challenging, as open hip joints and long adductors are required. Renewed emphasis on *Supta Padangushtasana* in the Primary Series will be helpful here. If necessary, progress slowly over months.

Place your right knee down on the floor gently, taking most of your weight into your arms. As your knee descends, strongly rotate the right femur internally. Having internally rotated the right femur, you can now engage the quadriceps on the right by gently pulling up on the kneecap, without the leg slipping out of half-lotus. The engaging of the quadriceps is used to protect the knee, which will be weight bearing in this posture. Balancing on a folded knee is a rather odd maneuver that is not performed in many postures (*Gorakshasana*, a posture not contained in the Ashtanga *vinyasa* system, would be another example). By engaging the quadriceps, we will press tibia and femur together to prevent forward travel of the tibia on the femur or vice versa, which can happen, especially if one of the bones is much longer than the other and presses into the floor more. Forward travel of either of the two bones here could lead to soft-tissue damage in the knee.

Be conscientious about performing both of these actions (inwardly rotating the femur and engaging the quadriceps) simultaneously to protect your knee. At the same time, release your hamstrings and adductors, as their action would suck the thigh back into the hip. Instead, let the femur reach out of the hip and down into the floor.

Once your knee is on the floor and its integrity is secured through medial rotation of the femur and engaging of the quadriceps by pulling up on the kneecap, gently move your knee toward the heel of the left foot. Ideally the right knee would touch the left heel, but it is suggested that you move slowly toward this ideal, if necessary over the course of months. Closing the gap between the right knee and the left heel requires great amounts of flexibility of the hip joint and a great degree of control over the medial rotators of the right femur. It is essential to adequately perform *Supta Vajrasana* and *Karandavasana* before attempting this posture, as they will produce the needed virtues.

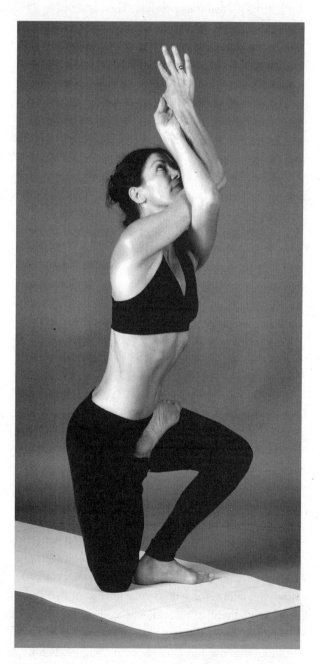

Vatayanasana

After having "closed the window" between the foot and the knee, bring your whole trunk, which might still lean forward, upright and lift your chest high. Lift your trunk not by arching your low back but by extending your hip joint on the right, which will inevitably intensify the workload of your right knee. Proceed sensibly.

Once your legs and trunk are in position, place your bent right arm on top of the left one, crossing above the elbow. Place the palms together and raise both arms up as far as possible. Then attempt to straighten them against the existing resistance. Now externally rotate both arm bones and draw the shoulder blades toward each other and down the back to release the pectoralis major and minor muscles. Look upward past your hands and hold *Vatayanasana* for five breaths.

Exhaling, release both arms and place your hands on the floor.

Vinyasa Eight
Inhaling, take the weight into your arms and lift up, keeping the right leg in half-lotus.

Vinyasa Nine
Exhaling, jump back into a *Chaturanga Dandasana*–like posture, repeating *vinyasa* four.

Vinyasa Ten
Inhaling, move into an Upward Dog–like posture, repeating *vinyasa* five.

Vinyasa Eleven
Exhaling, move into a Downward Dog–like posture, repeating *vinyasa* six. Gently take your right leg out of half-lotus, assisting with your left hand if necessary. Now bend your left leg and, assisting with your right hand, place it into half-lotus. Make sure that your foot is placed snugly up into your groin. Do not jump forward with your foot resting somewhere on your quadriceps; otherwise, you are applying lateral force onto your knee joint that can lead to ligament strain and eventually damage. To secure the knee up into the groin we use the same technique as used in *Karandavasana*. Slightly bend the straight right leg and then sweep the knee of the

folded left leg repeatedly out to the side and back toward the knee of the right leg. The pressure of the right leg will let your left foot slide up into the groin. If no movement is achieved, you need to again address the traction issue discussed already in this book under *Karandavasana* (p. 156) and previously in *Ashtanga Yoga: Practice and Philosophy* (p. 102).

Vinyasas Twelve to Sixteen
Repeat *Vatayanasana* on the left side.

Vinyasa Seventeen
Inhaling, from the Downward Dog–like position jump forward to standing, keeping your leg in half-lotus. With your left arm, quickly reach around your back, bind the big toe of the left foot, and look up. The binding of the toe is an important detail that seals the posture energetically. It is important that you bind before looking up and completing the inhalation.

Vinyasa Eighteen
Exhaling, bend forward, placing your left hand next to your left foot with your fingertips in line with your toes, a repetition of *vinyasa* two. Make sure that you continue to hold on to your big toe.

Vinyasa Nineteen
As with the transition performed when exiting *Ardha Baddha Padmottanasana*, here we come up in two stages. Inhaling, lift your chest and look up, keeping your right hand on the floor. Then exhale while holding this posture. This is a repeat of the position of *vinyasa* seventeen.

Vinyasa Twenty
Inhaling, come up to standing, keeping the left big toe bound in the process. *Vatayanasana* won't be completed until you stand completely upright with your leg still bound. Again you need to radically inwardly rotate the left femur to safely draw the foot high up into the right groin. If you do this properly, your lotus flexibility will benefit greatly from *Vatayanasana*.

Exhaling, replace the left foot on the floor and return to *Samasthiti*.

Please note: The *vinyasa* counts of the last four postures were concluded by a full *vinyasa* (coming to standing). From now on we go back to transiting through a simple half-*vinyasa*.

Parighasana

IRON CAGE POSTURE

Drishti Upward

OVERVIEW: After the excitement of the backbends, leg-behind-head, and arm balances, the calming effect of a forward bend continues the winding down of the series.

Vinyasa Count

Vinyasa One
Standing in *Samasthiti*, inhale, raise your arms, and look up.

Vinyasa Two
Exhaling, fold forward, placing your hands on either side of your feet.

Vinyasa Three
Inhaling, straighten your arms, flatten out your back, and look up.

Vinyasa Four
Exhaling, jump back into *Chaturanga Dandasana*.

Vinyasa Five
Inhaling, move into Upward Dog.

Vinyasa Six
Exhaling, move into Downward Dog. These first six *vinyasas* are identical with those of *Surya Namaskara* A.

Vinyasa Seven
Inhaling, jump through to sitting and assume a posture similar to *Triang Mukha Ekapada Pashimottanasana* in the Primary Series, only here draw your right knee 90 degrees out to the side. You may, as in *Krounchasana*, jump straight into the posture. Place your hands on your hips and square your torso toward the folded right leg.

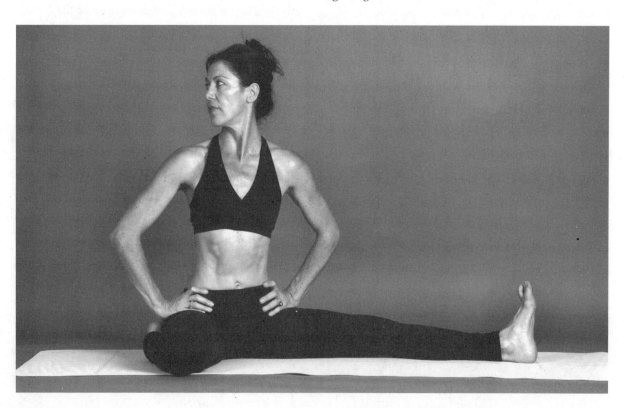

Parighasana, vinyasa seven

Vinyasa Eight

Exhaling, twist your torso laterally and fold down with the left side of your torso along your straight left leg, while your chest keeps facing your folded right leg. Take the inside of your left foot with your left hand and, bending your arm, place your left shoulder against the inside of your left leg. Reach now over your head with your right arm and take the outside of your left foot. Use both arms to twist more deeply, lifting the right shoulder back over the left one. Draw both shoulder blades down your back, turn your head, and look up to the ceiling. Take your left elbow off the floor.

Work both legs as if you were doing *Triang Mukha Ekapada Pashimottanasana*. Pull up on the left kneecap and draw the left heel into the floor. Extend out through the bases of all toes against the pull of both hands. Make sure that you do not actively flex (dorsi flex) your left foot, as this would put strain on the cruciate ligaments of your knee.

Unless your hamstrings on the left are extremely long, there will be a strong tendency to externally rotate your left thigh to escape the stretch of the two inner hamstrings (semimembranosus and semitendinosus). If this tendency is present, counteract it by vigorously rotating your left thigh internally.

Now strongly externally rotate your right thigh and work on grounding your right sit bone. This will lead to a formidable stretch of the right low back, particularly the quadratus lumborum on the right. The quadratus lumborum may tighten during backbending and leg-behind-head postures, especially when they are performed with excess fervor and lack of finesse.

Assist the stretching of the right low back by breathing into and elongating the right waist. The ability to elongate the waist is paramount not only in forward bending and backbending but also in leg-behind-head postures. It can be learned right here.

Look upward, past your right elbow, and take five deep breaths.

ACTIVE RELEASE TECHNIQUE: Draw your left heel into the floor by gently engaging your hamstrings, which will tend to lift you back out of the posture. Vigorously counteract and annul this tendency by using the iron cage of your arms to draw and twist your chest deeper into the posture.

Vinyasa Nine

Inhaling, let go of your foot and return to the upright position, placing both hands on your hips as in *vinyasa* seven, and exhale.

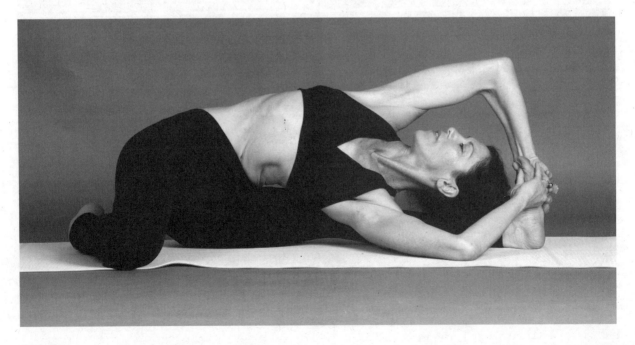

Parighasana

Vinyasa Ten

Place both hands on the floor and, inhaling, lift up.

Vinyasa Eleven

Exhaling, jump back into *Chaturanga Dandasana*.

Vinyasa Twelve

Inhaling, move into Upward Dog.

Vinyasa Thirteen

Exhaling, move into Downward Dog.

Vinyasas Fourteen to Twenty

Repeat *Parighasana* on the left side.

Gaumukhasana

COW FACE POSTURE

Drishti Nose and upward

OVERVIEW: *Gaumukhasana* opens the shoulders in anticipation of the concluding headstand series.

Vinyasa Count

Vinyasa Seven

Inhaling, jump through and, crossing the thighs, place the right thigh atop the left one. Now, crossing the shins, place the right foot to the left of the left foot, so that they are touching. Slowly lower down and balance on your heels, with both sit bones off the floor.

Do not mistake this posture for the one in which the Indian musicians sit for some ten hours a day — with their sit bones both touching the floor and the feet on either side. That would not provide enough challenge for somebody who is about to complete the Intermediate Series. The present posture is decidedly more difficult and it involves balancing. Here we have both feet next to each other under our sit bones. You will feel a significant stretch of the quadriceps on both sides. If the quadriceps is not stretched enough (even after being stretched in the intermediate backbends), *Gaumukhasana* will also be challenging for the knee joints. If this problem is present, sit every day in *Supta Virasana* for fifteen to

twenty minutes. (See *Ashtanga Yoga: Practice and Philosophy*, p. 57.)

Once the feet are close together, the foundation of the posture is very narrow; hence, you will need to balance. This is intended. Do not avoid it by placing your feet apart.

Reach with both hands around your right knee and interlock your fingers so that the bases of the fingers interlock, not just the fingertips. This will make the following action much more difficult. You could easily cheat, but consider one thing: Every yoga posture is a physical prayer to the Supreme Being. What sort of act do you want to offer to the Supreme Being? It should be an authentic and true offering; therefore, you are advised to perform the complete posture without cutting corners.

Lift your chest high and place your chin down on the manubrium (top part of the sternum), into *Jalandhara Bandha* position.[28] Draw the shoulder blades down the back and the lower abdomen in.

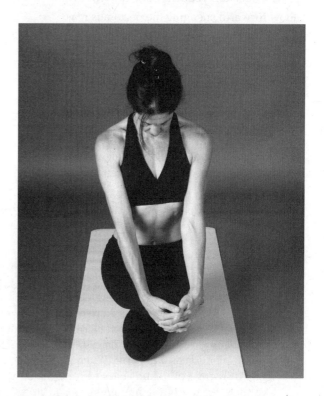

Gaumukhasana A

28 "*Jalandhara Bandha* position" refers to a position that externally looks identical to *Jalandhara Bandha*. However, the significant internal action of swallowing and consequently locking the throat for breath retention, done in *Jalandhara Bandha*, does not occur here.

Look toward the nose, which connects you to *Mula Bandha*. At the same time, the pelvic floor is intensely stimulated by your sitting on both heels. Stay in *Gaumukhasana* A for five breaths and gaze toward your nose.

Vinyasa Eight

Inhaling, reach up with your right arm, flex your elbows, and place your hand on your back.

With your left hand, reach behind your back and up between your shoulder blades and interlock with your right hand.

If your shoulders are very flexible, you can grab one or both wrists instead.

Bring your torso upright and draw your right elbow far back. Look up and draw your shoulder blades down your back. Hold *Gaumukhasana* B for five breaths and look upward.

ACTIVE RELEASE TECHNIQUE: Draw your right elbow forward, engaging the pectoralis major muscle. Pulling the right hand down the back using your left arm will deepen the stretch.

WARM-UP AND RESEARCH POSTURE: If you cannot interlock your hands at all, do one or both of the following exercises outside of your practice:

1. Stand in front of a table or chair and fold forward so that your elbows rest on the edge in front of you and place your hands together in prayer position. Let your chest

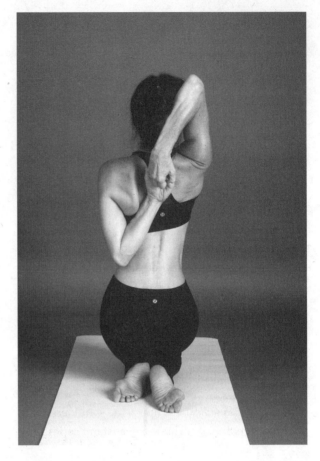

Gaumukhasana B

sink down toward the floor and feel the stretch in your shoulder joints.

2. Sit or stand upright and raise your right arm to your limit with your elbow flexed. With your left hand press your right elbow further back beyond your head.

PREPARING THE SHOULDERS FOR *GAUMUKHASANA*

Gaumukhasana promotes the complete flexion of the humerus. It particularly stretches the triceps muscle, which may have become shortened from the many repetitions of lowering down into *Chaturanga Dandasana*. The triceps perform elbow extension. They work eccentrically when entering *Chaturanga Dandasana* and concentrically on exiting the posture. If the triceps are tight, you will find the arm position of *Gaumukhasana* difficult. When performing *Virabhadrasana* A and *Utkatasana*, put more emphasis on drawing your hands back beyond the crown or even back of your head and thus out of view. Complete flexion of the humerus is also improved by drawing your sternum toward and over the imagined line going through both wrists when performing *Urdhva Dhanurasana* (backbending). Another way of opening the shoulders is to draw the chest down to the floor in Downward Dog. However, this action should be performed only by students with relatively stiff shoulders or high muscle tone. In a flexible student, the action would lead to collapsing behind the heart. If in doubt, let a qualified teacher assess the situation.

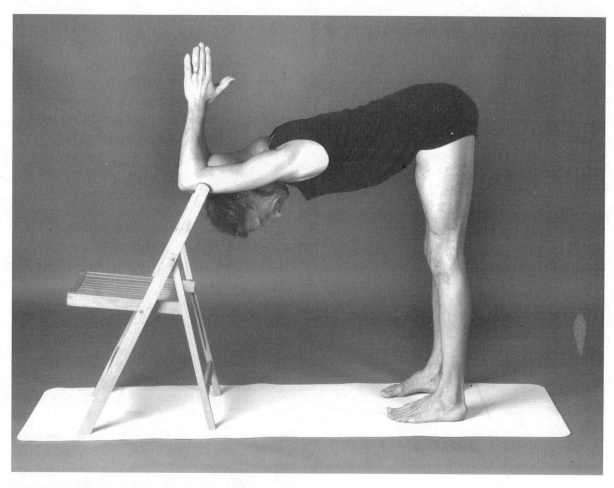

Shoulder warm-up 1

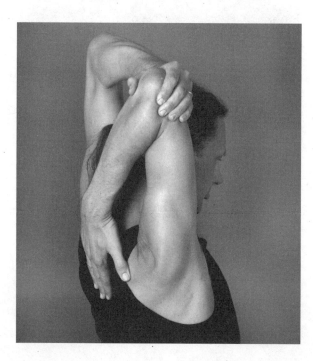

Shoulder warm-up 2

Vinyasa Nine

Exhaling, release your arms and place your hands down.

Vinyasa Ten

Inhaling, lift up into *Lollasana*.

Vinyasa Eleven

Exhaling, glide back into *Chaturanga Dandasana*.

Vinyasa Twelve

Inhaling, move into Upward Dog.

Vinyasa Thirteen

Exhaling, move into Downward Dog.

Vinyasas Fourteen to Twenty

Repeat *Gaumukhasana* on the left side.

175

Supta Urdhva Pada Vajrasana

RECLINING THUNDERBOLT POSTURE
WITH ONE FOOT UPWARD

Drishti Nose

OVERVIEW: This is a surprisingly difficult posture, as the binding of the half-lotus needs to be maintained during the transition. As usual, the key to success is to break down the posture into its constituent phases and isolate them.

CONTRAINDICATIONS: Knee injuries or tight adductors.

Vinyasa Count

Vinyasa Seven
Inhaling, jump through and, exhaling, lie down.

Vinyasa Eight
Inhaling, take both legs over into *Halasana* and place your right leg into half-lotus.

Exhaling, with your right hand reach around your back and bind your right big toe.

If you can't reach your big toe, try any or all of the following:

- Stretch your quadriceps by sitting in *Virasana* to deepen your lotus.
- Place more emphasis on internal femur rotation to deepen your lotus.
- Practice *Baddhakonasana* with renewed vigor for the same reason.
- Stretch your pectoralis minor with exercise 2 on page 111 for enhanced shoulder flexibility.
- Dispose of excess adipose tissue stored around your waist. The location of body fat has been shown to be a more accurate indicator of weight-related illness versus the total amount of body fat. Adipose tissue stored around the waist is known as abdominal obesity and is an indicator for the development of coronary heart disease via formation of arterial plaques through low density lipoprotein (LDL). The removal

of such tissue will not only improve your overall health but will also improve the likelihood of binding in the present posture.

With your left hand, bind the big toe of the still-straight left leg. Bring your right knee as close as possible to the left knee; ideally, both thighs would be parallel and the right femur would be radically internally rotated. Keeping the knees together is the key to the subsequent movement, which, although it looks quite easy, is one of the more difficult transitions in this series. Draw your right foot high up into your left groin and then bend your right arm, drawing your elbow as far out to the right as possible. In *vinyasa* nine, this will result in your forearm being at a right angle to your lumbar spine rather than over your elbow, allowing you to eventually roll over your forearm. If your forearm were instead over your elbow, your elbow would then be positioned diagonally across your low back and thus would impose all sorts of uncomfortable and unpredictable forces against your lumbar vertebrae.

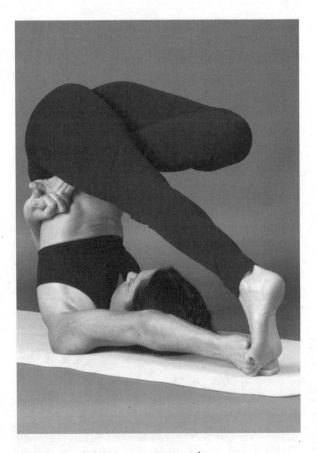

Supta Urdhva Pada Vajrasana, vinyasa eight

Vinyasa Nine

We will break this difficult *vinyasa* down into phases to make it accessible to those who are lacking extreme flexibility of the hip joints.

PHASE 1 — BENDING THE LEFT LEG

With the beginning of the inhalation, bend your left leg and place your left ankle just outside of your left hip joint. Change your grip and take the outside of your left foot with your left hand. Use this hand now to completely flex your knee joint by stretching your quadriceps. The relation of your left leg to your left thigh needs to be the same as if you were sitting in *Virasana* without any padding under your sit bones.[29] If you can't perform this position, don't attempt *Supta Urdhva Pada Vajrasana*, as this inability indicates that your quadriceps are not yet long enough to perform this posture safely.

PHASE 2 — DRAWING BOTH KNEES UP TO THE CEILING

Continuing the exhalation, draw both thighs together up to the ceiling by extending your hip joints. Do that by keeping your knees together and keeping both legs in position.

Keep your right foot bound and keep drawing your left leg into *Virasana* position. Once both knees point straight up to the ceiling, induce some lumbar arch, which will enable you to safely roll over your right arm. You are now in a shoulder stand–like position with one leg in half-lotus and the other folded. Both thighs, however, are vertical to the floor.

PHASE 3 — ROLLING DOWN

Exhaling, round your upper back somewhat (not your low back) and roll down over your arm, keeping your hip joints extended. Make sure that you keep your shoulders on the floor until both legs touch down. Keep your low back lordotic to reduce pressure on the spine and continue to draw your elbow out to the side while you flex it. Keep both knees together, as otherwise you will not be able to keep your right big toe bound. Before your knees and legs touch down, make sure that

you press your left leg up against your left thigh, point (plantar flex) your left foot and flex (curl under) your toes. Failing to do so could result in hurting or bruising your toes, particularly the left big toe.

PHASE 4 — LIFTING THE TORSO

Once your knees touch down, immediately initiate the inhalation, start to flex your hip joints, and use the existing momentum to come up to a sitting position. As you rock up, continue to draw your knees together and to rotate your right femur medially (inwardly), while keeping your right big toe bound.

Once you are upright, place your left hand under your right knee, palm facing down and fingers under the knee, as you would in *Bharadvajasana*. The difference is that here you keep your knees together while in the posture dedicated to Rishi Bharadvaja, you draw your knees far apart.

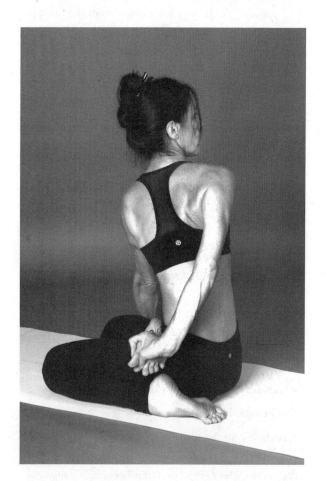

Supta Urdhva Pada Vajrasana

---

29 Anatomically, the term *leg* refers only to the part of the lower extremity from the knee to the ankle joint. The part above the knee joint is referred to as *thigh*.

Twist to the right and firmly ground your left sit bone. Lift the front of your chest and draw your shoulder blades down the back. As in all twists, drop your chin and lift your back of your head up to the ceiling.

Look toward your nose and take five breaths.

Exhaling, release your hands, swing around, and place your hands down ready for jump-back. Alternatively, you may straighten the right leg or even both legs if your knees feel sensitive to jumping out of half-lotus.

ACTIVE RELEASE TECHNIQUE: Same as in *Bharadvajasana*.

WARM-UP AND RESEARCH POSTURE: Assume the end version of *Supta Urdhva Pada Vajrasana* and then slowly lie down on your back while keeping your toe bound and both knees on the floor. You will have to transit through this posture for an instant on your way to the final posture. Arch your back away from the floor to improve your hold on the big toe. Feel how lumbar lordosis rather than kyphosis improves your grip.

Vinyasa Ten
Inhaling, lift up into *Lollasana*.

Vinyasa Eleven
Exhaling, glide back into *Chaturanga Dandasana*.

Vinyasa Twelve
Inhaling, move into Upward Dog.

Vinyasa Thirteen
Exhaling, move into Downward Dog.

Vinyasas Fourteen to Twenty
Repeat *Supta Urdhva Pada Vajrasana* on the left side.

Mukta Hasta Shirshasana

FREE HANDS HEADSTAND

Drishti Nose

OVERVIEW: The seven headstands energetically seal the Intermediate Series. A lot of energy has been created and released during the practice of the series. This energy now needs to be accumulated and stored. According to the yogic texts, the nectar of life (*amrita*) drizzles from the soft palate (the end of the *sushumna*), a place called the moon, downward, to then be burned by the sun of the gastric fire. Headstands reverse this process by placing the sun above the moon. The other reason for the headstands is that through their variety they offer the opportunity to closely study the subtle alignment of the shoulders. Understanding this alignment is necessary before the yogi practices the advanced arm balances of the third series.

Vinyasa Count — A Version

Vinyasa Seven
Inhaling, hop forward and land on your knees.

Exhaling, place your head and hands down in a three-point-headstand position, with your forearms perpendicular to the floor. Place the highest point of your head down. Most students have the tendency to balance too far toward the forehead, which unnecessarily compresses the neck. Of course, it is

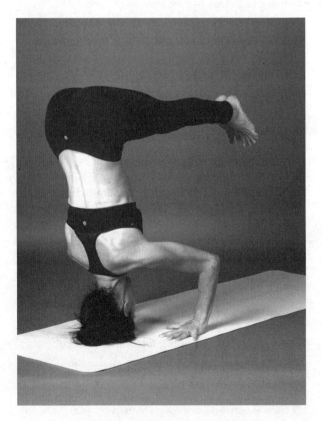

Entering headstand with straight legs, *vinyasa* seven

178

also possible to place the weight too much toward the back of the head. If this is done continuously over a long period, a reverse curvature may be induced in the cervical spine. If in doubt, ask a qualified instructor to assess your head position.

Once you have the head in the correct position, straighten your legs and walk your feet in toward your head as far as possible, without rounding your back. In fact, to achieve a headstand while keeping the legs straight, you will need to increase the lordotic curve in your low back. At this point your hips and buttocks will need to extend back beyond your spine for your feet to lift off the floor. This happens naturally and without effort when the hips are taken far enough back. To not lose your balance, simply keep your weight evenly distributed between your hands and the crown of your head.

Vinyasa **Eight**

Inhaling, slowly lift your straight legs together up into headstand. You need to be comfortable with transiting in and out of headstand with straight legs if you are practicing the Intermediate Series. This way of transiting is vastly superior to transiting with bent legs, as it creates more core strength, of which you will need copious amounts in many of the *asanas* in this and the next series. Avoid using the help of a wall for balancing in all headstand variations. As already explained, walls are *tamasic* objects that cannot supply feedback. (The same must, of course, be said about books and DVDs. They cannot provide feedback even if the knowledge enclosed in them is of a *sattvic* nature.) Students who do use walls are often stunted in their development. If you need help, a teacher who is able to analyze your postures can tell you exactly which actions in the posture you are not performing.

Firmly pressing your hands into the floor, lift your legs until your hip joints are completely extended and your body forms a straight line from head to toe. Point your feet and keep all leg and trunk muscles engaged lightly to prevent the sagging of blood toward the brain. Keep your *bandhas* firmly engaged and breathe slowly into the chest, keeping the diaphragm oscillating freely. Breathing in all inversions should always be slow, as rapid breathing would disturb your balance through

the resonance frequency created in the abdomen. This would lead to either the body swinging back and forth like a pendulum or so much energy being wasted on the suppression of this swinging that the student would fatigue quickly and fall out of headstand. All inversions therefore require slow and controlled thoraco-diaphragmatic breathing.

As in all headstand versions, engage lower trapezius to draw your shoulder blades up toward the ceiling, and attempt to carry most of your weight in your arms. However, the latter instruction is not as important here as in *Shirshasana*, since we hold these headstand versions for five breaths only. Take five breaths and look toward your nose.

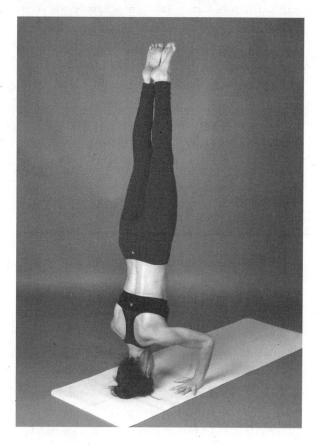

Mukta Hasta Shirshasana A

To transit out of this posture, we will use essentially the same method employed and described under *Pincha Mayurasana*. You need to transit out of these inversions on the peak of the inhalation but before you begin the exhalation. On the last inhalation, shift more weight from your head to your hands, become light, and when you are most buoyant, press your hands powerfully into the floor. The crucial moment to change your hand position is when you stop resisting gravity and allow your feet to fall toward the floor. Keep your body weight forward on your hands so that your feet land lightly and with minimal impact.

Vinyasa Nine

Exhaling, drop into *Chaturanga Dandasana* with both legs at the same time. If you cannot rely on your shoulder strength, then flex your hip joints slightly on the way down to use your hip flexors to soften the landing. If you are capable of performing half-*vinyasas* without touching your feet down, then on your way out of *Mukta Hasta Shirshasana*, draw your hands toward your waistline and suck your chest toward the front end of your mat. You can then lower down with your back slightly extended. This way you can fade out the movement and land lightly.

Whichever method you choose, to prepare for the impact make sure that your feet are flexed (dorsi flexed) and your toes are extended (curled up).

Vinyasa Ten

Inhaling, move into Upward Dog.

Vinyasa Eleven

Exhaling, move into Downward Dog.

Vinyasa Count — B Version

Vinyasa Seven

Inhaling, hop forward and land on your knees.

Exhaling, place your head and hands down as in *Mukta Hasta Shirshasana* A, but then straighten your arms and place your palms, facing up, on either side of your feet so that your arms are parallel to each other. Straighten your legs now and walk your feet in as far as possible. Engage the stabilizer muscles of the shoulder girdle strongly to secure the position of your shoulder blades. Make sure that you include the muscles in your back (latissimus dorsi, lower trapezius, rhomboids) and do not attempt to perform the stabilizing in the posture with your pectoralis major and minor only. This is a common mistake that in the long run leads to an

imbalance between the muscles on the front and back of the chest and shoulders.

Vinyasa Eight

Inhaling, maintain the pressure of the backs of the wrists and hands onto the floor, and slowly lift your straight legs together up into headstand. Follow all the instructions given for the previous headstand.

Firmly engage all the muscles of the shoulder girdle and arms to balance.

Take five breaths and look toward your nose.

On the last inhalation, hook the breath into the *bandhas* and become as light as possible.

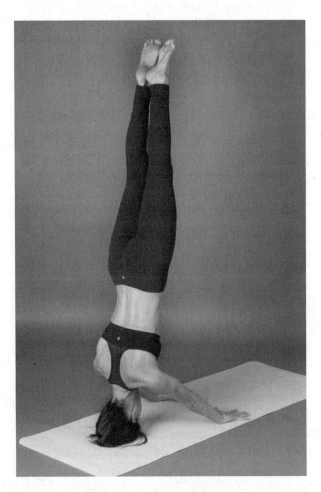

Mukta Hasta Shirshasana B

When you are most buoyant, quickly move your hands back into a three-point-headstand position (as in *Mukta Hasta Shirshasana* A), shift your weight toward your hands, and press them powerfully into the floor.

Vinyasa **Nine**

Exhaling, drop into *Chaturanga Dandasana*, as in the previous version.

Vinyasa **Ten**

Inhaling, move into Upward Dog.

Vinyasa **Eleven**

Exhaling, move into Downward Dog.

Vinyasa **Count — C Version**

Vinyasa **Seven**

Inhaling, hop forward and land on your knees.

Exhaling, place your head and hands down as in *Mukta Hasta Shirshana* A, then extend your arms out to the sides with palms facing downward. Ideally, your arms will be straight out, in line with your head, but if you are new to the posture, you will likely need to keep your arms 20 to 30 degrees further forward to train yourself to balance in this difficult variation. The wide arm position of this variation often leads to taking most of the body's weight on the head. Avoid this as much as you can by pressing your hands into the floor. However, this can lead to another problem: hyperextension of the elbow joints. If the insides of your elbows ache after doing the Intermediate Series, elbow hyperextension in *Mukta Hasta Shirshasana* C is most likely the culprit.[30] In this case, you need to slightly bend your elbows in this posture (if you were practicing in a very full class, you might have to do this anyway because of lack of space).

Straighten your legs and walk your feet in as far as possible.

Vinyasa **Eight**

Inhaling, slowly lift your straight legs together up into headstand. Follow all the instructions given for the previous versions.

Firmly engage all the muscles of the shoulder girdle and arms to balance. Create lightness in the core of your body and suck every cell of your body up toward the ceiling using the breath. It is possible; try it out. Stand tall. Imagine that you are carrying a

30 The other likely cause would be if you let the crease of your elbow face outward in *Ardha Matsyendrasana*.

heavy weight on your head. In that case, you would not slump down but would stand as tall under the weight as possible. If you were to slump, the curvatures in your spine and thus the gravitational force would increase. By standing tall you decrease the lumbar, thoracic, and cervical curves and thus use less muscle activity to carry the weight. Here, you especially need to reduce the cervical curvature right before you jump out of the posture.

Take five breaths and look toward your nose.

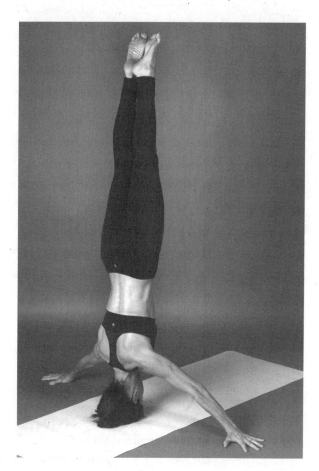

Mukta Hasta Shirshasana C

On the last inhalation, hook the breath into the *bandhas* and become as light as possible. When you are most buoyant, quickly move your hands into a three-point-headstand position (as in *Mukta Hasta Shirshasana* A), shift your weight toward your hands, and press them powerfully into the floor.

Vinyasa **Nine**

Exhaling, drop into *Chaturanga Dandasana*, as in the previous version.

Vinyasa Ten
Inhaling, move into Upward Dog.

Vinyasa Eleven
Exhaling, move into Downward Dog.

Baddha Hasta Shirshasana

BOUND HANDS HEADSTAND

Drishti Nose

OVERVIEW: See *Mukta Hasta Shirshasana*

Vinyasa Count — A Version

Vinyasa Seven
Inhaling, hop forward and land on your knees.

Exhaling, place your head and arms into the regular headstand position that is part of the cool-down sequence at the end of each series. Adjust the width of the elbows first by reaching with your hands around the opposite elbow. Then interlock your fingers and bring your wrists apart.[31] Place the back of your head against your hands and the highest point of the head down on the floor, remembering that the majority of students will balance too far on the forehead and thus create tension in the neck. Of course, you can also balance too far on the back of the head, a much less common error. This in time may lead to a flattening of the natural lordotic curve of the neck or even reverse the curvature (reducing the shock-absorbing quality of the cervical spine). If you are in doubt, the position needs to be assessed by a qualified teacher.

Straighten your legs and walk your feet in as far as possible, without rounding your back.

Vinyasa Eight
Inhaling, slowly lift your straight legs together up into headstand. Follow all the instructions given for the previous headstand.

Engage all the muscles of your shoulder girdle and your arms firmly to balance.

Take five breaths and look toward your nose.

31 Unless you use the short humeri/long neck version described in *Ashtanga Yoga: Practice and Philosophy*, p. 122.

The posture up to here will prove no challenge, as you are practicing it daily already. The only trick is to shift your hands quickly enough from the present position into the three-point-headstand position. You need to make sure that your hands are only loosely interlocked and that there is little or no weight on them just before you pull out.

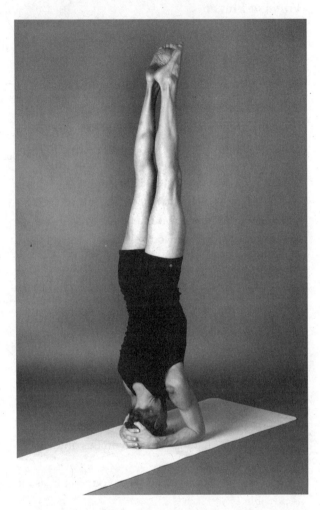

Baddha Hasta Shirshasana A

On the last inhalation, hook the breath into the *bandhas* and become as light as possible. When you are most buoyant, quickly move your hands into a three-point-headstand position (as in *Mukta Hasta Shirshasana* A), shift your weight toward your hands, and press them powerfully into the floor.

Vinyasa Nine
Exhaling, drop into *Chaturanga Dandasana*, as in the previous versions.

Vinyasa Ten

Inhaling, move into Upward Dog.

Vinyasa Eleven

Exhaling, move into Downward Dog.

Vinyasa Count — B Version

Vinyasa Seven

Inhaling, hop forward and land on your knees.

Exhaling, place your head and arms in exactly the same positions as in the previous posture. This time, however, after you place your head in the correct position, reach with your hands around your elbows and keep them clasped. The key to the position is the correct distance from the crown of your head to the line going through both elbows. It needs to be exactly the same as in your daily headstand.

Straighten your legs and walk your feet in as far as possible, without rounding your back.

Vinyasa Eight

Inhaling, slowly lift your straight legs together up into headstand. Follow all the instructions given for the previous headstand, trying as usual to carry most of the weight with your arms.

Take five breaths and look toward your nose.

The transition out of this posture is easier than that out of the previous one.

On the last inhalation, hook the breath into the *bandhas* and become as light as possible. When you are most buoyant, quickly move your hands into a three-point-headstand position (as in *Mukta Hasta Shirshasana* A), shift your weight toward your hands, and press them powerfully into the floor.

Vinyasa Nine

Exhaling, drop into *Chaturanga Dandasana*, as in the previous versions.

Vinyasa Ten

Inhaling, move into Upward Dog.

Vinyasa Eleven

Exhaling, move into Downward Dog.

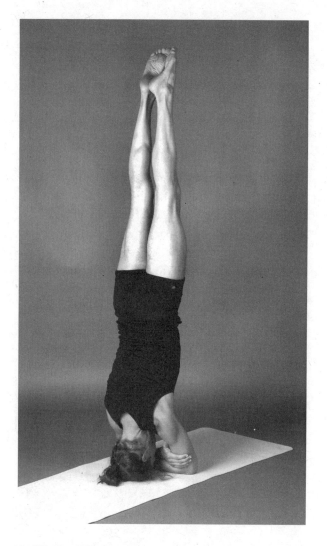

Baddha Hasta Shirshasana B

Vinyasa Count — C Version

Vinyasa Seven

Inhaling, hop forward and land on your knees.

Exhaling, place your head and arms in exactly the same positions as in *Baddha Hasta Shirshasana* A. This time, however, after you place your head in the correct position, let go of your hands and place your forearms parallel to each other, in a forearm-balance position. Again, the key to the position is the correct distance from the crown of your head to the line going through both elbows. It needs to be exactly the same as in your daily headstand. If you deviate from this ideal line in either direction, you will find it difficult to lift up into the posture.

Straighten your legs and walk your feet in as far as possible, without rounding your back.

Vinyasa Eight

Inhaling, slowly lift your straight legs together up into headstand. You will need considerable hamstring flexibility to do so, but resist the temptation to solve the problem by bending your legs. You will be rewarded with an increase in core stability if you perform the posture properly.

Follow all the instructions given for the previous headstands, trying as usual to carry a lot of weight with your arms. This posture is very similar to *Pincha Mayurasana*, with the difference that here your head touches the floor lightly. Externally rotate the humeri to prevent the wrists from moving together and the elbows from moving apart. The inability to perform this action is usually caused by a chronically short and tight infraspinatus muscle (for an illustration of the infraspinatus, see *Ashtanga Yoga: Practice and Philosophy*, p. 31). In this case

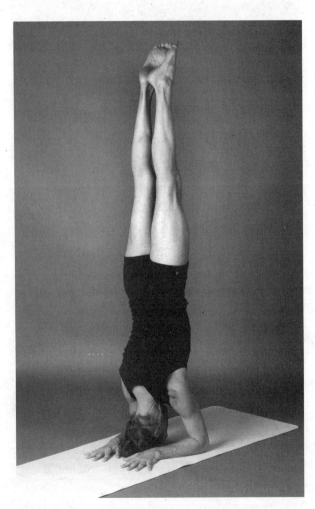

Baddha Hasta Shirshasana C

massage and/or trigger point (see p. 77) this muscle daily; to a certain extent you can do this yourself. A shortened infraspinatus is usually part of a general mis-tone and imbalance of the shoulder girdle. This needs to be addressed before you attempt advanced arm balances, as those postures would exacerbate an existing imbalance. To address shoulder imbalance, see the section on the shoulder joint (pp. 71–77).

Take five breaths and look toward your nose.

The transition out of this posture is the easiest out of all *Baddha Hasta Shirshasanas*.

On the last inhalation, hook the breath into the *bandhas* and become as light as possible. When you are most buoyant, quickly move your hands into a three-point-headstand position (as in *Mukta Hasta Shirshasana* A), shift your weight toward your hands, and press them powerfully into the floor.

Vinyasa Nine

Exhaling, drop into *Chaturanga Dandasana*.

Vinyasa Ten

Inhaling, move into Upward Dog.

Vinyasa Eleven

Exhaling, move into Downward Dog.

Vinyasa Count — D Version

Vinyasa Seven

Inhaling, hop forward and land on your knees.

Exhaling, place your head and arms in exactly the same positions as in the *Baddha Hasta Shirshasana* A. This time, however, after you place your head in the correct position, let go of your hands and place your palms on your back, so that you are balancing only on your head and your elbows. Rather than placing your hands on your trapezius muscle close to your neck, try to place them as far out on your shoulders as possible. Inability to do so is usually caused by stiff shoulders.

Also here, the key to the position is the correct distance from the crown of the head to the line going through both elbows. It needs to be exactly the same as in your daily headstand.

Straighten your legs and walk your feet in as far as possible, without rounding your back.

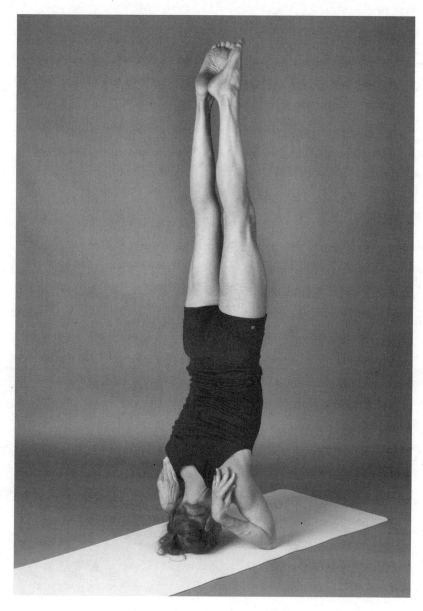

Baddha Hasta Shirshasana D

Vinyasa **Eight**

Inhaling, slowly lift your straight legs together up into headstand. The lifting is actually easier than in the previous version.

Follow all the instructions given for the previous headstands, trying as usual to carry a lot of weight with your arms. It is especially important here to draw the shoulder blades up to the ceiling.

Take five breaths and look toward your nose.

The transition is performed in the same way as in the previous postures.

Vinyasa **Nine**

Exhaling, drop into *Chaturanga Dandasana*.

Vinyasa **Ten**

Inhaling, move into Upward Dog.

Vinyasa **Eleven**

Exhaling, move into Downward Dog.

Vinyasa **Twelve**

Inhaling, jump through to *Dandasana*.
Exhaling, lie down.

BACKBENDING, COOL-DOWN, AND RELAXATION POSTURES

The backbending, cool-down, and relaxation postures following the Intermediate Series are the same as those following the Primary Series. They are described in detail in *Ashtanga Yoga: Practice and Philosophy* (pp. 111–30) and are as follows:

Urdhva Dhanurasana
Pashimottanasana
Sarvangasana
Halasana
Karnapidasana

Urdhva Padmasana
Pindasana
Matsyasana
Uttana Padasana
Shirshasana
Urdhva Dandasana
Baddha Padmasana
Yoga Mudra
Jnana Mudra
Utpluthi
Shavasana

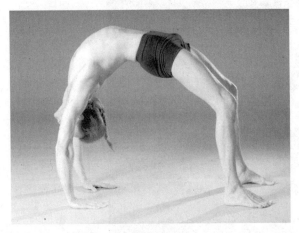

Urdhva Dhanurasana

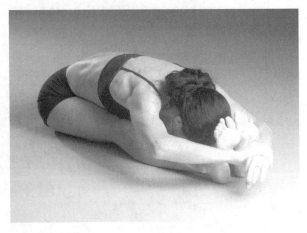

Pashimottanasana

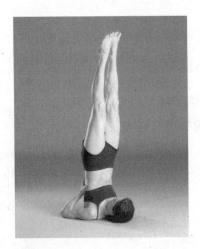

Sarvangasana

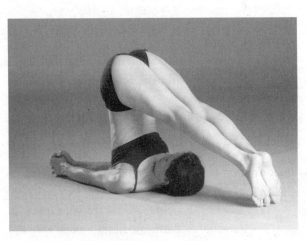

Halasana

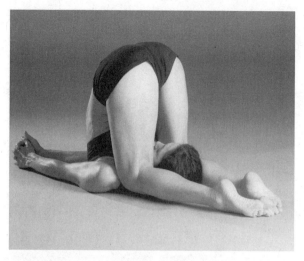

Karnapidasana

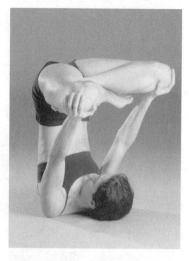

Urdhva Padmasana

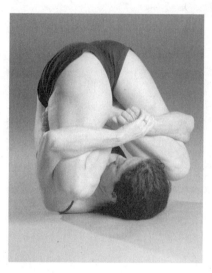

Pindasana

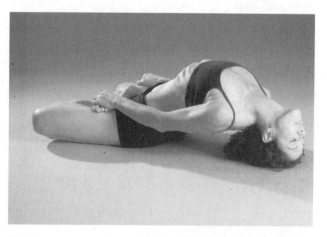

Matsyasana

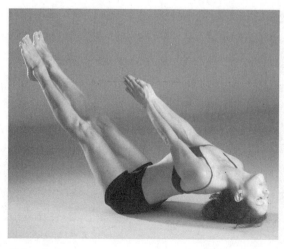

Uttana Padasana

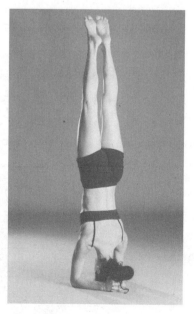

Shirshasana

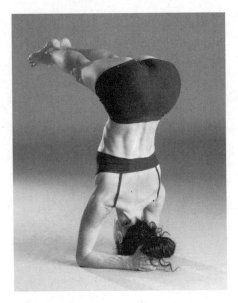

Urdhva Dandasana

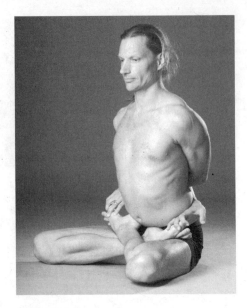

Baddha Padmasana

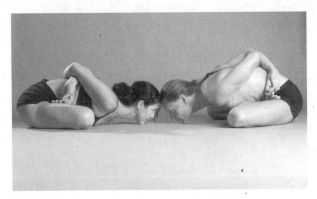

Yoga Mudra

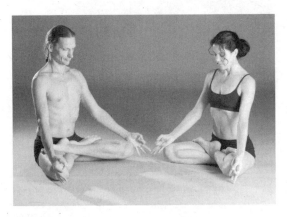

Jnana Mudra

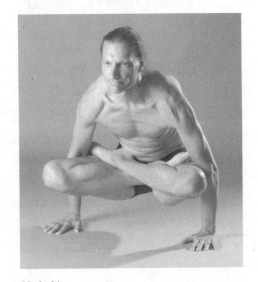

Utpluthi

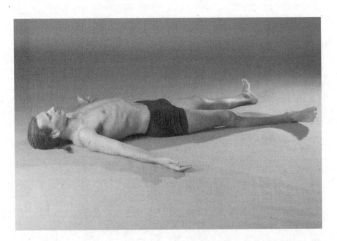

Shavasana

EPILOGUE

Lord Rama stated that the ancient sages went to heaven only after they had displayed an enormous amount of correct exertion.[1] At first sight, this statement appears to be at odds with Shankara's dictum that liberation cannot be attained by any sort of action.[2] Shankara denies any causal connection between actions such as *asana*, *pranayama*, ritual, meditation, or *samadhi* and the knowing of the *Brahman* (infinite consciousness). Since the *Brahman* is eternal and uncaused, it cannot be caused by any action. But Lord Rama does not speak of a causal connection; he speaks of a temporal connection. He says that the sages attained their coveted state after they had performed the required actions. The significant word here is *after*, which indicates a temporal connection between exertion and goal. The causal connection between the two, which Shankara denied, would have been indicated by the word *because*.

The difference between the two positions is one of perspective. Shankara speaks from the absolute truth of infinite consciousness. From this perspective, no act can produce or bring about this consciousness, because the *Brahman* never ceased to be. Lord Rama, on the contrary, speaks from the relative perspective of everyday conditioned existence. From this view, every being has to bring itself into shape, make itself fit for receiving the divine blessing of realizing the infinite consciousness. This is not done by sitting and thinking about it or claiming and believing that one has attained that state already. It is, as Lord Rama states, to be attained only through intense and correct exertion.

Yoga supplies us with the resources for such an exertion. With every step we take, we are rewarded with more energy, courage, and clarity. May we use it to travel onward on the trail blazed by the ancient sages.

1 *Ramayana, Ayodhya Kanda* 101:29; the reason Lord Rama speaks about "heaven" and not about "liberation," as Shankara did, is that the *Ramayana* is addressed to common humanity, whereas Shankara's commentary addresses the erudite.
2 *Brahma Sutra Commentary* I.I.4.

GLOSSARY

ABDUCTOR A muscle that draws a bone away from the midline of the body.

ACHARYA Teacher; one who has studied the texts, has practiced the methods, has achieved the results, and is capable of communicating them.

ADDUCTOR A muscle that draws a bone toward the midline of the body.

ADHIKARA Fitness; a set of criteria that determines whether a student is fit to follow the methods of a particular school of yoga, determined by the student's current level of spiritual growth.

ADI PARVA The first chapter of the *Mahabharata*.

ADVAITA VEDANTA Upanishadic philosophy founded by Acharya Gaudapada and developed by Acharya Shankara that propounds unqualified monism, holding that the individual self (*atman*) and the deep reality (*Brahman*) are identical.

AGNI Fire.

AHAMKARA Egoity; the source of identification as "I" or as the one who owns a perception; not to be mistaken with the Freudian term *ego*.

AJNA CHAKRA The sixth chakra, the third-eye energy center.

AKASHA Space, ether.

AKSHARA Syllable.

AMRITA The nectar of immortality.

ANAHATTA CHAKRA The fourth chakra, the heart energy center.

ANANDA Ecstasy, bliss.

ANANTA Infinity; a name of the serpent of infinity.

ANTERIOR Forward, in front of; opposite of posterior.

ANTEVERSION Angle or degree to which the head of the femur points forward when seen from above.

APANA Vital downward energy current.

APSARAS A celestial nymph and dancer whose duty is to use her eroticism to distract *rishis* from their ascetic practices, thus restoring the balance of the universe.

ARJUNA Hero of the *Mahabharata* who metaphorically represents the lower or phenomenal self.

ARTHAVEDA The *Upaveda* (ancillary *Veda*) pertaining to economy.

ASAMPRAJNATA Objectless *samadhi*, supercognitive *samadhi*.

ASANA Posture; the third limb of Ashtanga Yoga.

ASHRAMA The hermitage of an ascetic; also, the four stages of life, that is, *brahmacharya*, *grhasta*, *vanaprashta*, and *sannyasin*.

ASHTADHYAYI The treatise on Sanskrit grammar authored by Panini.

ASHTANGA VINYASA YOGA Ancient mode of Ashtanga Yoga that was revived in modern days by Shri T. Krishnamacharya.

ASIS Anterior superior iliac spine of the ilium.

ASMITA Literally, I-am-ness; egoism, one of the five forms of suffering; also, the form of objective *samadhi* that arises when pure I-am-ness is witnessed.

ASTRA A missile, an arrow released with a magical incantation.

ASURA A demon or anti-god; a powerful being overcome by the *tamas guna*.

ATHARVAVEDA One of the four *Vedas*.

ATMAN The true self, consciousness; the term Vedanta uses instead of *purusha*.

AVATARA Divine manifestation.

AVIDYA Ignorance.

AYURVEDA Ancient Indian medicine, one of the four subsidiary *Veda*s (*Upavedas*).

BANDHA Bond, energetic lock.

BEDA ABEDA Identity-in-difference doctrine; a doctrine held by Ramanuja that states that the individual soul is identical with the Supreme Being in the fact that it is pure consciousness, yet different in that the Supreme Being is omnipotent and the soul is not.

BHAGAVAD GITA Song of the Lord; the most influential of all *shastra*s, in which the Supreme Being in the form of Lord Krishna amalgamates the teachings of *Samkhya*, Yoga, and Vedanta.

BHAGAVATA PURANA Also called *Shrimad Bhagavatam*, a *Purana* that deals with devotion to the Supreme Being in the form of Lord Vishnu and describes some of the *avatara*s of Vishnu, including Krishna.

BHAKTI Devotion; from *bhaj*, "to divide," the belief that there is an eternal divide between the Supreme Being and the world that cannot be overcome through knowledge, and hence the Supreme Being must be met with an attitude of devotion.

BHAKTI YOGA Yoga of love, the practice of devotion to the Supreme Being.

BHARADVAJA A Vedic rishi.

BHOGA Consummation, experience, bondage.

BHUMIKA Stage; the stage of evolution of a practitioner, which determines his fitness (*adhikara*) for a particular practice.

BHUTA SHUDDHI Elemental purification; the traditional way of involuting by dissolving each element (*bhuta*) into the next higher element, thus climbing up the ladder of the chakras.

BIJA AKSHARA Root syllable; a mantra related to a particular chakra and element.

BONDAGE Erroneous identification with the transitory.

BRAHMA A five-headed deity; the creator, the first being that appears at the beginning of each universe and forms the universe based on its beings' subconscious conditioning — the Brahma of the current universe is called Prajapati (progenitor), the grandsire of humankind.

BRAHMACHARYA Recognition of *Brahman* in everything; also, celibacy.

BRAHMA, LORD A deity, the creator; the first being that arises at the beginning of each universe due to its subconscious desire and conditioning.

BRAHMAN Infinite consciousness, deep reality, the reality that cannot be reduced to a deeper layer.

BRAHMARANDHRA Gate of *Brahman*; the upper end of *sushumna*.

BRAHMA SHIRSHA ASTRA Brahma's head missile, the most destructive of all missiles.

BRAHMA SUTRA Principal treatise of the Vedanta, authored by Rishi Vyasa.

BRAHMA VIDYA An alternative name for Jnana Yoga; a Jnanin aims to recognize the identity between his self (*atman*) and the infinite consciousness (*Brahman*).

BRAHMIN One who serves God through his spirit; also, a member of the priest caste.

BRHAD ARANYAKA UPANISHAD Literally, "forest-dweller *Upanishad*"; the oldest and most revered *Upanishad*.

BUDDHI Intellect, seat of intelligence.

BUDDHI YOGA Yoga of intellect; a term generally applied to *Samkhya*.

CERVICAL SPINE The vertebrae of the neck.

CHAKRA Subtle energy center in the body.

CHARAKA SAMHITA Treatise on *Ayurveda*; the author, Charaka, is said to be an incarnation of Patanjali.

CHANDAS The *Vedanga* (Vedic limb) pertaining to meter.

CHIT Consciousness.

CHITTA The mind; the aggregate of intellect (*buddhi*), egoity (*ahamkara*), and thinking agent (*manas*).

COGNITION The effort of the mind to identify and interpret data supplied by the senses.

COGNITIVE *SAMADHI* Objective *samadhi*; *samadhi* whose arising depends on cognition of an object.

CONSCIOUSNESS That which is conscious, the observer, awareness; this definition is opposed to that of modern psychology, which sees consciousness as that which we are conscious of.

COUNTER-NUTATION Annulling of a forward-bowing movement of the sacrum.

DARSHANA View, system of philosophy. The *darshana*s are divided into orthodox and heterodox, depending on whether they accept or reject the authority of the *Vedas*. The orthodox *darshana*s are *Samkhya* (rational inquiry), *Yoga* (science of the mind), *Mimamsa* (science of action), *Nyaya* (logic), *Vaiseshika* (cosmology), and *Vedanta* (analysis of the *Upanishads*). These *darshana*s ideally do not compete with each other but solve different problems. The Yoga master T. Krishnamacharya had degrees in all six systems. The heterodox *darshana*s are *Jaina* (Jainism), *Baudha* (Buddhism), and *Charvaka* (materialism). A special case is Tantra, which is neither accepted as orthodox nor seen as heterodox. Shankara was probably the last human being to have mastered all ten systems of philosophy.

DEVA Celestial being, divine image, or divine form; often translated as "god."

DEVANAGARI City of the Gods; the script used to write Sanskrit.

DEVI SARASVATI The goddess of learning, art, and speech.

DHANURVEDA The *Upaveda* (ancillary *Veda*) pertaining to military science.

DHARANA Concentration; the sixth limb of Ashtanga Yoga.

DHARMA Characteristic, attribute; righteousness, virtue.

DHARMA SHASTRA Scripture dealing with right action.

DHYANA Generally translated as "meditation," an ongoing stream of awareness from the meditator toward the object of meditation and of information from the object toward the meditator; the seventh limb of Ashtanga Yoga.

DHYANA YOGA Yoga of meditation.

DOSHAS In Ayurveda, the three constitution types of the body, that is, *vata*, *pitta*, and *kapha*.

DRISHTI Focal point.

EIGHT LIMBS The eight constituents of Patanjali's yoga: *yama, niyama, asana, pranayama, pratyahara, dharana, dhyana,* and *samadhi*.

EKAGRA CHITTA Single-pointed mind, the mind fit to practice higher yoga.

ENTROPY The amount of disorder in a system; the second law of thermodynamics states that with the progress of time, the amount of entropy (disorder) in each system, such as the universe, increases, until the system breaks down.

EXTENSION Increasing the angle between two bones.

FEMUR Thighbone.

FLEXION Decreasing the angle between two bones.

FULL-*VINYASA* SYSTEM *Asana* practice in which one does a *vinyasa* to standing (the equivalent of performing Surya Namskara A) between sitting postures.

GANDHA Subtle earth element; quantum (*tanmatra*) of earth; smell.

GANDHARVAVEDA The *Upaveda* (ancillary *Veda*) pertaining to music.

GANESHA, LORD The first son of Lord Shiva and the Great Goddess Uma Parvati, the keeper of the gateway to heaven.

GAYATRI The most sacred of all mantras, conceived by the Rishi Vishvamitra.

GHERANDA SAMHITA A Tantric treatise describing Hatha Yoga.

GLENOID FOSSA The cavity of the shoulder joint.

GLENOID LABRUM The cartilage lining of the glenoid fossa.

GOVINDA A cowherd; also, a name of Lord Krishna, who was, when young, hidden in a rural village to escape the murderous wrath of his uncle Kamsa.

GREAT GODDESS The female aspect of the Supreme Being, known under many names, such as Uma, Durga, Parvati, Devi, and Shakti.

GUNAS The qualities or strands of *prakrti* that form, through their various intertwinings, all phenomena; the three *gunas* are *rajas*, *tamas*, and *sattva*.

HALF-*VINYASA* SYSTEM Practice in which one transits through *Chaturanga Dandasana*, Upward Dog, and Downward Dog between sitting postures.

HAMSA A swan; a metaphor for the soul; a vehicle of Lord Brahma; the name of the mantra by which *prakrti* permeates the universe.

HANUMAN, LORD Monkey-god, hero of the *Ramayana*, egoless superhero, and perfect devotee.

HATHA YOGA A Tantric school of yoga that was founded in approximately 1100 CE by the master Gorakhnath; literally, sun/moon yoga, it emphasizes balancing the solar and lunar energy channels in the body. Hatha Yoga shifted the focus away from the mysticism and philosophy of the older Upanishadic types of yoga toward using the body as a tool.

HATHA YOGA PRADIPIKA A Tantric treatise authored by Svatmarama.

HEART Sanskrit *hrdaya*, referring to the core of all phenomena, which according to the Vedanta is consciousness; if the term is used in an anatomical instruction, it refers to the core of the rib cage.

HUMERUS Arm bone.

HYPEREXTENSION Extension beyond 180 degrees.

IDA Lunar energy channel, connected to the left nostril.

INDRA, LORD Lord of Thunder, king of the heavens.

INSERTION OF A MUSCLE The end of the muscle that is distant from the center of the body.

INTELLECT Seat of intelligence.

ISHTADEVATA Meditation deity; a personal projection that enables one to establish a devotional relationship to the Supreme Being.

ISHVARA The Supreme Being, *Brahman*, with form.

ISOMETRIC EXERCISE Exercise in which the targeted muscle does not get shortened.

ISOTONIC EXERCISE Exercise that involves shortening a muscle.

ITIHASAS Scriptures that deal with what once was, history: the *Mahabharata*, the *Ramayana*, and the *Yoga Vashishta*.

JAGAT GURU A world teacher; an ephithet given to teachers such as Shankaracharya or Ramanujacharya.

JIVA Phenomenal self; an image of oneself that is formed through contact with the manifold phenomena of the material and subtle world; not the true self.

JNANA Knowledge; specifically, knowledge of the self.

JNANA YOGA Yoga that seeks to teach the identity of the individual self (*atman*) and the infinite consciousness (*Brahman*).

JNANIN Knower; specifically, a knower of the self.

JYOTISHA The *Vedanga* (Vedic limb) pertaining to astrology.

KADGA A sacrificial sword.

KALAKUTA A world poison, which appeared during the churning of the oceans by the *devas* and *asuras* and was imbibed by Lord Shiva to save the world from destruction.

KALI YUGA The current age, the age of darkness, which started in 3102 BCE with the death of Lord Krishna.

KALPA The *Vedanga* (Vedic limb) pertaining to ritual.

KAMADHENU A celestial wish-fulfilling cow, a symbol of giving and fertility.

KANDAS Portions; divisions of the *Vedas*.

KAPHA One of the three *ayurvedic* constitution types, sometimes translated as "phlegm."

KAPALIKA A skull carrier; a sect worshipping Lord Shiva.

KAPILA, RISHI Founder of *Samkhya*, the first systematic philosophy, noted in the *Bhagavad Gita* and *Bhagavata Purana* as a manifestation of the Supreme Being.

KARANA SHARIRA The causal body; the body of knowledge and intelligence.

KARMA Action.

KARMA KANDA OF THE VEDA The portion of the *Veda* that deals with action.

KARMA, LAW OF Law of cause and effect.

KARMASHAYA Karmic storehouse; place where the effects of our actions are stored.

KARMA YOGA Yoga of action; in its original Vedic sense, Karma Yoga is any yoga that employs ritualistic action, such as *asana*, meditation, or mantra, to produce spiritual gain. The term excludes Jnana Yoga and Bhakti Yoga, which are thought to operate beyond spiritual gain.

KARTIKEYA, LORD The second son of Lord Shiva and the Great Goddess Uma Parvati; a general of the celestial army, also called Murugan, Ayeppa, Subhramaniam, Kumara, or Skanda.

KATHA SARIT SAGARA A collection of Indian folktales and fables, attributed to Somadeva.

KRISHNA, LORD A form of the Supreme Being, *avatara* of

Lord Vishnu, teacher in the *Bhagavad Gita*; a metaphor for the divine self.

KRISHNAMURTI, JIDDU An outstanding teacher of the twentieth century who placed emphasis on sound reasoning and on the axiom that all initiation is self-initiation.

KRIYA YOGA Preliminary yoga consisting of simplicity (*tapas*), the reading of sacred texts (*svadhyaya*), and acceptance of the existence of a Supreme Being (*Ishvara pranidhana*); also, a Tantric mode of yoga using breath, mantra, and visualization.

KRODHA YOGA Yoga of hatred and aversion.

KSHATRIYA One who serves God through one's will; also, a member of the warrior caste.

KUMBHAKA Breath retention, an important *pranayama* method; sometimes used synonymously with *pranayama*.

KUNDALINI The obstacle that closes the mouth of *sushumna*; the rising of *shakti* in the *sushumna*.

KUNDALINI YOGA A mode of yoga that focuses on the raising of the life force.

KURUKSHETRA Field of action; the location of the battle of the *Mahabharata*; also, a metaphor for daily life.

KYPHOSIS Forward curvature of the spine.

LATERAL Sideward, away from midline of the body.

LATERAL ROTATION External rotation.

LAYA YOGA Yoga of concentration.

LIBERATION To recognize one's true nature as the eternal, immutable consciousness.

LORDOSIS Backward curvature of the spine.

LUMBAR SPINE The vertebrae of the low back.

MADHYAMA The third phase of sound; all subtle mantric sounds; the Sanskrit language.

MAHABHARATA The largest piece of literature created by humankind, authored by Rishi Vyasa and containing the *Bhagavad Gita*; *dharma shastra* (scripture dealing with right action), which comes to the conclusion that however hard you try, you can never be completely right.

MAHABHUTA Gross element, that is, earth, water, and so on.

MAHAPRALAYA A great dissolution of a cycle of world ages (*Maha Yuga*).

MAHAVRATA A great vow, a form of penance adopted by Lord Shiva after severing the head of Lord Brahma, which led to the rise of the Kapalika order.

MAHA YUGA Great *yuga*, consisting of the four ages, *Satya Yuga, Treta Yuga, Dvapara Yuga*, and *Kali Yuga*.

MALA A garland, often of prayer beads or flowers.

MANANA Contemplating.

MANDALA A circular drawing that exemplifies sacred geometry and serves as a meditation object.

MANIPURAKA The third chakra, the navel chakra, the fire energy center.

MANTRA A mystical syllable designed to create and alter reality by influencing the vibrational patterns that make up creation.

MANTRA YOGA A mode of yoga that focuses on the use of sound waves and incantations.

MATRYOSHKA Nested Russian dolls; a metaphor for the interrelationship of the eight limbs of yoga.

MEDIAL Toward midline of the body.

MEDIAL ROTATION Internal rotation.

MIMAMSA Ritualism.

MOKSHA Liberation from bondage.

MOKSHA SHASTRA Any scripture dealing with liberation.

MOUNT MERU The name of the world axis; the subtle equivalent of Mount Kailasha in Tibet.

MUDHA CHITTA A mind that is infatuated with materialistic concerns and therefore unfit to do yoga.

MUDRA An energetic seal, usually a combination of *asana, pranayama*, and *bandha*.

MUKHA Free, unbound.

MUKTI Liberation, emancipation.

MULA BANDHA Root lock; contraction of the pubococcygeus.

MULADHARA The first chakra, the base chakra, the earth energy center.

NADI Literally, river; an energy channel in the subtle body.

NADI SHODHANA Purification of the energy channels.

NARADA A rishi, author of the *Bhakti Sutra*, and attendant of the Lord Vishnu.

NIDHIDHYASANA To be permanently established in self-knowledge.

NIDRA Deep dreamless sleep, the third state listed in the *Mandukya Upanishad* (the others are waking state [*jagrat*], dream [*shushupti*], and consciousness [*turiya*]; also, the fourth fluctuation of the mind listed by Patanjali in Yoga Sutra I.6 (the others are correct cognition, wrong cognition, perceptualization, and memory).

NIRGUNA Formless, qualityless.

NIRGUNA BRAHMAN Formless *Brahman*, deep reality, infinite consciousness.

NIRODHA CHITTA A suspended mind; the natural state of mind; the goal of yoga.

NIRUKTA The *Vedanga* (Vedic limb) pertaining to etymology.

NIYAMA Observances; the second limb of Ashtanga Yoga.

NUTATION A forward-bowing movement of the sacrum or the Earth axis.

NYAYA The Vedic system of logic.

OBJECT Everything that is not the subject (consciousness), including ego, intelligence, and the universe.

OBJECT OF MEDITATION Any object of *sattvic* quality, such as a mantra, the symbol *Om*, a *yantra* or *mandala* (sacred geometry), a lotus flower, the breath, one's meditation deity, emptiness, the light or sound in the heart, the intellect, the subtle elements.

OBJECTIVE *SAMADHI* *Samadhi* whose arising depends on an object.

OBJECTLESS *SAMADHI* *Samadhi* whose arising does not depend on an object and therefore can reveal the subject, pure consciousness.

OM The sacred syllable emitted by the Supreme Being, the sound that produces all other sounds and into which all other sounds return.

ORIGIN OF A MUSCLE The end of the muscle that is closer to the center of the body.

PADA Foot; also, a subdivision of a text.

PANDAVAS The five sons of King Pandu: Yudhishthira, Bhima, Arjuna, Sahadeva, and Nakula.

PANINI Rishi and Sanskrit grammarian.

PARA The first phase of sound; divine intention; *shabda Brahman*.

PARAVAIRAGYA Supreme surrender or detachment, total letting go.

PASHUPATA Lord of the Beasts; a name of Lord Shiva; an ancient school of Shiva worshipers.

PASHYANTI The second phase of sound; the sacred syllable *Om*.

PATANJALI The author of the *Yoga Sutra* and treatises on Sanskrit and *Ayurveda*; a manifestation of the serpent of infinity.

PINGALA Solar energy channel.

PITTA One of the three *ayurvedic* constitution types, sometimes translated as "bile."

POSTERIOR In back of; opposite of anterior.

PRAKRTI Procreatress, procreativeness, nature; the matrix or womb that produces the entire subtle and gross universe apart from consciousness.

PRANA Life force or inner breath; also, sometimes refers to anatomical or outer breath; also, vital upward energy current.

PRANAYAMA Breath extension, breathing exercises to harmonize the flow of life force; the fourth limb of Ashtanga Yoga.

PRASHTHANA TRAYI Triple canon of authoritative texts: the *Upanishads*, *Bhagavad Gita*, and *Brahma Sutra*.

PRATYAHARA Independence from sensory stimuli; the fifth limb of Ashtanga Yoga.

PRITHVI Gross earth element.

PURANA Literally, ancient, pure; the word that gave rise to the English word *pure* and contains the concept that things are purest at their outset or origin.

PURANAS Sacred texts that relate mysticism and philosophy, in the form of allegories and stories.

PURUSHA Pure consciousness, which is eternal and immutable; term used by *Samkhya* and yoga instead of *atman*.

RAJAS Frenzy, energy, dynamics; one of the *gunas* of *prakrti*.

RAJA YOGA Royal yoga; a term generally applied to the three higher limbs of Ashtanga Yoga, that is, *dharana*, *dhyana*, and *samadhi*.

RAMA, LORD Sixth *avatara* of Lord Vishnu; hero of the *Ramayana* who proves that however great the mess, if you always give your best, you will end up okay.

RAMANA MAHARSHI An important Jnana Yogi of the twentieth century.

RAMANUJA, ACHARYA One of the world teachers; a teacher of Bhakti Yoga, the founder of Visishtadvaita Vedanta, the propounder of the identity-in-difference doctrine, and the author of Shri Bhashya commentary on the *Brahma Sutra*.

RAMAYANA Literally, Rama's way; an ancient epic (*itihasa*) that describes the life of Rama, an *avatara* of Lord Vishnu.

RIGVEDA One of the four *Vedas*.

RISHI A Vedic seer, a liberated sage, one who through suspension of the mind can see to the bottom of his heart.

SACRUM The triangular bone that forms the base of the spine, consisting of several fused vertebrae; in ancient Greece, it was thought to contain the soul, hence the name "sacred bone."

SADHU One who practices a religious *sadhana* (discipline).

SAGUNA With form, with quality.

SAGUNA BRAHMAN The Supreme Being, *Brahman*, with form.

SAHASRARA The seventh chakra, the crown chakra, the energy center of consciousness.

SAMADHI Absorption, ecstasy; the eighth limb of Ashtanga Yoga.

SAMADHI YOGA Yoga of absorption.

SAMAPATTI The mind's identity with an object; the state of the mind during objective *samadhi*.

SAMAVEDA One of the four *Vedas*.

SAMKHYA The oldest system of philosophy, founded by Rishi Kapila; an analysis of the constituents of creation; a way to achieve liberation by means of intellectual reflection.

SAMKHYA KARIKA The treatise authored by Ishvarakrishna describing the *Samkhya* system of philosophy. The *Karika* is of great importance, since it is the oldest surviving text describing the *Samkhya* on which yoga is based. One needs to keep in mind, however, that this text is younger than the *Yoga Sutra* and is not representative of older and more original forms of *Samkhya*.

SAMPRAJNATA Objective *samadhi*, cognitive *samadhi*.

SAMSARA Conditioned existence, the endless round of rebirths.

SAMSKARA Subconscious imprint.

SAMYAMA Combined application of *dharana*, *dhyana*, and objective *samadhi*.

SANATANA DHARMA Eternal teaching, nowadays mistakenly referred to as Hinduism, the teaching of Hindustan.

SANSKRIT The programming language used to write the

operating system of the subtle body; the language of the gods.

SAPTARISHIS The group of the seven most prominent rishis.

SARASVATI The goddess of learning, art, and speech; also, an ancient river.

SAT Truth; according to Indic thought, only what is permanent is true — all else is appearance; the term *sat*, therefore, applies to pure consciousness only.

SATTVA Light, wisdom, intelligence; one of the *gunas* of *prakrti*.

SATYA YUGA The golden age, the age of truth; the first of the four *yugas*.

SAVITRI Sun god.

SHABDA Sound; the entirety of all vibrational patterns.

SHABDA BRAHMAN Brahmic sound; divine intention.

SHAIVITE A worshiper of Shiva.

SHAKTI The Great Goddess, the consort of Lord Shiva; personification of *prakrti*; energy, life force, *prana*.

SHANKARA, ADI World teacher, yoga master, propounder of Jnana Yoga and Advaita Vedanta; author of commentaries on the *Brahma Sutra*, the *Upanishads*, the *Bhagavad Gita*, and thirty other texts; founder of ten monk orders and four large monasteries whose abbots today still carry the title Shankaracharya. His dates are disputed. Western academics often place him at 800 CE. Tradition places him at 1800 BCE. Also known as Shankaracharya or Shankara Bhagavatpada.

SHASTRA Scriptures, good books; path to truth.

SHATAPATHA BRAHMANA Vedic text describing rituals.

SHATKRIYA Literally, "six actions," a set of purifying actions used in Hatha Yoga to restore the balance among the three constitution types (*doshas*) of the body.

SHIKSHA The *Vedanga* (Vedic limb) pertaining to phonetics.

SHIVA, LORD A name of the Supreme Being, pure consciousness, *Brahman* with form.

SHLOKA Verse, stanza; also, Sanskrit grammar.

SHOKA Grief, the sentiment that led to the composition of the *Ramayana*.

SHRAVANA Listening to the instruction of an authentic teacher.

SHRUTI Literally, "that which is heard"; revealed scriptures of divine origin, which are seen or heard by a *rishi*, that is, the *Vedas* and *Upanishads*

SIDDHA A perfected being; a yoga master who has become an immortal, ethereal being.

SIDDHIS Perfections, supernatural powers, proof.

SKANDA, LORD General of the celestial army, Lord of War, second son of Lord Shiva and the Godmother Uma Parvati.

SKANDA PURANA The largest *Purana*, dedicated to Lord Skanda.

SMRTI Sacred tradition, scriptures conceived by the human mind that explain the revealed *shruti*; memory, one of the five fluctuations of the mind.

SOMA, LORD Lord of the Moon; lunar deity.

STHULA SHARIRA The gross body, the body visible to the senses.

STUTI Praise, advertising, glorification; the sometimes-confusing tendency of the *shastras* to exaggerate the effectiveness of the means propounded therein.

SUBTLE Something real but not perceptible to the senses; able to be perceived directly in objective *samadhi*.

SUPERCOGNITIVE SAMADHI *Samadhi* beyond cognition of object, objectless *samadhi*, *samadhi* that reveals the subject, the consciousness.

SUPREME BEING An alternative term for God that is less loaded.

SUSHUMNA The subtle body's central energy channel; Hatha Yoga's metaphor for the heart.

SUTRA A short aphorism.

SVADHISHTHANA The second chakra, the lower abdominal chakra, the water energy center.

SVADHYAYA Study of sacred texts.

TAPAS The ability to sustain one's practice in the face of adversity; also, austere practices, an ancient precursor to yoga.

TAMAS Dullness, inertia, mass; one of the *gunas* of *prakrti*.

TANMATRA Subtle element or essence; quantum; infra-atomic potential.

TANTRA The system that focuses on the precise performance of actions rather than mystical speculation; also, the treatise in which this system is described.

TANTRA YOGA A category of yoga modes based on Tantric texts, including Hatha Yoga, Laya Yoga, Kundalini Yoga, and Mantra Yoga, among others.

TEJAS Inner glow, luster.

THORACIC SPINE The vertebrae of the rib cage.

THORACO-DIAPHRAGMATIC BREATHING Breathing that includes both the thorax and the abdomen without restricting the diaphragm.

TIBIA Shinbone.

TIRTHA A sacred bathing spot, visited for purification.

TIRTHA YATRA A pilgrimage to a sacred bathing spot.

TITTIBHA An insect; also, the name of an *asura*.

TRIPURA The three demon cities that were destroyed by Lord Shiva's arrow.

UDDIYANA A precursor to Nauli, which is one of the *Shatkriya*s of Hatha Yoga; sucking of the abdominal contents up into the thoracic cavity during *Kumbhaka*, not to be confused with *Uddiyana Bandha*.

UDDIYANA BANDHA Elevating lock, lower abdominal lock; drawing of the lower abdominal contents in against the spine.

UJJAYI PRANAYAMA Literally, "victorious stretching of life force"; a breathing exercise that makes the breath and its subtle equivalent long and smooth.

UMA PARVATI Another name for Shakti; the Godmother; the female form of the Supreme Being.

UPANISHADS Ancient scriptures revealed to the *rishis*, out of which all systems of Indian philosophy developed. The *Upanishad*s are called *shruti*, "that which is heard." As all knowledge and in fact the whole universe, according to the *Vedas*, consists of sound or vibratory patterns, mystical knowledge needs to be heard. Such knowledge can, of course, be conceived only by the *rishis* (seers), those who can listen and see to the bottom of their hearts, as that's where the knowledge is.

UPASANA KANDA OF THE VEDA The portion of the *Veda* dealing with worship, which gave rise to Bhakti Yoga.

UPAVEDA An ancillary *Veda*, of which there are four: *Ayurveda* (medicine), *Arthaveda* (economy), *Dhanurveda* (military science), and *Gandharvaveda* (art / music).

VAHANA A vehicle, a carrier of a celestial being.

VAIKHARI The fourth phase of sound; gross sound, including sounds that are inaudible to the human ear.

VAIKSHESHIKA The Vedic system of cosmology.

VAISHNAVITE A worshiper of Vishnu.

VAJRA Adamantine; a celestial weapon; a thunderbolt.

VAMANA, RISHI An ancient seer, the author of the *Yoga Korunta* and Ashtanga Vinyasa Yoga; tradition places him at 2000 BCE.

VARUNA Lord of the Ocean.

VASANA Conditioning; an accumulation of subconscious imprints.

VASISHTA, RISHI The author of portions of the *Veda* and the *Yoga Vashishta*, the court priest of King Dasharatha, and the father of Lord Rama in the *Ramayana* epic.

VATA One of the three *ayurvedic* constitution types, sometimes translated as "wind."

VAYU Literally, wind, vital air current; also, Wind god.

VEDANGAS Limbs or adjuncts of the *Veda*. They are *Vyakarana* (grammar), *Jyotisha* (astrology), *Nirukta* (etymology), *Shiksha* (phonetics), *Chandas* (meter), and *Kalpa* (ritual).

VEDANTA Literally, the end of the *Veda*; analysis of the content of the *Upanishads*, its main treatise being the *Brahma Sutra*. Several schools developed (Advaita Vedanta, Visishtadvaita Vedanta, Dvaita Vedanta).

VEDAS The oldest sacred texts of humankind. Rishi Vyasa divided the one *Veda* into four: the *Rigveda*, *Yajurveda*, *Samaveda*, and *Atharvaveda*, all of which are subdivided into *Samhita* (hymns), *Brahmana* (ritual), *Aranyaka* (worship), and *Upanishad* (mysticism). There are four ancillary *Vedas* (*Upavedas*), which are *Ayurveda* (medicine), *Arthaveda* (economy), *Dhanurveda* (military science), and *Gandharvaveda* (art / music). The *Veda* has six limbs (*Vedangas*), which are *Vyakarana* (Sanskrit grammar), *Jyotisha* (astrology), *Nirukta* (etymology), *Shiksha* (phonetics), *Chandas* (meter), and *Kalpa* (ritual, duty). Early

hymns of the *Rigveda* are in excess of eight thousand years old. According to tradition, the *Vedas* are eternal and are seen at the beginning of each world age by the *rishis*.

VIDYA Correct knowledge; the opposite of ignorance (*avidya*).

VIDYAS Sciences.

VIKSHIPTA CHITTA The oscillating or confused mind; it has glimpses of true knowledge and is therefore the mind fit to commence practice of yoga.

VINYASA Sequential movement that links postures together to form a continuous flow. It creates a movement meditation that reveals all forms as being impermanent and for this reason unnecessary to hold on to.

VISHNU, LORD A name of the Supreme Being; *Brahman* with form.

VISHUDDHA The fifth chakra, the throat chakra, the space (ether) energy center.

VISHVAMITRA, RISHI The seer who saw the *Gayatri*, the most sacred of all mantras. Vishvamitra never hesitated to take hardship on himself, performing the severest and longest austerities of all the *rishis*. He could never say no to the downtrodden if they approached him for help; this earned him his name, which means "friend of the world."

VISHVARUPA Cosmic manifestation of the Lord Vishnu.

VISISHTADVAITA VEDANTA An Upanishadic philosophy developed by the Acharya Ramanuja that propounds qualified monism, holding that the individual self (*atman*) and the deep reality (*Brahman*) are identical yet different.

VRTTI Literally, whirls, fluctuations, or modifications of the mind.

VYAKARANA The *Vedanga* (Vedic limb) pertaining to grammar.

VYASA, RISHI The divider of the *Veda* and the author of the *Mahabharata*, *Brahma Sutra*, *Yoga Commentary*, and *Purana*s.

YAGNA A Vedic sacrifice.

YAJNAVALKYA, RISHI The most prominent of the Upanishadic *rishis*, he formulated the core doctrine of the *Upanishads*: that all appearances are nothing but *Brahman*.

YAJURVEDA One of the four *Vedas*.

YAMA Restraints; the first limb of Ashtanga Yoga.

YANTRA A sacred drawing that is eventually visualized; a meditation object used in the school of Tantra.

YOGA CHIKITSA Yoga therapy; the fruit of the Primary Series of Ashtanga Vinyasa Yoga.

YOGA KORUNTA The treatise on sequential yoga authored by Rishi Vamana.

YOGA NIDRA Yogic sleep, a state between sleep and *samadhi*; the state of Lord Vishnu in which he absorbs the universe between Great Dissolution and Big Bang.

YOGA SUTRA The defining ancient text on yoga, authored by Patanjali.

YOGA TARAVALI A text on Hatha Yoga composed by Shankaracharya.

YUGA A world age or epoch.

BIBLIOGRAPHY

Aranya, Swami Hariharananda. *Yoga Philosophy of Patanjali*. Albany: State University of New York Press, 1983.

Avalon, Arthur. *Kularnava Tantra*. Delhi: Motilal Banarsidass, 1965.

Baba, Bangali, trans. *Yogasutra of Patanjali*. Delhi: Motilal Banarsidass, 1976.

Bader, Jonathan. *Meditation in Sankara's Vedanta*. New Delhi: Aditya Prakashan, 1990.

Banerjea, Akshaya Kumar. *Philosophy of Goraknath*. Delhi: Motilal Banarsidass, 1983.

Bharati, Agehananda. *The Tantric Tradition*. New York: Anchor Books, 1970.

Briggs, George Weston. *Goraknath and the Kanphata Yogis*. Delhi: Motilal Banarsidass, 1938.

Bronkhorst, Johannes. *The Two Traditions of Meditation in Ancient India*. Delhi: Motilal Banarsidass, 1993.

Calais-Germain, Blandine. *Anatomy of Movement*. Seattle: Eastland Press, 1993.

Coulter, H. David. *Anatomy of Hatha Yoga*. Honesdale, PA: Body and Breath, 2001.

Dasa, Bhumipati, trans. *The Harivamsha Purana*. Vrindaban, India: Rasbihari Lal & Sons, 2005.

Dasgupta, Surendranath. *A History of Indian Philosophy*, 5 vols. Delhi: Motilal Banarsidass, 1975.

———. *Yoga Philosophy in Relation to other Systems of Indian Thought*. Delhi: Motilal Banarsidass, 1974.

De Michelis, Elizabeth. *A History of Modern Yoga: Patanjali and Western Esotericism*. London: Continuum International, 2005.

Desikachar, T. K. V., trans. *Nathamuni's Yoga Rahasya*. Chennai, India: Krishnamacharya Yoga Mandiram, 1998.

———. *Yoga Taravali*. Chennai, India: Krishnamacharya Yoga Mandiram, 2003.

Dikshitar, Ramachandra. *The Purana Index*. Delhi: Motilal Banarsidass, 1951.

Feuerstein, Georg, Subhash Kak, and David Frawley. *In Search of the Cradle of Civilization*. Delhi: Motilal Banarsidass, 2005.

Freeman, Richard. *The Yoga Matrix: The Body as a Gateway to Freedom*. Louisville, CO: Sounds True. 6 compact discs or 1 MP3 download.

Gambhirananda, Swami, trans. *Bhagavad Gita with Commentary of Sankaracarya*. Kolkata, India: Advaita Ashrama, 1997.

———. *Brahma Sutra Bhasya of Sri Sankaracarya*. Kolkata: Advaita Ashrama, 1965.

Ganguli, Kisari Mohan, trans. *The Mahabharata*. 12 vols. New Delhi: Munshiram Manoharlal, 2001.

Godman, David, ed. *Be as You Are: The Teachings of Sri Ramana Maharshi*. New Delhi: Penguin Books India, 1985.

Goldman, Robert P., ed. *The Ramayana of Valmiki*. 7 vols. Delhi: Motilal Banarsidass, 2007.

Goswami, Shyam Sundar. *Layayoga: The Definitive Guide to the Chakras and Kundalini*. Rochester, VT: Inner Traditions, 1999.

Haldeman, Scott. *Principles and Practice of Chiropractic*. New York: McGraw-Hill, 2005.

Hoppenfeld, Stanley. *Physical Examination of the Spine and Extremities*. Upper Saddle River, NJ: Prentice-Hall, 1976.

Jacobs, Alan. *Ramana, Shankara and the Forty Verses*. Delhi: Motilal Banarsidass, 2005.

Jois, Sri K. Pattabhi. *Ashtanga Yoga with K. Pattabhi Jois*, 2nd series (video). Santa Monica, CA: Yoga Works Productions, 1996.

———. *Yoga Mala*. New York: Patanjala Yoga Shala, 1999.

Kak, Jaishree. *Mystical Verses of Lalla*. Delhi: Motilal Banarsidass, 2007.

Krishnamurti, J. *Krishnamurti to Himself*. San Francisco: HarperCollins, 1993.

———. *Krishnamurti's Journal*. Chennai, India: Krishnamurti Foundation Trust India, 2003.

Larson, Gerald James. *Classical Samkhya*. Delhi: Motilal Banarsidass, 1969.

Lester, Robert C. *Ramanuja on the Yoga*. Madras, India: Adyar Library and Research Centre, 1976.

Liebenson, Craig. *Rehabilitation of the Spine*. Baltimore: Lippincott Williams & Wilkins, 2007.

Madhavananda, Swami, trans. *The Brhadaranyaka Upanisad*. Kolkata: Advaita Ashrama, 1997.

Maehle, Gregor. *Ashtanga Yoga: Practice and Philosophy*. Novato, CA: New World Library, 2007.

Mani, Vetam. *Puranic Encyclopedia*. Delhi: Motilal Banarsidass, 1975.

Miele, Lino. *Ashtanga Yoga*. Rome: International Federation of Ashtanga Yoga Centres, n.d.

Mohan, A. G., trans. *Yoga Yajnavalkya*. Chennai, India: Ganesh & Co., n.d.

Monier-Williams, Monier. *A Sanskrit-English Dictionary*. Delhi: Motilal Banarsidass, 2002.

Mueller, Max, ed. *The Laws of Manu*. Delhi: Motilal Banarsidass, 1964.

———. *The Shatapatha Brahmana*. Delhi: Motilal Banarsidass, 1963.

———. *Vedic Hymns*. Delhi: Motilal Banarsidass, 1964.

Neumann, Donald A. *Kinesiology of the Musculoskeletal System*. St. Louis: Mosby, 2002.

Nikhilananda, Swami, trans. *The Mandukya Upanishad with Gaudapada's Karika and Sankara's Commentary*. Kolkata: Advaita Ashrama, 1987.

O'Flaherty, Wendy Doniger. *Shiva: The Erotic Ascetic*. London and New York: Oxford University Press, 1981.

Osborne, Arthur. *Ramana Maharshi and the Path of Self-Knowledge*. Tiruvannamalai, India: Ramanasramam, 2002.

Powell, Robert, ed. *The Experience of Nothingness: Sri Nisargadatta Maharaj's Talks on Realizing the Infinite*. Delhi: Motilal Banarsidass, 2004.

———. *The Nectar of Immortality: Sri Nisargadatta Maharaj's Discourses on the Eternal*. Delhi: Motilal Banarsidass, 2004.

Radhakrishnan, Sarvepalli, trans. *The Bhagavad Gita*. New Delhi: HarperCollins Publishers India, 2002.

Raja, K. Kunjunni, trans. *The Hatha Yoga Pradipika of Swatmarama*. Adyar, India: Adyar Library and Research Centre, 1972.

Ramakrishnananda, Swami. *Life of Sri Ramanuja*. Madras, India: Sri Ramakrishna Math, 1977.

Saraswati, Prakashanand. *The True History and the Religion of India*. Delhi: Motilal Banarsidass, 2001.

Saraswati, Swami Yogeshwaranand. *First Steps to Higher Yoga*. New Delhi: Yoga Niketan Trust, 2001.

———. *Science of Divinity*. New Delhi: Yoga Niketan Trust, 1973.

Shastri, J. L., ed. *The Linga Purana*. Delhi: Motilal Banarsidass, 1973.

———. *The Narada Purana*, 5 vols. Delhi: Motilal Banarsidass, 1980.

———. *The Shiva Purana*, 4 vols. Delhi: Motilal Banarsidass, 1970.

Sinh, P., trans. *The Hatha Yoga Pradipika*. Delhi: Sri Satguru Publications, 1915.

Sørensen, Søren. *An Index to the Names in the Mahabharata*. Delhi: Motilal Banarsidass, 1904.

Subramaniam, Kamala, trans. *Srimad Bhagavatam*. Mumbai: Bharatiya Vidya Bhavan, 1997.

Swahananda, Swami, trans. *Chandogya Upanisad*. Madras, India: Sri Ramakrishna Math, 1956.

Sweeney, Matthew. *Astanga Yoga As It Is*. N.p.: Yoga Temple, 2005.

Tagare, Ganesh Vasudeo, trans. *The Skanda Purana*. 20 vols. Delhi: Motilal Banarsidass, 1993.

Tawney, Charles Henry, trans. *Somadeva's Katha Sarit Sagara*. 10 vols. New Delhi: BRPC, 2001.

Tyagisananda, Swami, trans. *Narada Bhakti Sutras*. Madras, India: Sri Ramakrishna Math, 1983.

Vasu, Srisa Chandra, trans. *The Gheranda Samhita*. Delhi: Sri Satguru Publications, 1986.

———. *The Siva Samhita*. Delhi: Sri Satguru Publications, 1984.

Venkatesananda, Swami, trans. *The Supreme Yoga [Yoga Vashishta]*. 2 vols. Shivanandanagar: Divine Life Society, 1995.

Vimuktananda, Swami. *Aparokshanubhuti of Sri Sankaracharya*. Kolkata, India: Advaita Ashrama, 1938.

Vireswarananda, Swami, trans. *Brahma Sutras According to Sri Sankara*. Kolkata, India: Advaita Ashrama, 1936.

Whicher, Ian. *The Integrity of the Yoga Darsana*. New Delhi: D. K. Printworld, 2000.

Whitney, W. D. *The Roots, Verb-Forms and Primary Derivatives of the Sanskrit Language*. Delhi: Motilal Banarsidass, 1963.

Woodroffe, John. *Introduction to Tantra Shastra*. Madras: Ganesh & Co., 1973.

———. *Principles of Tantra*. Madras: Ganesh & Co., 1991.

———. *Sakti and Sakta*. Madras: Ganesh & Co., 1994.

———. *The Serpent Power*. Madras: Ganesh & Co., 1995.

Yogananda, Paramahansa. *God Talks to Arjuna*. Kolkota: Yogoda Satsanga Society of India, 2002.

———. *The Yoga of Jesus*. Los Angeles: Self-Realization Fellowship, 2007.

INDEX

Page numbers in *italic* type refer to illustrations. Page numbers in **bold** type refer to material contained in sidebars or tables.

on *samadhi*, power of, 6

on *vajra*, as yogic quality, 39

yoga obstacles listed by, xx–xxi, 9

See also eight limbs of Ashtanga Yoga; *Yoga Sutra*

patella, 109, 109n13

pectoralis major, **124**, 161, 165

pectoralis minor, 111, **124**, 165

pelvis

torqued, **125**, 125n16

twisted, 137, 144, **145**, 145n24

Pincha Mayurasana (feathers of the peacock posture)

anatomical focus of, **63**

contraindication, 152

drishti/overview, 152

mythology of, 48

posture category, **31**

as prerequisite for *Karandavasana*, 155

prerequisite posture for, 152

vinyasa count, 152–55

Pindasana, **145**, 187

pingala (energy channel), xix–xx, 38, 83, 89

Pingala (*rishi*), 26

power, 164, 164n26

Prahlada (demon emperor), **30**, 34, 35–36

Prajapati (deity), 35n11, 45n33

prakrti (unmanifest state), 22

prana (divine energy), 9, 23

ambiguous meaning of, 81

ascent of, **9**, 89

blockage of, 82–83

breath as gross expression of, 79

psychological equivalent of, 106

reduced stability of, 145n24

use of term, 106n12

pranayama (breath extension)

in Ashtanga Yoga, xv, xvi–xvii, 9

effects of, 9

kumbhaka and, 83n14, **125**

as "mind control," 83n12

misconceptions about, 83n14

subtle breath anatomy and, 81–84

Ujjayi, 84, 88

Vedanta advice against practice of, 28

Prasarita Padottanasanas A–D (warm-up postures), 99

prashthana trayi, 17

See also Bhagavad Gita; Brahma Sutra; Upanishads

pratyahara (internal focus), xv, xvi, 9–10, 88

Primary Series, 93, 94

correct practice of, as prerequisite for Intermediate Series, xx, xxi

dosha-harmonizing/detoxifying effects of, **84**

goal of, xx

Intermediate Series vs., xix

leg-behind-head postures, 128

posture categories, 29

as practice foundation, 89–90

warm-up postures, 95

Prithu, 50

proprioception, 112

proprioceptive neuromuscular facilitation (PNF), **111**

psoas, 68, *68*, 116

pubis, 65–66, 69

pubococcygeal muscle, 85

Puranas, 16, 25, 34, 87

Q

quadratus lumbatorum, 172

quadriceps, 109n13, 112, 116, 117, 118, 173

R

rajas (energy particle), 22, 29

rajas (frenzy), xviii, xviiin5

Raja Yoga, 7

Rama, Lord

asuras and, **30**

in posture mythology, 38, 48

as Vishnu *avatara*, 35n9

weapon of, 38

Ramana Maharshi, 4–5, 13, 83

Ramanuja, 5

Ramayana

asuras in, **30**

authorship of, 43

Ayodhya Kanda, 43

on heaven attained through correct exertion, 189, 189n1

mythical origins of, 35

posture mythology in, 33, 38, 43, 48, 50

in Sanskrit tradition, 25

Saptarishis listed in, 43

Ravana (demon king), 50

rectus femoris, 109n13, 112

Reich, Wilhelm, 106

religion, true, 19

respiration. *See* breath/breathing

rhomboid muscles, 72–74, *73*, *75*, *77*, 165

rigidity, 82

Rigveda, 3, 25, 39–40, 43, 53

rishis (Vedic masters), 30, 43

See also specific rishi

rotator cuff muscles, 71–72, 74, 76

S

sacroiliac joints

asanas focusing on, **63**, 65

cerebrospinal fluid pulse in, 67–68, *68*

composition of, 66

function of, 66

iliacus in relation to, *69*

injuries to, 70–71, 137, 144

movements of, 66–68, *66*, 67n10, *68–69*, **69**

as part of pelvic girdle, 65–66

psoas and, 68, *68*

sacrum, 65–68, *69*, 112

saguna Brahman, 17

sahasrara chakra, 22, 24, 82

samadhi (ecstasy), 88

in Ashtanga Yoga, xv, xvi, 11–13

cognitive, 7n9

ecstasy of, 11, **12**

goal of, 11–12

understood through Indian spirituality, 13–14

use of term, 11n15

Samadhi Yoga, 7

Samasthiti (warm-up posture), 95, 96, 98

Samaveda, 3, 25, 53

Samkhya (creation), 53, 53n1, 88n2

Samkhya Karika (Vedic text), 4, 4n3

samskaras (subconscious imprints), 23, 85

Sanaka (*rishi*), 34

Sanatana Dharma, 26

Sanatkumara (*rishi*), 34

Sanskrit language

English vs., **24**

forms of, 25–26

letters of, 23

as mantric language, 21, 88

practice using, 88

pronunciation of, 25

About the Author

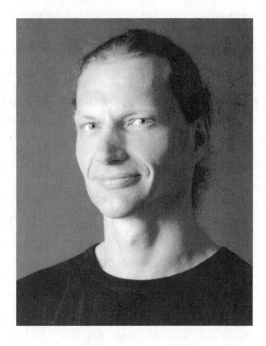

Gregor Maehle has studied history, comparative religion, philosophy, and Indology. He gained his understanding of anatomy by obtaining a German health practitioner license. During the 1980s and 1990s he lived for several years in India, where he studied the many branches of yoga under various masters, including K. Pattabhi Jois, B.N.S. Iyengar and B.K.S. Iyengar. In 1996, with his wife, Monica, he founded 8 Limbs Ashtanga Yoga in Perth, Australia. In 2006 he published the comprehensive textbook *Ashtanga Yoga: Practice and Philosophy,* which was subsequently republished in the United States, India, Japan, and Finland. For Gregor's teaching and workshop schedule, go to

www.8limbs.com

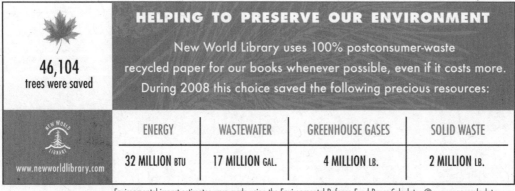